▼   ▼   ▼   ▼   ▼   ▼

Atlas of Laparoscopic Pelvic Surgery

▼ ▼ ▼ ▼ ▼ ▼ ▼ ▼ ▼

Atlas of Laparoscopic Pelvic Surgery

NICHOLAS KADAR,
MD, MA (Oxon), Grad IS MRCOG
Clinical Associate Professor
UMD-Robert Wood Johnson Medical School
Consultant, Perinatal Research Branch
National Institute of Child Health and Human Development
Director of Gynecologic Oncology
Jersey Shore Medical Center
Neptune, New Jersey

With contributions on Single Puncture Technique from
MARCO A. PELOSI, MD
Director of Obstetrics and Gynecology
Bayonne Hospital
Clinical Associate Professor
New Jersey School of Medicine
Bayonne, New Jersey

Illustrated by
ROBERT MCBRIDE
Manager of Education Media
UMDNJ School of Osteopathic Medicine
Stratford, New Jersey

b
Blackwell
Science

Blackwell Science

EDITORIAL OFFICES:
238 Main Street, Cambridge,
    Massachusetts 02142, USA
Osney Mead, Oxford OX2 0EL, England
25 John Street, London WC1N 2BL, England
23 Ainslie Place, Edinburgh EH3 6AJ, Scotland
54 University Street, Carlton, Victoria 3053, Australia

OTHER EDITORIAL OFFICES:
Arnette SA, 1 rue de Lille, 75007 Paris, France

Blackwell-Wissenschaft's-Verlag GmbH,
Kurfürstendamm 57,
10707 Berlin, Germany

Blackwell MZV, Feldgasse 13, A-1238 Vienna, Austria

Typeset by BookMasters, Ashland, OH
Printed and bound by Printek s.a., Bilbao, Spain
© 1995 by Blackwell Science, Inc.

95 96 97 98 5 4 3 2 1

Acquisitions: Michael Snider
Development: Gail Segal
Production: Michelle Choate
Manufacturing: Paul Lansdowne

Notice: The indications and dosages of all drugs in this book have been recommended in the medical literature and conform to the practices of the general medical community. The medications described do not necessarily have specific approval by the Food and Drug Administration for use in the diseases and dosages for which they are recommended. The package insert for each drug should be consulted for use and dosage as approved by the FDA. Because standards of usage change, it is advisable to keep abreast of revised recommendations, particularly those concerning new drugs.

DISTRIBUTORS:

North America
Blackwell Science, Inc.
238 Main Street
Cambridge, Massachusetts 02142
(Telephone orders: 800-759-6102 or 617-876-7000)

Australia
Blackwell Science (Australia) Pty Ltd
54 University Street
Carlton, Victoria 3053
(Telephone orders: 03-347-5552)

Outside North America and Australia
Blackwell Science, Ltd.
c/o Marston Book Services, Ltd.
P. O. Box 87
Oxford OX2 0DT
England
(Telephone orders: 44-865-791155)

Library of Congress Cataloging-in-Publication Data

Kadar, Nicholas.
    Atlas of laparoscopic pelvic surgery / Nicholas Kadar ;
  with contributions from Marco Pelosi ; illustrated by Robert
  McBride.
        p.   cm.
    Includes bibliographical references and index.
    ISBN 0-86542-417-9
    1. Generative organs, Female—Endoscopic surgery—
  Atlases. 2. Laparoscopic surgery—Atlases I. Pelosi,
  Marco. II. Title. [DNLM: 1. Genital Diseases, Female
  surgery—atlases. 2. Hysterectomy—methods—atlases.
  3. Surgery, Laparoscopic—methods—atlases.
  WP 17 K105a   1995]
  RG104.7.K33   1995
  618.1'059—dc20
  DNLM/DLC   94-13680
  for Library of Congress   CIP

To Nicola, Emily,
James and Harriet,
My patient family,
who never asked, "are you finished yet?"

Contents

A Tribute to Harry Reich

Many have contributed to the genesis of advanced laparoscopic pelvic surgery. Kurt Semm made numerous technical innovations essential to its development. The French, spearheaded by Professor Bruhat's team in Clairmont-Ferrand, broke more new ground in its clinical applications than anyone else, and included important breakthroughs in oncology by Dargent and Salvat. In the United States, Nezhat popularized the use of video laparoscopy and elevated laser dissection a fine art, Marco Pelosi developed single puncture techniques, and many others became expert laparoscopic surgeons who championed, or were the first to perform many operations laparoscopically. But peerless among these pioneers is Harry Reich, the complete laparoscopic surgeon. Master of every laparoscopic technique and undaunted by any laparoscopic undertaking, Reich has been a tireless champion of laparoscopic surgery: invincible in the operating room, magnanimous in sharing his knowledge, and unstinting in his support for others. But he will always be remembered not so much for his boundless energy or technical elan as for his surgical daring. This set him apart from others and imbued laparoscopic surgery with panache and unshakable resilience; it emboldened others and sustained its development against fierce and, at times, even brutal criticism. If the laurel of history for the development of laparoscopic surgery belongs to any one individual, that individual must surely be Harry Reich.

Nicholas Kadar

Preface

The relative status of laparoscopic cholecystectomy and laparoscopic hysterectomy accurately reflects the extent to which gynecology has been overshadowed by general surgery for innovation in endoscopic surgery. Laparoscopic cholecystectomy is a very successful operation that has replaced open cholecystectomy as the preferred method of removing the gall bladder in most patients, whereas laparoscopic hysterectomy is an operation that is mired in controversy. There are numerous reasons for this, some inherent in the nature of pelvic surgery, some self-inflicted.

Self-inflicted problems stem from the preoccupation of gynecologists with the technology that wedded laparoscopic pelvic surgery to new energy sources and instruments rather than sound surgical techniques. The importance attached to lasers, ultrasonic scalpels, argon beam coagulators, and the like has far overshadowed the thought and discussion given to either the precise anatomic relationships between pelvic structures or the fundamental surgical techniques of sharp-scissor dissection and blunt development of tissue planes that hold the key to laparoscopic pelvic dissection. Laparoscopic surgery came to be regarded as an entirely new kind of surgery that required special and altogether different skills from those needed for open techniques, skills that perhaps not every surgeon possessed. The truth is, however, that laparoscopic surgery is not difficult in the sense that playing Chopin's heroic polonaise is, and it does not take years to master. Its challenges are far more intellectual than mechanical, for their solution requires a deeper understanding of pelvic anatomy and the use of different strategies, rather than the acquisition of a technical ability not already held by the surgeon.

Inherent problems stem from the fact that laparoscopic hysterectomy has a much narrower therapeutic ratio than laparoscopic cholecystectomy, and it is also the more difficult operation. Abdominal hysterectomy is a less morbid operation than open cholecystectomy, and an abdominal incision can be avoided in many cases without laparoscopy by removing the uterus vaginally. Laparoscopic hysterectomy is more difficult because the attachments of the uterus cannot be simply clipped as in the case of the gall bladder, and the pelvis is much more difficult to dissect because tissues are hard to keep on tension. The most important difference by far, however, is that the same basic technique can be used to remove the gall bladder laparoscopically as is used in an open operation, whereas the technique used for abdominal hysterectomy does not lend itself well to a laparoscopic approach.

The desire to write this book had its genesis partly in the fevor unique to converts, and partly in the desire to dispel two myths: that laparoscopic surgery is a gimmick, and that it is a new kind of surgery that depends for its success on complex technology and ever more fanciful gadgets. I, too, started laparoscopic surgery as a skeptic, but discovered to my utter amazement, that it is a quintessentially traditional surgical art. Lasers, argon beam coagulators, ultrasonic scalpels, Roeder loops, weird implements and gadgets were entirely peripheral to it, totally irrelevant. This was not a gimmick, but the queen and servant of surgery, demanding precise anatomic knowledge, exacting a meticulous technique, mercilessly unforgiving.

There can be no serious question that laparoscopic surgery represents a momentous surgical advance that will eventually alter the way most pelvic operations are performed. But laparoscopy is merely a method of visualization, and what is done under laparoscopic visualization must be good surgery, and this is achieved by using sound surgical techniques, not new energy sources. There is nothing mysterious or particularly difficult about laparoscopic surgery except that it requires a better knowledge of anatomy, more extensive dissection of the pelvis, and the use of a more meticulous technique of dissection than many gynecologists have grown accustomed to. The real challenge in learning laparoscopic surgery is as much the challenge of performing meticulous, anatomical dissections as it is learning to use new types of instruments and to operate watching monitors.

Performing an operation laparoscopically is not an end in itself, something to be persued at all cost to a successful conclusion, but simply a means to reduce morbidity. Unless morbidity is reduced there is no virtue whatsoever in doing a procedure laparoscopically. This has two important corollaries. If laparoscopic surgery is to realize its full potential it must be applicable to patients who are difficult surgical candidates rather than confined to selected individuals whose morbidity from an open approach is already very low. Conversely, if there is a simpler way to achieve the same result i.e. by the vaginal route, laparoscopy must be eschewed altogether. Therefore, we regard the vaginal and laparoscopic routes as complementary, not competing, approaches to the pelvis, a symbiotic relationship brought to greatest fruition in the laparoscopic treatment of early invasive carcinoma of the cervix.

This book is based on the philosophy that simple and proven surgical techniques are the basis of endoscopic surgery, which relies for its success more on the surgeon's skills than on high technology. Thus, readers will find a very detailed discussion of pelvic anatomy, of how to dissect the retroperitoneum, and of how to morcellate an enlarged uterus, but they will find almost nothing about lasers, for which we have no use.

Laparoscopic surgery does, of course, have certain unique characteristics which must be fully understood and mastered. These are discussed in detail, including how to position the patients, where to put the trocars and the monitors, how to use electrosurgery, how to suture and ligate tissues, and the distinction between them. The reader must also understand instrumentation, and this is also discussed at length. However, instruments are the servants of surgical technique, not the other way around, and they cannot substitute for anatomical knowledge or sound surgical technique any more than lasers can. Finally, laparoscopic surgery depends for its success on a number of other individuals besides the surgeon, and to a much greater extent than is true for open cases. An uncooperative anesthesiologist or circulation nurse, whose failure or refusal to acknowledge the benefits of laparoscopic surgery because he or she is not involved with the patient once the operation is over, can be more instrumental in prolonging operating time or undermining a surgeon's morale and enthusiasm than even the foulest pelvic pathology. Suggestions for dealing with this very real and uni-

versal problem are discussed together with credentialling and training guidelines.

I have asked Dr. Marco Pelosi to describe his single puncture techniques for this atlas for a number of reasons. First, his is a unique approach and he is a master of it. Single puncture techniques antedated the modern multiple puncture approach, which had few advantages over its single puncture counterpart prior to the advent of the microchip camera. Second, Dr. Pelosi's approach to endoscopy is philosophically deeply rooted in a traditionalist approach to surgery, and which is the raison d'etre of this atlas. Anyone familiar with Dr. Pelosi's background, which includes a two year fellowship in gynecologic oncology, and has witnessed his creativeness in the operating room, will not be surprised that this master vaginal surgeon and laparoscopist should have invented almost an entire system of endoscopic surgery that is nonetheless in the traditional mold. For him, the laparoscope is but an extension of the vaginal hand, and his accomplishments with the technique are formidable. My hope is that vaginal surgeons who are reluctant to abandon an approach that has served them well will study these techniques carefully and see them to be not a new method of surgery, but an extension of the old, an entre' into a new world that is not nearly as strange as they might have imagined.

I hope, therefore, that this book will cover the needs of all practicing gynecologists, even if not everyone will wish to perform all the operations described. Anyone who can learn gynecological surgery can learn to do it laparoscopically, if they wish to do so. To the open-minded, knowledgeable and experienced gynecologic surgeon who is eager to incorporate endoscopy into his or her surgical repertoire, the learning curve is relatively short, interesting, enjoyable and ultimately rewarding. The transition period may be more difficult for others, and the only advice I can offer them is not to attempt the transition unless and until they are committed to it. I am quite certain, however, that as more and more residents are taught the techniques in their training, advanced laparoscopic procedures will eventually become part of routine gynecology, just as vaginal surgery and diagnostic laparoscopy have, despite being considered at one time "specialized" procedures. In fact, I confidently predict that laparoscopic surgery will do much to raise the overall standard of gynecologic surgery, and if this book assists that process it have more than served its purpose.

Nicholas Kadar

▼　　▼　　▼　　▼　　▼　　▼　　▼　　▼　　▼

Acknowledgments

This atlas could not have been produced in the record time of three months without the help and patience of a number of individuals. Foremost among these is my family, who cheerfully put up with me as almost every nook and cranny of our house became a repository for seemingly endless stacks of paper, reprints, books, photographs and drawings. My office was not much better, and my nurse Eleanor and secretary Laura bore the consequences with equal equanimity. There was no time of day or night when the long-suffering Manny Meno of M Video Medical Productions was not prepared to resume our quest to capture the perfect picture from one of my videos, or Marco Pelosi could not take a picture of an instrument for me and have it delivered within an hour. Clearly, without the practical and emotional props they provided this atlas could not have been produced.

I also owe a large debt of gratitude to a number of individuals who have in one way or another sustained me during my quest to gain mastery over the laparoscopic techniques that are described in this atlas. Even those who have perused the editorials and letters written on this subject or have heard the early pioneers recount their spine chilling tales, however funny in hindsight, cannot know the full extent of the acrimony and humbug we have all had to endure in our quest for the Holy Grail. I hope I belong to the last generation of gynecologists that has had to learn their newfound craft in an atmosphere of cynicism and adversity. The great aria, Nessum Dorma, in Turandot ends with Calaf singing, "*Vincero, Vincero*" (I will conquer, I will conquer). If I can sing along with Calaf today it is only because of the camaraderie and support of Bill Logue, Luc Lemmerling, Susan McCoy, Ekkehard Kemmann, my former resident Joe Castelli, and, of course, Harry Reich and Marco Pelosi.

It is a particular pleasure for me to express my thanks to my Publisher, Blackwells, a name that brings back many fond memories to every old Oxonian. Without the support of Mike Snider and the painstaking work of Michelle Choate, the tangled web of this manuscript with its countless diagrams and photographs would never have been organized into its present form.

Nicholas Kadar

Glossary

Abbreviations used in figure legends are as follows:

Figure 2.10c	**PVS**—paravesical space
	OHA—obliterated hypogastric artery
Figure 6.14a	**Ur**—ureter
	Ov—ovary
Figure 6.14b	**PRS**—pararectal space
	EIA—external iliac artery
	EIV—external iliac vein
	OvnR—ovarian remnant
Figure 6.14c	**EIA/EIV**—external iliac artery/ external iliac vein
	Ps—psoas muscle
	Ur—ureter
Figure 7.2b	**Ur**—ureter
Figure 9.1	**Ut**—uterus
	Ov—ovary
	FT—tube
Figure 9.3b	**Ur**—ureter
	UtA—uterine artery
Figure 11.2	**RoL**—round ligament
	EIA—external iliac artery
	IPL—infundibulopelvic ligament
Figure 11.5	**EIA**—external iliac artery
	Ur—ureter
	IPL—infundibulopelvic ligament
Figure 11.6	**Rt(L)PVS**—Right (lateral) paravesical space
	IPL—infundibulopelvic ligament
	OHA—obliterated hypogastric artery
	Ur—ureter
Figure 11.7	**OHA**—obliterated hypogastric artery
	Lt(L)PVS—left (lateral) paravesical space
	LtEIA—left external iliac artery
Figure 11.8	**LPVS**—lateral paravesical space
	UtA—uterine artery

	MPVS—medial paravesical space
	OHA—obliterated hypogastric artery
	Ur—ureter
	PRS(un)—pararectal space (unopened)
Figure 11.9	**Ur**—ureter
	SVA—superior vesical artery
	OHA—obliterated hypogastric artery
	UtA—uterine artery
	RiPrS—right pararectal space
Figure 11.10	**LgUrA**–Laproclips on right uterine artery
Figure 11.12	**Ur**—ureter
	UtsL—uterosacral ligament being divided
Figure 11.13	**HPM**—hub of Pelosi mobilizer
	DPVW—divided posterior vaginal wall
Figure 12.2a	**Cx**—cervix
Figure 12.2c	**UtC**—uterine corpus
Figure 12.2d	**UtALt**—uterine artery/left
Figure 12.2e	**UtC**—uterine corpus
Figure 12.2f	**CIS**—cervical stump
Figure 12.2g	**Cx**—cervix
	ACC—anterior calpotemy closure
Figure 12.5b	**BvUs**—bivalving of the uterus
Figure 17.3	**My**—myoma
	Ut—uterus
	PdMy—pedunculated myoma
Figure 17.4a	**Ut**—uterus
	My—myoma
	Ov—Ovary
Figure 17.4b	**Ut**—uterus
	My—myoma
Figure 17.4c	**Ut**—uterus
	My—myoma
Figure 17.7	**My**—myoma
	BpN—bipolar needles
	Pit—pitressin injection
Figure 18.2a	**TVF**—transverse vesical fold
Figure 18.4	**PtO**—peritoneal opening into the space of Retzius

Part A
Basic Considerations

Chapter 1
Laparoscopic Surgery: Rationale, Results, Reply to Critics

A clash of doctrines is not a disaster—it is an opportunity.—Whitehead

RATIONALE

The reason for performing any operation laparoscopically can be simply stated: it is to avoid making an abdominal incision, thereby reducing operative morbidity, hospital stay, and time to full recovery. A laparoscopic operation does not have to be more effective than its open counterpart to justify the laparoscopic approach, and traditional measures of morbidity, e.g., pulmonary embolus, pneumonia, fistulas, etc., need not necessarily be reduced for the laparoscopic approach to be deemed worthwhile.

There are three important corollaries. First, one cannot use traditional measures of outcome to determine whether a laparoscopic operation is valuable or not. If one does, evidence to support its use will always be "Class IIIC" (i.e., inadequate, but selection may be made on other grounds). This fact seems to have been overlooked, for example, by the panel recently selected by the American College of Obstetrics and Gynecology to evaluate laparoscopic surgery (1,2).

Although the panel recognized that postoperative recovery and the cost of therapy are important variables to consider when choosing between two equally effective operations, it ignored these variables and based its assessment, of the laparoscopic treatment of endometriosis, for example, entirely on postoperative conception and surgical complication rates. Because laparoscopic and "open" operations did not differ with respect to these variables, it was concluded that there was "no evidence to recommend operative laparoscopy over laparotomy" (2). The same conclusion was drawn with respect to adnexectomy despite the acceptance that "those undergoing laparoscopy had significantly shorter hospital stays and recuperation periods" (1). On this logic, one could argue that there is no evidence to recommend lumpectomy and radiation over radical mastectomy for the treatment of breast cancer because these operations yield similar survival rates.

Second, if morbidity from conventional surgery is already very low, little will be gained from a laparoscopic approach. This needs to be borne in mind when comparative studies are designed. For example, to evaluate laparoscopic hysterectomy, Summit et al. (3) not only chose to compare the operation with vaginal hysterectomy but did so in a select group of women who were amenable for same day discharge. The alternative hypothesis of this study is simply not credible because the selection criteria used ensured that surgical morbidity would be extremely low in both its arms, leaving no realistic chance for the study to reach a result opposite to the one obtained. No competent laparoscopic pelvic surgeon would wish to treat women who are candidates for vaginal hysterectomy and same day discharge by a laparoscopic hysterectomy.

Third, because the value of laparoscopic surgery is judged on the basis of variables that have a large subjective component, e.g., when a patient is discharged from hospital, returns to work, etc., bias from treatment comparisons cannot be eliminated by simply randomly assigning treatments to a group of patients. It is well recognized that subjective outcome measures can be influenced by knowing which treatment the patients received, and blinding must be used to guard against such biases. It is self-evident that a comparative study involving laparoscopy and laparotomy cannot be blinded. Both the demands for and the interpretation of randomized trials involving such comparisons should be tempered by this knowledge.

RESULTS

Results pertaining to specific operations will be discussed more fully in subsequent chapters, but it is useful to have a broad, general perspective on what has been achieved by a laparoscopic approach to pelvic surgery from the very outset. To draw conclusions from what would otherwise be simply a catalogue of disparate observations, it is first necessary to establish some "rules for evidence." Some have suggested that evidence favoring a particular form of therapy can be categorized into a meaningful hierarchy that gives more weight to observations derived from randomized studies than observational ones. We will not adopt such an approach because in our view it is a simplistic one that ignores, among other things, that the evidentiary strength of data is context dependent. For example, as evidence for the effectiveness of the drug, the original observations on the effects of penicillin would be assigned a value of four, on a scale of one to five, five being the lowest.

Many questions need to be answered before the laparoscopic approach is accepted as the standard way to perform pelvic surgery, but the nature of these questions varies with the type of operation. For extirpative operations, such as hysterectomy, the issue of effectiveness is resolved as soon as the specimen is removed, and the merits of the laparoscopic approach must be judged from the reduction in morbidity, hospital stay, and recovery time that results.

For operations performed for pain, infertility, incontinence, or cancer, reduction in morbidity is still the goal, provided the success of the operation is not compromised. It is easy to demand that this be demonstrated by randomized trials without considering the feasibility of such an undertaking or what the results are likely to show. Those so tempted would do well to reflect on the fact that even a large organization, such as the Gynecologic Oncology Group, has been unable to complete a simple randomized trial to determine the value of pelvic radiation following radical hysterectomy in women with cervix cancer and pelvic lymph node metastases.

Although they have become almost de rigueur, unthinking calls for randomized trials to address each and every question pertaining to laparoscopic surgery should be replaced by a more thoughtful and considered approach. Take for example the concern that pelvic lymphadenectomy may not be as effective when it is carried out laparoscopically rather than in the conventional way. Even if 20% of women with operable, early stage carcinoma of the cervix had pelvic lymph node metastases, and they do not, and performing the lymphadenectomy laparoscopically rather than conventionally reduced the survival rate of those with pelvic lymph node metastases by 50%, i.e., from 50% to 25%, approximately 85 patients with positive nodes would need to be randomized to each of two treatment groups to detect such a large detrimental effect, which translates into a need to have randomized over 800 women into one of two treatment groups. Is it likely that a randomized study designed to evaluate laparoscopic lymphadenectomy would yield a positive result, or if a null result was obtained, that this would reassure skeptics? We think the sober reality is that, like the recent RADIUS study of routine ultrasound in pregnancy, any trial of this nature is much more likely to end as a multimillion dollar failure convincing no one (4).

We would argue that although long-term results must be scrutinized, deductions about treatment efficacy can be made on the basis of technical considerations. After all, we are not dealing with "new" operations so much as performing operations about which a great deal is known with a different method of exposure. Is it likely, then, that a laparoscopic pelvic lymphadenectomy that involved the same steps as an open operation, achieved the same anatomical result verified by photodocumentation, and yielded the same number of lymph nodes would be less effective than a conventional lymphadenectomy? We very much doubt it; but, more importantly, even if it was less effective, a randomized trial would be unlikely to show it. Similar considerations apply to many other operations, such as colposuspension.

Thus, in our view, there are no compelling reasons to believe that an operation performed laparoscopically would yield different results from its open counterpart if performed in exactly the same way and judged to have been satisfactorily executed by accepted criteria, e.g., a colposuspension from the number, position, and security of the knots, a lymphadenectomy from the number of nodes recovered, and so on. We also do not believe that randomized trials are required to demonstrate that a laparoscopic operation reduces morbidity if dramatic differences are observed in this regard. For example, no one could be discharged home the day after an extraperitoneal aortic lymphadenectomy, whereas almost all women are discharged the day after laparoscopic aortic lymphadenectomy. Randomized trials were never developed to prove the self-evident, and some treatment effects are self-evident.

Recent data pertaining to major laparoscopic pelvic operations will be examined from this point of view, and we shall have more to say about randomized trials in Chapter 25.

Laparoscopic Hysterectomy

It has been apparent from many case series that laparoscopic hysterectomy is a less morbid operation than abdominal hysterectomy (5), and this has now been confirmed in randomized trials (6,7). Women can be discharged sooner, they require less pain medication, and they recover more quickly as reflected by earlier return to work. There are no such advantages of a laparoscopic hysterectomy over a vaginal hysterectomy (3,8), nor would any be expected from the nature of the respective procedures.

Operating time and hospital costs are significantly greater for laparoscopic than for abdominal hysterectomy, but several factors influence these variables. Operating time varies with how it is defined, the type of pathology present, and, independent of pathology, by the type of laparoscopic hysterectomy (see Chapter 10) carried out (9). Operating time falls with the experience of the surgeon and does so significantly after 10–20 cases (10). It is presently unclear whether laparoscopic hysterectomy will, by its nature, always take much longer than abdominal hysterectomies.

The longer operating times associated with laparoscopic hysterectomy translate into higher hospital costs, but the reduction in hospital stay counterbalances this (11,12). Clearly, whether laparoscopic or abdominal hysterectomy costs more will depend, among other things, on the relative cost of staying longer in hospital or in the operating room (12). The use of disposable instruments, particularly staplers, and lasers increases the cost of laparoscopic hysterectomy and these are the variables to target to reduce costs. If staplers and lasers are not used, laparoscopic hysterectomy is only marginally more expensive than abdominal hysterectomy (12).

Informative though these studies have been, they have not nor can they answer the question that has become a rallying point of criticism against laparoscopic hysterectomy, namely, "How do you know the hysterectomies could not have been done vaginally?" This question is rhetorical, if not disingenuous, given that only about 5% of hysterectomies performed for indications other than prolapse are removed vaginally (13), but the question is deferred until Chapter 10.

Laparoscopic Operations for Gynecological Malignancies

Long-term results pertaining to the laparoscopic treatment of gynecological malignancies are not yet available, but there is no evidence that the short-term survival of patients with endometrial or cervical cancer treated laparoscopically might be drastically reduced, including those treated for relatively advanced pathology (14). There is, however, in our view, incontrovertible evidence that morbidity is dramatically reduced by the laparoscopic approach. There have been no significant complications associated with over 200 published cases of laparoscopic pelvic lymphadenectomy (15–18). There have been only two instances of caval injury in over 100 laparoscopic aortic lymphadenectomies (17,19), and almost all women have been discharged within one to two days after surgery (17,20,21). Experience with laparoscopic radical hysterectomy is more limited. One case of ureteric injury has been reported (14), and hospital stay has averaged about three days, significantly less than for historical controls undergoing radical abdominal hysterectomy (22,23).

Laparoscopic Operations for Incontinence

Laparoscopic operations for incontinence have been confined to the Burch procedure, with some modifications made to the manner of suture placement. To judge by the abstracts presented at international meetings, the procedure is being widely adopted. Complications have been largely confined to inadvertent cystotomies that were repaired laparoscopically without sequelae. Blood loss, duration of hospitalization, and time taken to return to work have all been significantly less than for historical controls undergoing abdominal colposuspension (24). Short-term results have been equivalent to those reported for abdominal colposuspension; although long-term results are obviously lacking, there isn't much long-term data available for the open operation either. Liu and Nezhat et al. report a combined short-term cure rate of 94% (158/169) with 5% of the patients developing de novo detrusor instability (24,25).

Miscellaneous Operations

Many other operations are associated with a reduction in morbidity if they are performed laparoscopically rather than in the conventional way. As even critics agree, these include salpingostomy and salpingectomy for tubal pregnancies, excision of moderate to severe endometriosis, adnexectomy, and ovarian cystectomy, and, more controversially, appendectomy and presacral neurectomy. They will be considered in more detail in later chapters. Reservations about the appropriateness of a laparoscopic approach center on two operations: laparoscopic tubal reanastomosis and laparoscopic myomectomy. The concerns stem from the fact that the techniques presently used for endoscopic suturing, even in the hands of the most proficient endoscopist, can never achieve the results obtained with conventional suturing, and in certain circumstances, although not all, e.g., colposuspension, this affects results. In other words, just as the ability to perform a laparoscopic operation in exactly the same way as at laparotomy has reassured us about its efficacy, the inability to replicate laparoscopically what is done at laparotomy has given cause for concern. The concern over the laparoscopic treatment of intramural fibroids is discussed in Chapter 17 and justification for the concern over laparoscopic tubal reanastomosis was provided by Reich et al. (26), who recently reported a pregnancy rate of only 35% following laparoscopic reversal of sterilization.

REPLY TO CRITICS

Laparoscopic surgery has evinced much criticism, often of an ad hominem nature, from several quarters (2,27–30). It has been claimed that laparoscopic surgery is of unproven value and potentially unsafe, but the arguments are unsound in our view.

Lack of Evidence

Some have concluded that the use of operative laparoscopy for the extended indications to be described in this atlas has only anecdotal rather than scientific support (1,2,27). We believe the data reviewed above show otherwise. Factors that may have contributed to this false impression are (1) premature evaluation of the techniques, (2) refusal by editors to publish relevant data, and (3) failure to separate the indications and inherent effectiveness of an operation from the merits of performing it laparoscopically rather than by the conventional route. Laparoscopy is simply a method of visualization: it cannot legitimize unindicated or ineffective surgery, nor does an unindicated operation become more heinous for having been performed laparoscopically. An unindicated laparoscopic hysterectomy, for example, is grounds for criticizing the indications, not the laparoscopic approach.

The distinction between when and how best to perform an operation is most easily blurred if the indications for an operation are in dispute. It is then all too easy to equate an argument against performing the operation with evidence that the laparoscopic approach is not beneficial. Good examples of this can be found in the opinions that have been expressed about the laparoscopic treatment of endometriosis and pelvic pain. These conditions have always been difficult to manage and the best way of doing so a hotbed of controversy. Yet, once a laparoscopic approach was adopted for their management, it seemed to provide an outlet for decades of therapeutic frustration and uncertainty, and the laparoscope was made a scapegoat.

Gant (2), for example, undertook a "comparison of pregnancy outcomes with laparotomy versus laparoscopic techniques" for treating endometriosis and concluded that there was no evidence that minimal endometriosis required treatment at all, an entirely separate point that was equated with evidence against treating minimal endometriosis laparoscopically. The evidence for treating minimal endometriosis rests on the observation that (1) minimal endometriosis impairs fertility (31), and can cause pain, and (2) if left untreated, endometriosis probably progresses (32). One may or may not accept this as a justification for treating minimal endometriosis discovered at diagnostic laparoscopy, but that is not to say that if it is to be treated at all, it is better to treat it laparoscopically. Preliminary results of an ongoing randomized trial do, in fact, show a benefit from treating minimal endometriosis associated with pain (33).

Before it was carried out laparoscopically, presacral neurectomy was a controversial addendum to conservative operations for pain associated with endometriosis, which many reputable academics favored because retrospectively controlled data appeared to show some benefit (34,35). The practice seemed to have been vindicated by a recent prospective, randomized study, which was so suggestive that neurectomy was beneficial that the study was prematurely terminated by the monitoring committee, (36) until a more recent prospective, randomized, but unblinded trial provided contradictory evidence (37). Exactly where such conflicting "Class I" evidence from randomized trials that were supposed to settle the matter leaves one is open to debate, and will be discussed further in Chapter 19, but that does not mean that the best way to perform a neurectomy is equally debatable. Case series have shown quite unequivocally that women treated laparoscopically for endometriosis obtain the same degree of pain relief but go home much sooner than historical controls subjected to a laparotomy and that laparoscopic presacral neurectomy is as safe and anatomically as extensive and complete as the open operation (38).

Laparoscopic Surgery is Unsafe

Every successful laparoscopic operation is associated with fewer complications and a quicker recovery than its abdominal counterpart, but there can be no doubt that an occasional patient has had to pay the price for this achievement. In his 1993 presidential address to the AAGL, Dr. Brian Cohen said, "There can be no learning curve for the patient." This is a noble sentiment, which we all wish were true. The history of surgery, however, clearly shows that inchoate operations are associated with an increased complication rate, and, unfortunately, laparoscopic operations are no exception.

With that said, complication rates invariably fall as experience with new operative techniques increases, and it is, in fact, astonishing how low the complication rate associated with most major laparoscopic pelvic operations has been from the very outset. In a French multicenter collaborative study involving 8343 minor and 9178 major or advanced laparoscopic procedures, the nonfatal complication rate was 1.08/1000 minor cases and 5.23/1000 major or advanced cases (39). The main exception has been laparoscopic hysterectomy, which, even in the hands of experienced pelvic surgeons, such as gynecologic oncologists (40–42) and expert laparoscopists (43), has placed the ureter at risk of injury. The reason for this, in our opinion, is that laparoscopic hysterectomy cannot be approached in the same way as an abdominal hysterectomy. But, this is simply an argument for developing specific laparoscopic techniques for ureteric dissection and simple hysterectomy not a cause for abandoning an otherwise useful operation.

This is not to deny that safety issues overshadow in importance all other considerations pertaining to laparoscopic surgery. Whatever the advantages of laparoscopic surgery may be, if they cannot be made as safe as open procedures, they will and should be discarded. The need for training, credentialling, and audit must be recognized and implemented, and these issues will be discussed in Chapter 24.

CONCLUSIONS

There is considerable evidence that most laparoscopic operations are beneficial, but the information has been slow to appear in print because editors have been reluctant to publish manuscripts dealing with laparoscopic surgery in the belief that they are serving the common good. For example, in 1992, a major ob/gyn journal lamented that a recent literature search had identified only two cases of laparoscopic or laparoscopically assisted hysterectomy (27). The lament was disingenuous, however, for shortly thereafter the journal declined to publish a report on almost 600 laparoscopic hysterectomies (Reich, personal communications)!

There is also considerable evidence that laparoscopic operations are safe, although not innocuous. The ureteral injuries that have occurred with laparoscopic hysterectomies are particularly worrying, but because the causes of the injuries are being identified and new techniques for hysterectomy developed, there is every reason to hope that these injuries can and will be reduced to a minimum.

There is no evidence that the option of a laparoscopic approach has enticed gynecologists into performing operations that they would otherwise not have performed, a possibility that some have found especially disturbing (27), not unless one wishes to categorize lysis of adhesions during diagnostic laparoscopy in this way rather than as a bonus from a diagnostic procedure. In a consecutive series of 62 laparoscopic hysterectomies reported by Hasson (44), only 19% of patients had no pathological abnormality in the surgical specimen; in our own series of 24 obese (≥200 lbs) women undergoing laparoscopic hysterectomy only three (12.5%) had no pathological abnormality in the surgical specimen. These figures are no different from those reported by others for abdominal hysterectomy.

We would, therefore, reply to our critics by saying that laparoscopic surgery is not a technical gimmick of unproven value but the most significant development in surgery in recent times that will forever change the way many operations will be performed in the future.

REFERENCES

1. Grimes DA. Frontiers of operative laparoscopy: a review and critique of the evidence. Am J Obstet Gynecol 1992; 166:1062–1071.

2. Gant NF. Infertility and endometriosis: comparison of pregnancy outcomes with laparotomy versus laparoscopic techniques. Am J Obstet Gynecol 1992;166:1072–1081.

3. Summit RL, Stoval TG, Lipscomb GH, Long FW. Randomized comparison of laparoscopically assisted vaginal hysterectomy versus standard vaginal hysterectomy in an outpatient setting. Obstet Gynecol 1992;80:895–901.

4. Goncalves LF, Romero R. A critical appraisal of the RADIUS study. The Fetus 1993;3:7–17.

5. Liu CY. Laparoscopic hysterectomy. Gynaecol Endosc 1993;2:73–75.

6. Phipps JH, Nayak MJS. Comparison of laparoscopic versus vaginal hysterectomy and bilateral salpingo-oophorectomy with conventional abdominal hysterectomy and bilateral salpingo-oophorectomy. Br J Obstet Gynaecol 1993;100:698–700.

7. Auld BJ, Raju KS. A randomized prospective study of laparoscopically assisted vaginal hysterectomy versus abdominal hysterectomy in patients undergoing hysterectomy with bilateral salpingo-oophorectomy (Abstract). Presented at the 22nd Annual Meeting of the American Association of Gynecologic Endoscopists, San Francisco, CA, November 10–14, 1993.

8. Richardson RE, Broadbent M, Boumas N, Magos L. Randomized control trial of laparoscopically assisted against conventional vaginal hysterectomy (Abstract). Presented at the 2nd European Congress in Gynecological Endoscopy, Heidelberg, October 21–23, 1993; 106.

9. Richardson RE, Broadbent M, Boumas N, Magos L. What factors influence operating time at laparoscopically assisted hysterectomy? (Abstract) Presented at the 2nd European Congress in Gynecological Endoscopy, Heidelberg, October 21–23, 1993, 104–105.

10. Treger MA, Brody SA. Modification of surgical technique of LAVH based on preoperative clinical assessment (abstract). Presented at the 22nd Annual Meeting of the American Association of Gynecologic Endoscopists, San Francisco, CA, November 10–14, 1993.

11. Demco LA, Logan BS. Laparoscopic hysterectomy, a comparison to abdominal and vaginal hysterectomy. Presented at the 2nd European Congress in Gynecological Endoscopy, Heidelberg, October 21–23, 1993; 34.

12. DePrest J. "BELCOHYST": Two years experience of the Belgium National Register of Laparoscopic Hysterectomy (Abstract). Presented at the 2nd European Congress in Gynecological Endoscopy, Heidelberg, October 21–23, 1993; 34–35.

13. Vessey MP, Villard-Mackintosh L, McPherson K, Coulter A, Yeates D. The epidemiology of hysterectomy: findings in a large cohort study. Br J Obstet Gynaecol 1992;99:402–407.

14. Kadar N, Reich H. laparoscopically assisted radical Schauta hysterectomy and bilateral pelvic lymphadenectomy for the treatment of bulky Stage IB carcinoma of the cervix. Gynaecol Endosc 1993;2:135–142.

15. Querleu D. Laparoscopic para-aortic lymph node sampling in gynecologic oncology: a preliminary experience. Gynecol Oncol 1993;49:24–29.

16. Kadar N. Laparoscopic pelvic lymphadenectomy for the treatment of gynecological malignancies: description of a technique. Gynaecol Endosc 1992;1:79–83.

17. Childers JA, Hatch KD, Tran AN, Surwit EA. Laparoscopic para-aortic lymphadenectomy in gynecologic malignancies. Obstet Gynecol 1993;82:741–747.

18. Fowler J, Carter J, Carlson J, et al. Lymph node yield from laparoscopic lymphadenectomy in cervical cancer: a comparative study (Abstract). Gynecol Oncol 1993; 49:129.

19. Spirtos NM, Schlaerth JB, Spirtos TW, Kimball RE. Laparoscopic bilateral aortic and pelvic lymph node sampling: a new technique (Abstract). Gynecol Oncol 1993;49:137–138.

20. Kadar N. Laparoscopic resection of fixed and enlarged aortic lymph nodes in patients with advanced cervix cancer. Gynaecol Endosc 1993; 2:217–221.

21. Kadar N, Pelosi MA. Can cervix cancer be adequately staged by laparoscopic aortic lymphadenectomy? Gynaecol Endosc (in press).

22. Kadar N. Laparoscopic vaginal radical hysterectomy: an operative technique and its evolution. Gynaecol Endosc 1994;3:109–122.

23. Querleu D. laparoscopically assisted radical vaginal hysterectomy (Abstract). Presented at the 22nd Annual Meeting of the American Association of Gynecologic Endoscopists, San Francisco, CA, November 10–14, 1993.

24. Liu CY, Paek W. Laparoscopic retropubic colposuspension (Burch procedure). J Am Assoc Gynecol Laparoscop 1993;1:31–35.

25. Nezhat C, Nezhat C, Nezhat F, Bess O. Laparoscopic retropubic urethropexy (Abstract). Presented at the 22nd

Annual Meeting of the American Association of Gynecologic Endoscopists, San Francisco, CA, November 10–14, 1993.

26. Reich H, McGlynn F, Parente C, Sekel L, Levie M. Laparoscopic tubal anastomosis. J Am Assoc Gynecol Laparoscop 1993;1:16–19.

27. Pitkin RM. Operative laparoscopy: surgical advance or technical gimmick? Obstet Gynecol 1992;72:441–442.

28. Grimes DA. Laparoscopic surgery: experiment or expedient? Reply to letter. Am J Obstet Gynecol 1993; 168:1333–1334.

29. Trope C, Inversen T. Laparoscopic radical hysterectomy: technical gimmick or surgical advance? Gynaecol Endosc 1993;2:83–84.

30. Chandler JA. Laparoscopic pelvic surgery. Better? Safer? (letter). Am J Obstet Gynecol 1994;170:253–254.

31. Jensen RPS. Minimal endometriosis and reduced fecundability: prospective evidence from an artificial insemination by donor program. Fertil Steril 1987;47:40–48.

32. Mahmood TA, Templeton A. The impact of treatment on the natural history of endometriosis. Human Reprod 1990;5:965–970.

33. Garcia CR, David SS. Pelvic endometriosis: infertility and pelvic pain. Obstet Gynecol 1977;129:740–747.

34. Polan ML, DeCherney A. Presacral neurectomy for pelvic pain and infertility. Fertil Steril 1980;34:557–560.

35. Tjaden B, Schlaff WD, Kambel A, Rock JA. The efficacy of presacral neurectomy for the relief of midline dysmenorrhea. Obstet Gynecol 1990;76:89–91.

36. Candiani GB, Fedele L, Vercellini P, Bianchi S, Di Nola G. Presacral neurectomy for the treatment of pelvic pain associated with endometriosis: a controlled study. Am J Obstet Gynecol 1991;67:100–103.

37. Ewen SP, Sutton CJG, Whitelaw N, Haines P. Prospective randomized double blind controlled trial of the treatment of minimal to moderate endometriosis with laser laparoscopy (Abstract). Presented at the 2nd European Congress in Gynaecologic Endoscopy, Heidelberg, October 21–23, 1993; 44.

38. Nezhat CR, Nezhat FR. A simplified method of laparoscopic presacral neurectomy for the treatment of central pelvic pain due to endometriosis. Br J Obstet Gynaecol 1992;99:1659–1663.

39. Querleu D, Chevallier L, Chapron C, Bruhat MA. Complications of gynecological laparoscopic surgery. A French multicenter collaborative study. Gynaecol Endosc 1993;2:3–6.

40. Kadar N, Lemmerling L. Urinary tract injuries during laparoscopically assisted hysterectomy: causes and prevention. Am J Obstet Gynecol 1994;170:47–48.

41. Hunter RW, McCartney AJ. Can laparoscopic assisted hysterectomy safely replace abdominal hysterectomy? Br J Obstet Gynaecol 1993;100:932–934.

42. Childers JA, Brzechffa PR, Hatch KD, Surwit EA. laparoscopically assisted surgical staging (LASS) of endometrial cancer. Gynecol Oncol 1993;51:33–38.

43. Hourcabie JA, Bruhat M-A. One hundred and three cases of laparoscopic hysterectomy using endo-GIA staples and a device for presenting the vaginal fornices. Gynaecol Endosc 1993;2:65–72.

44. Hasson HM. Experience with laparoscopic hysterectomy. J Am Assoc Gyn Laparoscopists 1993;1:1-11.

Chapter 2
Preliminaries: Positioning the Patient and Equipment, Entering the Abdomen

Thinking is more interesting than knowing, but less interesting than looking.—Goethe

The importance of achieving optimal working conditions cannot be exaggerated. When things do not go smoothly in the operating room, it is almost always due to a concatenation of factors that militate against an optimal working environment, most commonly because

1. the patient and/or the equipment has not been properly prepared or positioned,
2. essential equipment, almost always the electrosurgical unit or the camera-monitor system, is malfunctioning,
3. essential equipment is not available, almost always because the hospital has refused to buy it or because the wrong equipment has been purchased, or
4. instrumentation of the abdomen has gone awry, usually because
   (i)   there is bleeding from the trocar insertion site,
   (ii) the peritoneum has been dissected away from the anterior abdominal wall during trocar insertion,
   (iii) the trocars have not been placed in the right positions, or
   (iv) a pneumoperitoneum has not been obtained.

PREPARING THE PATIENT

Proper patient preparation in the operating room requires correct positioning on the operating table, insertion of an orogastric tube, avoidance of nitrous oxide, and heating of the inspired air. Obviously, the cooperation of the anesthesiologist is required to achieve this, but endoscopic techniques are new for anesthesiologists too, and they may be reluctant participants in the undertaking to the extent that optimal working conditions are not always achieved, and the operation may be compromised.

There is controversy over whether the use of nitrous oxide, by causing bowel distention, impairs operative exposure. It is well recognized that nitrous oxide will cause an increase in the volume of gas in a closed space according to the formula:

$$100/(100-\%N_2O)$$

Therefore, if the patient is receiving 50% nitrous oxide, within about two hours, her bowel gas will increase by $100/50=2$, i.e., it will double; if she is receiving 75% nitrous oxide, her bowel gas will quadruple. There is no dispute over this point.

What is disputed, however, is the extent to which these considerations are relevant to unobstructed bowel. The volume of gas in the unobstructed bowel may be only about 100 ml, and even if this volume is doubled, this may not result in clinically significant bowel distention. It has also been argued that the unobstructed bowel does not constitute a closed space, but this is only true if the patient passes gas (which is uncommon under anesthesia) or a rectal tube is inserted and kept in place during surgery. Apparently, nitrous oxide does not cause sufficient bowel distention during laparoscopic cholecystectomy to interfere with the operation in most cases, but this is a rather

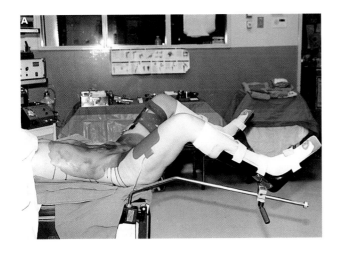

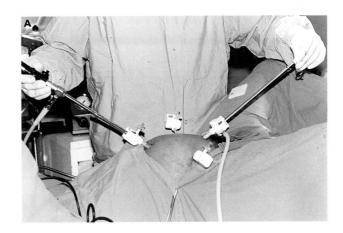

Figure 2.1A   Inadequate extension of the hips will interfere with manipulation of the lower abdominal trocars.

short operation, which is over before the nitrous oxide can be expected to exert its maximal effect on bowel distention. All in all, it is clear from first principles that nitrous oxide may impede a prolonged operation by causing sufficient bowel distention in some, even if not in all, patients, and it would seem prudent to avoid its use.

The problem of hypothermia and its prevention will be discussed in Chapter 5.

POSITIONING THE PATIENT ON THE OPERATING TABLE

For pelvic operations, patients are placed in Allen stirrups with the knees flexed, thighs abducted but not flexed at the hips. It is very important not to flex the hips; otherwise the thighs will limit the range of motion of instruments inserted through the lower abdominal trocars (Figure 2.1A). Thus, the angle between the torso and the upper thigh, in our opinion, should not be 150° but 180° (Figure 2.1B). Avoidance of the lithotomy position also mitigates the cardiopulmonary changes that take place during laparoscopic surgery by removing one of the factors that increases intra-abdominal pressure (see Chapter 5). Patients should be positioned while awake to ensure that undue stresses are not placed on the back and joints.

Shoulder braces should be used, especially in obese patients, because steep Trendelenburg position (20–30°) is often required. These need to be placed over the acromioclavicular joint and not over the soft tissues, to avoid injury to the brachial plexus.

The arms should not be placed in the "crucifix" position, and, under no circumstances, should they be abducted more than 90°. The ideal position is to have both arms tucked under the patient to minimize the risk of brachial plexus injury, with ulnar pads to protect the ulnar nerve. This ideal is often not attainable because of resistance from the anesthesiologists or because the patient is obese and there is simply insufficient room on the operating table to place both arms by the patient's sides. Under these circumstances, one arm should be abducted and the patient's head should be turned toward the side of the abducted arm to minimize stretching the brachial plexus (Figure 2.1B).

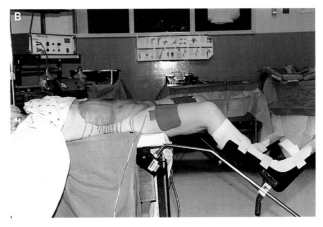

Figure 2.1B   Correct extension of the hips through 180°. Note that the patient's head has been turned toward the extended arm (which should always be the side the assistant stands on).

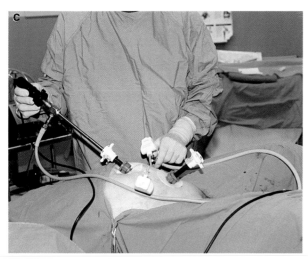

Figure 2.1C *The operating table should be lowered to waist height.*

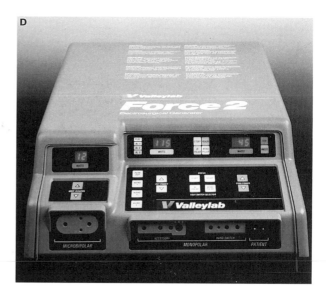

Figure 2.1D *Valley Lab Force 2 electrosurgical generator, showing bipolar and monopolar circuit attachment sites.*

Unless the surgeon is exceptionally tall, the operating table should be as low to the ground as it will go so that the surgeon's hands are at waist height, and the shoulder never has to be abducted during surgery; otherwise the deltoids will fatigue (Figure 2.1C). If the surgeon is short or the patient obese, the surgeon should stand on a low foot stool to ensure that the hands are at waist height. The foot pedals for the electrosurgical unit (unipolar and bipolar) are placed on a separate foot stool next to the one the surgeon is standing on. The amount of head-down tilt required will vary from case to case, and the minimum necessary should always be used.

Some electrosurgical units, such as those designed by Valley Lab, have two sets of pedals, one designed for the unipolar mode, and the other for the bipolar mode, and the surgeon can pick whichever mode he wishes to use by simply stepping on the appropriate pedal (Figure 2.1D). On other units, a switch has to be thrown by the circulating nurse to select the desired mode. If this is the only type of electrosurgical generator available, two generators should be used, one set to the unipolar mode and the other to the bipolar mode. Otherwise, the surgeon is dependent on the circulating nurse to switch from one mode to the other, and this is inefficient, causes delays, and can lead to errors because it is difficult to see from the operating table which mode has been selected.

SITES USED FOR TROCAR PLACEMENT

Trocar placement sites are, to some extent, a matter of personal preference and also, to some extent, tai-

lored to suit the circumstances of individual patients, i.e., size of patient, site and type of pathology present. Nonetheless, the same basic setup suffices for most major pelvic operations. We use four trocars placed in the following positions (Figure 2.2).

❶ A 10-mm trocar is placed infraumbilically and is used for the laparoscope.

❷ A secondary trocar is placed approximately one finger's breadth above the symphysis pubis. A 5-mm trocar is used for benign cases, and a 10-mm one for radical surgery. The general tendency is to place this port too high for fear of injuring the bladder. It should almost always be placed lower than a Pfannenstiel incision.

❸ Two additional 5-mm trocars are placed at a point just above the line joining the anterior superior iliac spines, and just lateral to the rectus sheath, which is approximately four inches either side of the midline.

At the end of the operation the fascia should be closed at trocar sites ≥10 mm; otherwise, there is a risk of hernia formation (1).

ANATOMY OF THE INFERIOR EPIGASTRIC ARTERY

The inferior epigastric artery is a branch of the external iliac artery just above the inguinal ligament. It runs upward and medially along the medial border of the deep inguinal ring to pierce the transversalis fas-

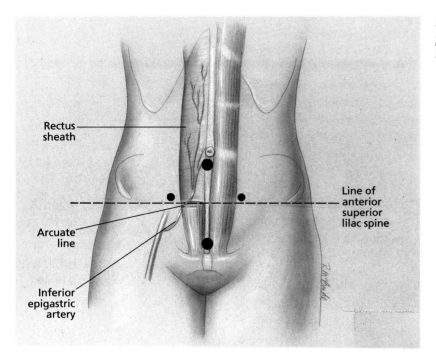

Figure 2.2 *Standard 4-mm trocar positions used for most major laparoscopic operations.*

Rectus sheath

Line of anterior superior lilac spine

Arcuate line

Inferior epigastric artery

cia and enter the rectus fascia at the arcuate line. The surface marking of the arcuate line is a line joining the anterior superior iliac spines (Figure 2.2). It is essential to avoid injury to the inferior epigastric arteries during insertion of the lateral trocars, and this can be achieved by placing the trocars lateral to the rectus sheath and above the line joining anterior superior iliac spine. Direct visualization of the epigastric is only helpful if the insertion site is below the level of the anterior superior iliac spine because, above that point, the epigastric

artery lies within the rectus sheath and is no longer visible through the peritoneum.

ESTABLISHING THE PNEUMOPERITONEUM

Insertion of the Veress Needle

Fat between the transversalis fascia and the parietal peritoneum is found predominantly in the triangle formed by the dome of the bladder and the two umbilical ligaments (Figure 2.3). The distance between the

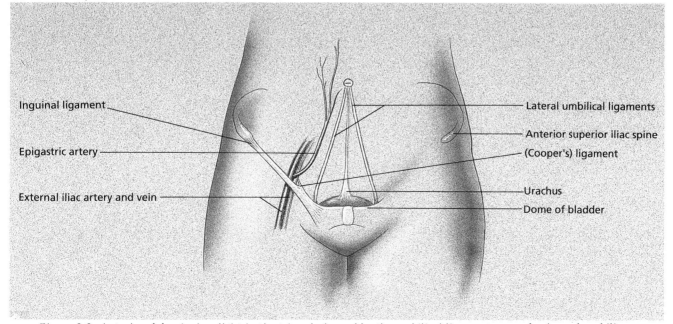

Inguinal ligament

Epigastric artery

External iliac artery and vein

Lateral umbilical ligaments

Anterior superior iliac spine

(Cooper's) ligament

Urachus

Dome of bladder

Figure 2.3 *Anterior abdominal wall fat in the triangle formed by the umbilical ligaments, symphysis, and umbilicus.*

skin and peritoneum is greatest within this area, and it is, therefore, not an ideal one for inserting the Veress needle. The shortest distance between the skin and peritoneum is at the umbilicus, where the skin, deep fascia, and peritoneum are fused. If this is used as the insertion site, extra long needles will not be required, even in obese patients, and the parietal peritoneum will not tent away from the Veress needle as it is being inserted.

Other sites have been used to insert the Veress needle when extensive adhesions involving the anterior abdominal wall were likely to be present. This can occur whenever a low midline incision is extended as far as the umbilicus or beyond, particularly if there have been multiple prior operations and if they have been complicated by or performed for infection. Under no circumstances should the Veress needle be inserted through such a scar. Rather, either the open technique must be used or the Veress needle inserted

1. at Palmer's point, approximately 3 cm below the left costal margin in the midclavicular line,
2. through the posterior vaginal wall,
3. through puncture of the uterine fundus, or
4. through the left ninth intercostal space in the midclavicular line, with a trocar subsequently placed just below the costal margin.

Technique of Insertion

The inferior wall of the umbilicus is incised with a scalpel either horizontally or transversely depending on the orientation of the natural skin fold. A No. 11 blade is preferred by this author, but whatever blade is used, the incision should be made with the blade parallel and not vertical to the skin, and it should be superficial. On no account should a stab incision be made because this can easily penetrate the peritoneal cavity and cause a bowel or large vessel laceration.

There are several techniques for inserting the needle, but this author still prefers to insert the Veress needle on the inferior wall of the umbilicus rather than at its base and to elevate the lower abdominal wall below the insertion site rather than vertically into the elevated umbilicus (Figures 2.4A,B). The purpose of this is to ensure that the course of the Veress needle will pass at right angles to the anterior wall. Elevation of the lower anterior abdominal wall does not create a space between the abdominal wall and the underlying tissues but simply positions the anterior wall at right angles to the path of insertion. Before inserting the Veress needle, the anterior superior iliac spines should

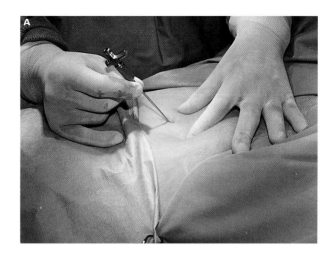

Figure 2.4A Infraumbilical insertion of the Veress needle at 45°.

be palpated and an imaginary line drawn to join them. The line will be at the level of the L4 vertebra, the usual site for the aortic bifurcation. This line, rather than the umbilicus, should be used for orientation because the position of the umbilicus is variable. The Veress needle is then inserted following an imaginary line to the midpelvis aiming toward the uterine fundus. This line should make a 45° angle with the long axis of the patient, but a shallower angle with the ground, because the patient will be in Trendelenburg position. Vertical insertions are, in this author's opinion, dan-

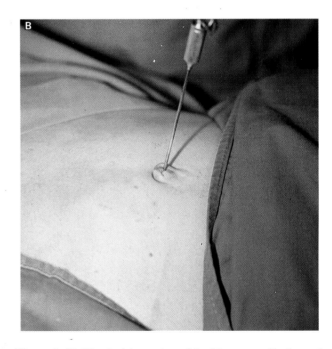

Figure 2.4B Vertical insertion of the Veress needle through the umbilicus.

Responses to issues brought forward by Dr. Prakash's deposition

1. As to his assertion that the initial scalpel incision "could not have caused the injury", this is both historically and as pertains to this case, alse. There have been multiple case reports of large vessel injury with the initial scalpel incision cited in both journals and textbooks. There is no absolute "correct" way of making the initial incision (i.e. no absolutely foolproof blade or technique); a textbook of surgery or a teaching physician such as myself would only say "make an incision through the skin". That statement implies not into the peritoneal cavity, which is certainly possible with a stabbing type of incision as was made in this case. Dr. Prakash is fully aware that his incision went beyond "the abdominal wall" (and I wonder if he recalls his statement at the immediate spurt of bright red blood—"Oh God, what have I done?". I remember this statement because this was such an exceptional case.) At no other time during the case (i.e. at the time of Verres needle insertion or trocar insertion) was unusual bleeding seen through or around the instrument. In addition, the extent of the retroperitoneal hematoma and the changes in vital signs all clearly point to the time of injury as the initial incision time.

2. The teaching and supervising physician wouldtypically stand to the right of the patient in cases such as this. This is where I was standing throughout the case to my tion. Even if I had inserted the Verres needle myself from this side, this is not "wrong". It may be slightly more difficult or awkward, but it is not "wrong". After the Verres needle insertion, I performed my usual procedures to check placement including observing the tip pressure, which was normal in this case; aspiratingg from the needle tip with a saline filled syringe (which woould clearly demonstrate blood if it was lodged in the aorta), anda hanging drop test which again was normal.

3. This statement seems strange in that he already said that his incision did not cause the injury. At that time, I would typically spread the umbilical creases open with an OPEN Kelly clamp to make it easier for the resident to see the incision placement. There was no "clamping of the skin" or undue pressure on the abdomen.

I also wonder if Dr. Prakash remembers my statement to him just before we started the procedure that in thin patients such as the one in this case, there were reports of vessel injury even at the initial incision and great care must be taken. This was my first time operating with Dr. Prakash (to the best of my recollection), and I also remember in our conversations both before and after the case that he emphasized that he had done many such procedures during his training in India.

gerous and risk injury to the aorta or vena cava even in experienced hands.

Correct positioning of the Veress needle is done by feel, and with experience, the operator will know when the Veress needle has been correctly placed. For this reason, those accustomed to the original reusable Veress needles should give some thought before switching to disposable ones and be mindful of the fact that these have completely different mechanisms of action, and consequently, the tactile sensation during insertion is entirely different from the one the surgeon may have grown accustomed to. Parenthetically, the same is, of course, true for different types of disposable trocars, which have different tip designs. The force required to insert these can vary enormously, and the sensation felt when the trocar is in the right place may vary considerably from one trocar to another. In this author's opinion, therefore, patient care is potentially compromised by the indiscriminate switching from one type of trocar to another that operating room administrators frequently foist on surgeons, ostensibly out of fiscal considerations that surgeons are in no position to verify for they are not privy to the terms of such arrangements. The various syringe tests that have been advocated to check on Veress needle placement are entirely nonspecific. If the Veress needle has been placed extraperitoneally, the space will easily accommodate 5–10 cc of fluid, and it is uncommon for fluid to be reaspirated with extraperitoneal insertion. This author does not consider these tests helpful and does not use them, nor does he twist the Veress needle in various directions to check its position. In the unlikely event that a viscus or, worse still, a large vessel has been perforated, manipulation of the needle will only worsen the damage, and if the needle is in the peritoneal cavity, moving it around in different directions can cause a vasovagal response.

Another indicator of correct needle placement is end **insufflation pressure,** which should be ≤ 15 cm/H_2O. The pressure measured during insufflation is the insufflation pressure, but this is only slightly higher than end insufflation pressure when the insufflation rate is less than 1 L/min. After about 500 ml of gas have been insufflated, there should be percussion resonance over the right hypochondrium. A much more helpful check, however, is the "watered sign," the name given to the wave-like fluctuation of the entire abdominal wall as it is successfully pressed and released suprapubically.

Direct Trocar Insertion

Direct trocar insertion is the method of insufflation now favored by the author except in patients at high risk for periumbilical adhesions, in which case Hasson's open technique is used.

The actual technique of trocar insertion is identical to that used to insert a Veress needle. A horizontal or vertical skin incision about 1 cm in length is made in the inferior wall of the umbilicus with a No. 11 blade. The abdominal wall is grasped in the midline halfway between the umbilicus and the symphysis and elevated. With the patient in Trendelenburg position, a 10-mm trocar is inserted into the peritoneal cavity along an imaginary line that makes an angle of about 45° with the long axis of the patient and meets the uterine fundus in the pelvis (Figure 2.5A). One smooth thrust is used, and the index finger is placed far down the shaft of the trocar to guard against unduly deep penetration, although this is less important if trocars with safety shields are used (Figure 2.5B).

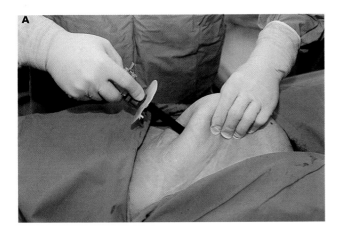
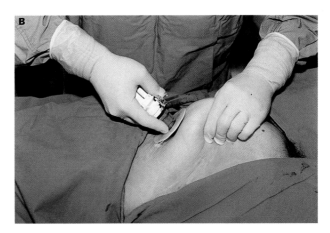

Figure 2.5A,B Direct insertion of a 10-mm Surgiport with an attached Endopatch used for trocar stabilization.

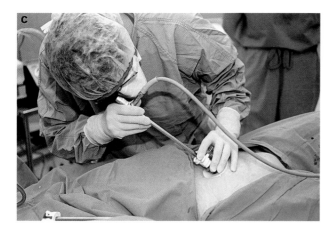

Figure 2.5C *The trocar position is checked laparoscopically prior to insufflation.*

Once the trocar has been inserted, under no circumstances is its position changed before it has been checked laparoscopically. The laparoscope is introduced and the abdominal wall elevated to check that the trocar has been placed intraperitoneally (Figure 2.5C). The abdomen is then insufflated using the highest flow rate available.

We have switched to using this technique because it is not only faster but, we believe, theoretically less dangerous. Trocar injuries end in calamity when they are recognized late or not at all. If the trocar is inserted into the peritoneal cavity and its position is not altered, any injury to a viscus or a vessel that may have occurred during insertion should, in principle, be identified immediately by the laparoscopic check on trocar location. Indeed, in one reported case of a trocar injury to the transverse colon, this is precisely how the injury was recognized and promptly repaired without sequelae (2). In one randomized trial, failed insertions occurred three times more frequently with the Veress needle technique than after direct trocar placement (2). Although this was not confirmed in a subsequent study, direct insertions were certainly as safe as the Veress needle technique (3).

OPEN LAPAROSCOPY

Open laparoscopy provides a completely different method of gaining access to the peritoneal cavity and eliminates the surprisingly small but definite risks inherent in the conventional, "blind" approach. We now use it exclusively in women who have had previous operations that place them at risk of having significant periumbilical adhesions and when the uterus is greatly

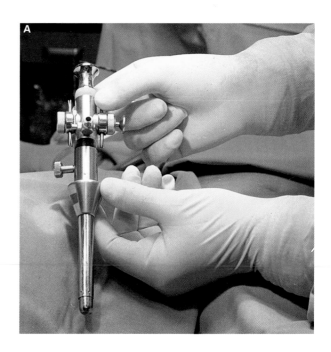

Figure 2.6A *The Hasson cannula.*

enlarged (see Chapter 13). The technique was developed by Dr. Harrith Hasson, who designed a special cone with V-shaped flanges for suture attachment to fit over the sleeve of a 10-mm trocar (Figure 2.6A). After opening the peritoneal cavity under direct vision, the trocar is introduced into the peritoneal cavity with a blunt obturator. It is then held in place by means of the Hasson cone, which is screwed tightly onto the trocar and fixed to the abdominal fascia by means of stay sutures in the fascia (Figure 2.6B). Hasson made the in-

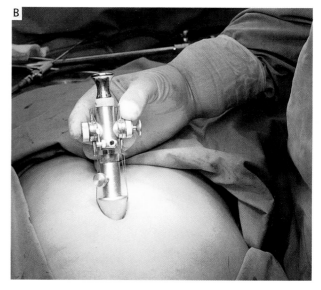

Figure 2.6B *The Hasson cannula secured in position.*

cision intraumbilically to take advantage of the fact that here the peritoneum and fascia fuse with the skin, and there is no intervening adipose tissue, even in obese patients. The incision can, however, be made extraumbilically.

The skin is picked up with Allis clamps and a 1– to 2–cm incision in made vertically in the umbilicus at the 6 o'clock position. The Allis clamps are then placed on the skin edges and, after separating the subcutaneous tissues by blunt scissor dissection, the deep fascia at the top of the incision is grasped with Kocker clamps and the fascia cleaned further (Figure 2.6C). A second Kocker clamp is placed on the fascia vertically below

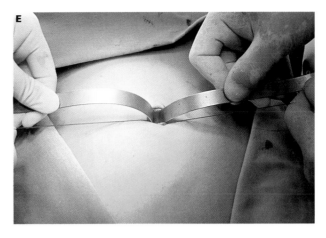

Figure 2.6E The peritoneal cavity is exposed with S-shaped retractors.

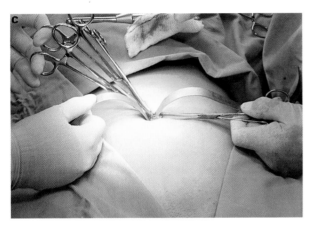

Figure 2.6C The skin has been incised and the fascia picked up and cleaned of overlying fat.

the first one, the fascia is incised transversely, and the opening is enlarged by spreading the jaws of a Kelly clamp. Each fascial edge is tagged with a zero polyglycolic acid suture (Figure 2.6D), and if the peritoneum was not entered with the Kelly clamp, it is now picked up and incised between two Kelly clamps. Small deaver-like ("S-shaped") retractors are placed in the peritoneal cavity for exposure (Figure 2.6E). The Hasson cone is slipped over a blunt-ended trocar and fastened into a position adjusted to the thickness of the abdominal wall (Figure 2.6F). The trocar and cone are

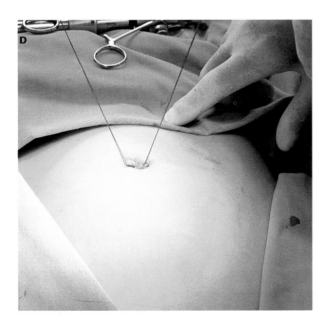

Figure 2.6D The fascial edges are tagged with sutures.

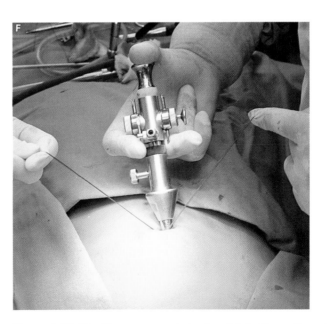

Figure 2.6F The Hasson cannula is placed into the peritoneal cavity and adjusted to the thickness of the anterior abdominal wall.

placed into the peritoneal cavity, the S-shaped retractors withdrawn, and the stay sutures threaded around the V-shaped flanges of the cone to secure the trocar in place (Figure 2.6B). When the incision is closed at the end of the operation, the stay sutures are tied to each other and then tied down as a horizontal mattress stitch. Different trocar systems have been designed for open laparoscopy. One we find particularly useful is shown in Figure 2.6G, which makes use of a retention device similar to that used for the Dexide trocars, and has a cover for the incision, which prevents loss of the pneumoperitoneum (Figure 2.6G).

Choice of Trocars

Numerous trocars are available, usually in three different sizes, 5-mm, 10/11-mm, and 12-mm, and they fall into two broad categories, reusable and disposable. The only advantage of a reusable trocar is its lower cost, although proper cost comparisons have not been carried out, and the actual cost saved by using reusable instead of disposable trocars is a matter for speculation. The disadvantages of reusable trocars compared with disposable ones is that they do not have spring-loaded protective shields, and they become dull with use and require greater force for in-

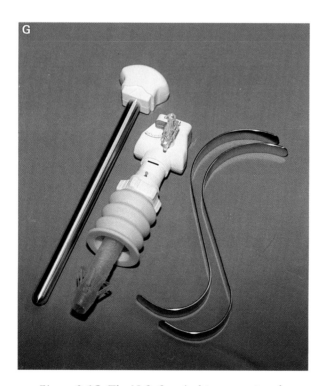

Figure 2.6G The U.S. Surgical trocar system for open laparoscopy.

sertion. Both these features increase the risk of injury to the underlying abdominal structures during insertion of the first trocar.

Whichever type of trocar is used, the one that requires the least amount of force to insert should be selected. We consider the Ethicon Tristar trocar to be particularly dangerous precisely because it requires a great deal of force to insert. Unfortunately, the company was slow to recognize this deficiency and surgeons' complaints were met with the rejoinder that the wrong technique of insertion was being used. This was, of course, quite untrue as reflected by the fact that the company is finally replacing these potentially dangerous trocars. Trocars that require a great deal of force to insert also tend to dissect the peritoneum away from the anterior abdominal wall, which can lead to problems with exposure.

A major problem that remains unresolved is how to fix the trocar sleeve in position for the duration of the operation. Trocar sleeves are frequently pulled out from the peritoneal cavity during instrument exchanges. This causes loss of the pneumoperitoneum and delays the operation. If the trocar is not reinserted through its original path, gas can escape through the first puncture site, cause subcutaneous emphysema, and dissect the peritoneum away from the anterior abdominal wall, leading to problems with exposure. On the other hand, if the trocars are pushed in too deeply, this can interfere with the surgery and prevent instruments from opening properly.

The U.S. Surgical Corporation was the first to introduce a screw-fixing device to fit onto trocar sleeves to hold them in place. This has become the most popular method of trying to fix trocars in place, and some manufacturers have incorporated the thread into the trocar sleeve. Although the method may work for short, simple operations, we have not found it to work well for major cases requiring extensive dissection and manipulation of the trocar. The thread of the screw-fixing device soon works loose and enlarges the trocar tract, which has already been enlarged by the screw-fixing device. In our opinion, this predisposes to hernia formation because the distal end of the trocar tract will become enlarged by the manipulation of instruments (1).

Although our experience with it is still limited, the Dexide self-stabilizing trocar seems promising (Figure 2.7A). After the trocar is inserted, an umbrella-like device is opened, which resembles a mushroom or Malencot catheter (Figure 2.7B). This is pulled up against the anterior abdominal wall, and a collar is pushed

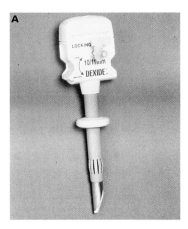

Figure 2.7A The Dexide trocar.

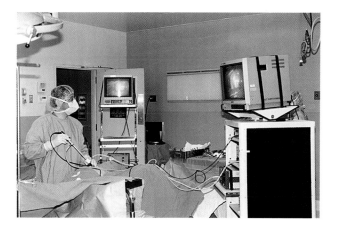

Figure 2.8 The video monitors are placed at 4 and 8 o'clock positions. (Patient's head is at 12 o'clock.)

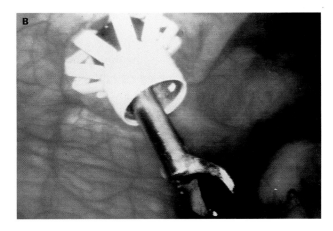

Figure 2.7B The Dexide trocar showing the "umbrella" retention device.

down onto the skin to prevent the trocar from slipping too far into the peritoneal cavity. We have also not had an adequate opportunity to evaluate the new Endopatch designed by the Autosuture company (Figures 2.5A,B), but the few times we have been able to use it, the Endopatch has worked extremely well and stayed in place even during long, complicated operations requiring extensive dissection (one radical hysterectomy and bilateral pelvic lymphadenectomy, and one aortic lymphadenectomy and simple hysterectomy).

POSITIONING THE VIDEO MONITORS

Three-dimensional space is projected onto two dimensions in the videoscopic display of endoscopic procedures. However, provided that the video monitor being observed by the operating surgeon is positioned in the line of the laparoscope, little difficulty will be encountered with hand-eye coordination (Fig-

ure 2.8). Depth perception is gained from the relative position of the operating instrument to the structures in the pelvis. At any given level in the pelvis, movements in two dimensions will correspond exactly to the two-dimensional movements observed on the video monitor. However, if a line drawn perpendicular to the monitor being observed makes an angle with a line parallel to the direction in which the laparoscope is pointing, difficulties with hand-eye coordination will at first be encountered.

The situation is best likened to steering a remote controlled toy car. As long as the car is traveling away from the driver, steering will not present a problem, but if the car is traveling toward the driver, he or she will find it extremely difficult to steer the car at first. Steering is made much easier if the controls are turned upside down, the surgical parallel of which is changing sides on the operating table. The secret of ridding oneself of the need to change sides during surgery is mentally to picture where the instruments being viewed on the monitor are in the patients. Without this mental effort, the brain treats the video image as the real world. However, if the mind's eye tells it where the instruments actually are, the image on the video screen will be interpreted by the brain as the place only to view the real world.

For pelvic operations, the monitors are best positioned at the foot of the operating table at the 4 and 8 o'clock positions (Figure 2.8). If the laparoscope is inserted through the suprapubic trocar, so that the direction of "vision" is toward the patient's head (Figure 2.9), the monitors are best placed above the level of the umbilicus at approximately the 2 and 10 o'clock positions. This arrangement is usually required for aortic lymphadenectomy and presacral neurectomy.

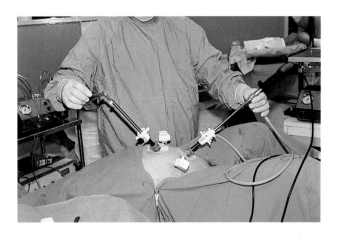

Figure 2.9 The laparoscope is inserted suprapubically for aortic lymphadenectomy and presacral neurectomy, and the cameras are placed above the surgeon at 2 and 10 o'clock.

Trouble-Shooting the Video System

The video system is to laparoscopic surgery what exposure is to laparotomy. Failure to invest in a superlative camera-light-cable-monitor system is the most foolish of false economies. Operations are needlessly prolonged if the surgeon cannot see properly because of glare, inadequate light, or interference from the electrosurgical unit. These problems are the most common causes of equipment malfunction and cause operations to be prolonged more than any other factor.

Glare

Glare is not merely an annoyance or inconvenience. It can be a distinct hazard and slow the operation down considerably (Figure 2.10A). Try to imagine dissecting the external iliac vein out of its areolar sheath when there is a bright reflection from the overlying artery. The vein wall can, as it is, merge imperceptibly with the surrounding areolar tissue, and the added incumbrance that glare imposes can be very troubling to the surgeon, not to say potentially dangerous for the patient.

Those who operate at more than one hospital will have the advantage (or some might consider disadvantage) of working with a variety of cameras, light cables, etc. It becomes readily apparent that sophisticated though these video cameras all are, some of much better than others because they cause less glare or provide sharper, more natural colors.

Glare is a function of the sensitivity of the camera, which is measured in lux, a concept entirely analogous to the sensitivity or "speed" of the photographic film used for everyday photography. The more sensitive the camera, the less light is required for the same clarity of image, and the less light is reflected back to the camera. However, just as the use of photographic film that is too fast for a given purpose will yield an overexposed picture, glare may result if the sensitivity of the camera, its light source, and the feedback system (automatic iris) that regulates the amount of light delivered to the field are not properly balanced. Unfortunately, it is not easy for surgeons to discover where the problem lies, and sales representatives are not ready to disclose potential deficiencies in their systems.

Dark Image

If the image on the video camera-monitor system is too dark, the likely cause will depend on whether

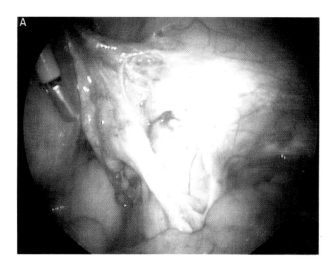
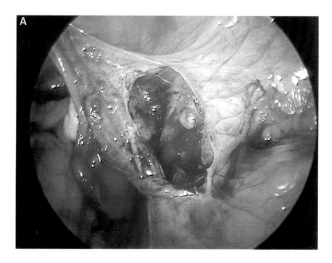

Figure 2.10A Photograph of opened pelvic sidewall triangle (left) taken with the Laprocam (Stortz) and (right) the Stryker 3-chip camera. Notice that in addition to the glare in the first photograph, the rest of the field is dark, and the colors unnatural.

this is a recent problem in a system that was previously functioning satisfactorily or one that is constant (Figure 2.10B). When confronted by a dark image, the surgeon should first check that the high-gain switch on the light source has been turned on. The light cable should be checked next by holding one end of it up to the operating room light and looking down its other end. Burned out fibers will appear as black specks, and if more than about 20% of the area contains damaged fibers, the cable should be replaced. If the surgeon is constantly working with a dark image, the problem may lie anywhere along the "circuit," from light source to laparoscope, camera, and monitor.

The light source may be inadequate, although this is unlikely for all video camera systems are now equipped with 300–400-W halogen light sources. (The most powerful light source currently available is the 300-W xenon light source.) After checking the optical fibers in the cable, its size should be checked to ensure that a 4.8- or 6-mm rather than the standard 3.5-mm cable is being used. The wider cables have more quartz fibers and transmit significantly more light. It should be a simple matter to replace. The laparoscope should also be checked by holding it to one's eye to determine both the clarity and brightness of the image. The lens system can be damaged by repeated sterilization, particularly the lens coating, so that much of the light delivered to the laparoscope will not be transmitted. Finally, the camera or the monitor may simply be insensitive, and the only solution to poor quality image is to replace them.

There is little question in this author's mind that the Stryker 3-chip camera linked to a 600-line Sony monitor provides the best image currently available in terms of brightness and color quality. In addition to the camera's greater sensitivity, 3-chip cameras use analogue signals and require less signal processing than single-chip cameras and provide a far superior overall image. The image is bright, there is little glare, and the colors are faithful and do not "bleed" (Figure 2.10C). Single-chip cameras convert the analogue signals from the charge-coupled device (CCD) into digital signals, which are processed with respect to brightness and color and then converted back into an analogue image that is projected onto the video monitor. The quality of the chip as well as the processing can probably affect the final image, but it is impossible for surgeons to predict simply from the specifications of the system which system will perform better. For example, a brand new ACMI-Circon video camera system was recently installed at one of the hospitals where the author operates as a consulting gynecologist, and a laparoscopic hysterectomy with which he was assisting a gynecologist actually had to be abandoned because the image was so red that extraperitoneal structures could not be discerned, and the problem, which has resurfaced on other occasions since, could not be corrected by adjusting the controls on the video monitor.

Interference

Electrical signals from the electrosurgical generator can be picked up on the video monitor, and this usually interferes significantly with the surgeon's ability to see and slows the pace of surgery consider-

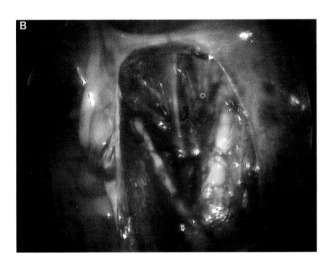

Figure 2.10B Photograph of the right pelvic sidewall taken with the Laprocam (Stortz). The field is dark and the colors unnatural.

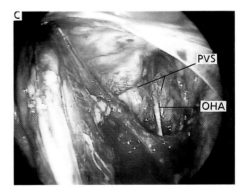

Figure 2.10C Photograph of the right paravesical space taken with the Stryker 3-chip camera. Compare the image quality with Figure 2.10B.

ably. The causes of this problem seem not to be well understood by biomedical engineers, much less surgeons. The most popular view is that there is "cross talk" between the electrical leads connecting the monitor and other equipment and that the problem can be resolved by connecting the video system to a socket separate from those into which other electrical equipment in the operating room are plugged. This tactic has certainly not solved the problem at one of the hospitals where the author operates as a consulting gynecologist.

Another view is that electrical interference reflects a fault in one or more of the condensers of the electrosurgical unit. Electricity "leaks" out and is picked up by the connecting wires of the video monitor, which act as an antenna. Whichever view is correct, and they may both be, it is clear that such interference should not be allowed to be treated merely as a nuisance. It compromises the quality of the surgery and may, in fact, reflect a potentially hazardous problem with the electrosurgical generator. It should be the responsibility of the director of the operating room to see to it that the hospital's biomedical engineers solve the problem.

Fogging

Fogging is caused by condensation of water vapor on the end of the laparoscope. The condensation occurs because the gas in the peritoneal cavity is warm and moist and the end of the laparoscope is cold. The solution lies in warming the end of the laparoscope by either dipping it into warm water or touching it against the peritoneum.

Magnification

Finally, mention should be made of the effect of magnification of the laparoscope on image characteristics. Full-screen laparoscopes magnify the image 20- to 25-fold, and the image fills the entire video monitor screen. Laparoscopes that magnify only 12- to 16-fold provide an image that does not fill the entire screen but appears within a black circle. These latter are preferable in our opinion. Full-screen laparoscopes force the surgeon to work too close to the tissues, and they also do not have such good depth of focus.

REFERENCES

1. Kadar N, Reich H, Liu CY, Manco GF, Gimpleson R. Incisional hernias following major laparoscopic gynecological procedures. Am J Obstet Gynecol 1993;168: 1493–1495.

2. Borgatta L, Gruss L, Barad D, Kaali SG. Direct trocar insertion versus Veress needle use for laparoscopic sterilization. J Reprod Med 1990;35:891–894.

3. Nezhat FR, Silfen SL, Evans D, Nezhat C. Comparison of direct insertion of disposable and standard reusable laparoscopic trocars and previous pneumoperitoneum with Veress needle. Obstet Gynecol 1991;78:148–149.

Chapter 3
Principles and Uses
of Electrosurgery

Everything should be made as simple as possible; but not more so.—Einstein

ELECTROSURGERY VERSUS LASER SURGERY

The ability to coagulate and cut tissues with an electric current is indispensable to laparoscopic surgery regardless of the basic technique of dissection used. All laparoscopic surgeons must, therefore, become adept at electrosurgery, and to do so, they must understand how electrosurgery works and produces its tissue effects (both desirable and undesirable). However, in the strict sense, very little physics is required for such an understanding.

Although surgeons must meet stringent credentialling guidelines before they are allowed to use lasers in the operating room, no credentialling is required for the use of electrosurgical instruments. Classic gynecological texts, such as Te Linde's *Operative Gynecology,* devote an entire chapter to lasers but have not a word to say about the principles of electrosurgery. This is alarming, for in no sense is electricity less "technical," easier to use, or safer than laser light. If anything, the opposite is true.

We have purposefully chosen to say little about lasers in this atlas because they are entirely peripheral to art and craft of laparoscopic pelvic surgery, and situations in which a laser is indispensable simply never arise in the way they do, for example, in ophthalmology. Nonetheless, the public still thinks of laparoscopic surgery as "laser surgery," an emphasis that is grotesquely misplaced. If the same amount of thought, time, and money had been spent on the technology of endoscopic suturing or the design of oper-

ating tables, for example, as have been spent on lasers, laparoscopic surgery would probably be far further advanced than it is today.

A laser simply uses light (photons) to achieve what electricity achieves with electrons, and the many advantages claimed for lasers (more precise cutting, less tissue damage, better surgical results) have never been objectively demonstrated. Laser surgery is much more expensive and slower and produces more plume than a technique based on sharp scissor dissection complemented by electrosurgical coagulation and cutting. In our experience, most surgeons who rely exclusively on lasers for laparoscopic dissection never become very adept at sharp scissor dissection during laparotomy.

The surgeon who has mastered sharp scissor dissection will rarely, if ever, have need for lasers. He or she will certainly not find them to provide a more precise way of cutting tissues than scissors, especially not when endoscopic visualization is used, or to allow as complete or clean a dissection of vital structures, such as the vena cava or iliac vessels, as scissor dissection. Moreover, lasers that cut "precisely," i.e., the CO_2 laser, are not very hemostatic, especially not when used down the laparoscope for their focal length is then long and essentially fixed, the beam cannot be defocused, and only the tiniest of blood vessels can be coagulated. The truth of this was underscored in an otherwise excellent recent article (1) on the "laseroscopic" treatment of endometriosis by an essayist who suggested that presacral neurectomy should only be performed if, *inter alia,* an argon beam coagulator is available to control the hemorrhage, which can be considerable! Solid state lasers that are more hemostatic are also less "precise," and no laser can achieve the same degree of hemostasis as can be achieved with bipolar coagulation.

There is also no objective evidence for the claim that lasers produce less tissue damage or better surgical results than electrosurgery. After controlling for power density (see below), lasers and electric currents produce similar amounts of acute tissue damage, subsequent fibrosis, and adhesion formation (2). Pregnancy rates after lysis of adhesions, salpingostomy, and ablation of endometriosis are also similar regardless of whether electrosurgery or a laser is used (3,4). For all these reasons the routine use of lasers during operative laparoscopy should be discouraged in our opinion.

Properties of Electrosurgical Generators

▶ Current Characteristics

Frequency: For domestic and commercial use, electricity is supplied as an alternating, sinusoidal current with a frequency of 50 Hz (Europe) or 60 Hz (USA). In other words, this is what enters an electrosurgical generator when it is plugged into the mains. The current (electrons) flows in one direction until the maximum voltage is reached, falls to zero, and then flows in the reverse direction until it reaches the same peak voltage, whereupon the cycle repeats itself (Figure 3.1).

The frequency of the current is the number of times it changes direction per second, and this is measured in Hertz (Hz). One Hz = 1 cycle per second; 1 kilohertz (KHz) equals a thousand Hz, and 1 megahertz (MHz) equals a million Hz. Electrosurgical generators convert the incoming 60-Hz current into high frequency (usually 500 KHz to 3 MHz) current to prevent depolarization of nerves and muscles.

When an electric current is applied to tissues, charged particles within the electrical field move toward the pole that is of opposite charge. When an alternating current is applied, the polarity of the active electrode constantly changes sign, and charged particles move toward and then away from it as the current flow changes direction.

When an electrical current is applied to a nerve, sodium ions move out of the nerve and it is depolarized. Alternating currents with frequencies >10 KHz will not, however, depolarize nerves because the electrical field is unidirectional for <1/5000 of a second, and this is not sufficient to cause depolarization. The current frequencies produced by modern electrosurgical generators are much higher than necessary to prevent depolarization, but there are no known added advantages associated with such high frequencies. (Because the current frequency is in the same range as radiowaves, the terms radiofrequency current and radiofrequency electrosurgical generators are sometimes used.)

Type of Current: Electrosurgical generators provide two types of current, unmodulated and modulated (each, of course, is still a high frequency, alternating current). For many years, these two types of current were, unfortunately, referred to as "cutting" and "coagulating" currents, respectively, and these misnomers caused much confusion and engendered many misconceptions about electrosurgery. Cutting and coagulation are tissue effects, not types of current, and as we shall see, each effect can be produced by both an unmodulated and a modulated current.

The difference between a cutting and a coagulating current is quite simply the length of time for which the current actually flows while the generator is activated (Figures 3.2A–C). An unmodulated ("cutting") current flows continuously throughout the time the generator is activated (Figure 3.2A), whereas a modulated current flows for only part of the time. By convention, a "coagulation" current is one that flows for 10% of the time that the electrosurgical generator is activated (Figure 3.2B); blended currents flow for time periods that are in between these extremes, for example, 30%, 50%, or 70% of the time that the electrosurgical generator is activated (Figure 3.2C). (Those with a penchant for lasers may wish to liken an unmodulated current to the continuous lasing mode and a modulated current to the superpulse mode.)

The wave form of a modulated and blended current is also, in fact, slightly different from that of an unmodulated current, but this is an unimportant detail. The difference stems from the fact that the current does not instantaneously stop and start with each transition between the "on" and "off" periods. Instead, the

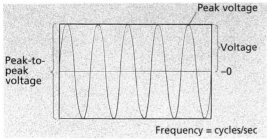

Figure 3.1 Characteristics of an alternating, sinuisoidal current.

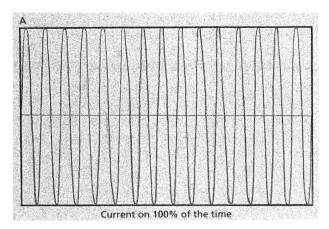

Figure 3.2A Unmodulated or "cutting" sinusoidal current flows throughout the time that the electrosurgical unit is activated.

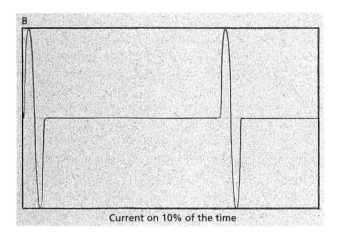

Figure 3.2B Modulated or "coagulation" current is one that, by convention, flows for only 10% of the time that the electrosurgical unit is activated

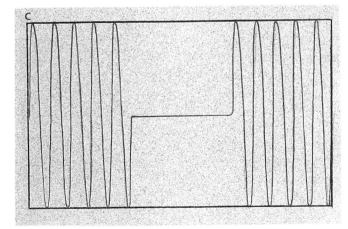

Figure 3.2C An example of a blended current flowing for about 70% of the time that the electrosurgical unit is activated.

voltage decreases rapidly but in a stepwise manner before the current flow is extinguished.

▶ **Power Output:** In addition to these qualitative differences between the electric currents produced by a generator, there are also quantitative differences that, colloquially speaking, reflect differences in current strength or intensity. The "intensity" of a current is measured in amps, and it is determined by the rate of electron flow, just as the rate of flow of water is determined by volume per time. Force is required to drive electrons along a wire or tissues, just as head of pressure is required for water to flow. This force is called the electromotive force, and it is measured in volts.

The voltage of a sinusoidal current can be expressed as the peak or peak-to-peak voltage, also called the "tension" of the current (Figure 3.1). Peak voltage is measured from zero to the peak, and peak-to-peak voltage is the difference between two peaks, i.e., twice the peak voltage. The amount of current flow produced by a given electromotive force depends on the resistance to current flow, and this is expressed by Ohm's law:

$$\text{Force (volts)} = \text{Current flow (amps)} \times \text{Resistance (ohms)}$$

This relationship expresses the fact that more force is required to generate the same flow of current as resistance is increased.

Just as a car going at a given speed must do more work to go up an incline than along the flat, an electrosurgical generator must do more (electric) work to generate a given current (in amps) with a higher voltage. The electrical work done by a generator is called its power output, and it is measured in watts. Thus,

$$\text{Power (watts)} = \text{Force (volts)} \times \text{Current flow (amps)}.$$

The power output (wattage) of most electrosurgical generators are calibrated in arbitrary units, on an arbitrary scale, which is nonlinear and bears no relationship to the scale used to calibrate a different machine. What this means is that if the power output of two machines is arbitrarily calibrated from 1 to 10, the power output of one generator set to "5," say, bears no relationship to the output of another generator set to "5." Moreover, if the setting is increased from 5 to 6, it does not follow that the watts generated will increase by 10%, or that the power output of two different machines will increase by the same number (or proportion) of watts. Generators that specify the power output in watts, e.g., from Valley Lab, are to be preferred.

The characteristics of modulated and unmodulated currents of equal power (watts) have different characteristics. An unmodulated current flows continuously; it has higher amperage and lower voltage. Modulated currents, however, have lower amperage and higher voltage, and the more the current is modulated, the higher the voltage per watt. High voltages, as we shall see, are a liability because they determine the ability of a current to spark or "jump." Modern electrosurgical generators now have much lower peak voltages than they had at one time and are, therefore, much safer.

▶ **Circuitry:** In order for an electric current to flow, a pathway must exist for the electrons to return to their site of origin, i.e., an electric circuit must be made. This can be achieved in several ways, but each type of circuit involves an active electrode from which the current emanates, and a second electrode through which the electrons are returned to the generator. The various circuits that are used for electrosurgery differ in the nature of this secondary electrode, and the manner in which the current is routed back to the generator (Figures 3.3A–C).

There are two entirely different basic arrangements, the monopolar and the bipolar. Each mode must be used with instruments specifically designed for that type of circuit, i.e., bipolar instruments must be used with the bipolar mode, and monopolar instruments with the monopolar mode. All generators used for laparoscopic surgery are equipped with each type of circuit, and the surgeon can select either one.

The fundamental difference between monopolar and bipolar circuits lies in the number of poles or electrodes physically present at the site where the current is applied to the tissues. In the monopolar mode, only one, the active, pole is present, and this is true even if the instrument used has two prongs, such as the monopolar forceps once used for sterilization. The other electrode is at a site remote from the active electrode (usually the thigh), and it is also different in size and much larger. There is a considerable distance between the two electrodes, and tissues other than those to which the current is applied are included in the circuit. The resistance to electron flow (impedance) in this type of circuit is high, and a high power output is required.

There are two types of monopolar circuits called the grounded and the isolated. In a grounded circuit, the second electrode, called the ground plate, is placed

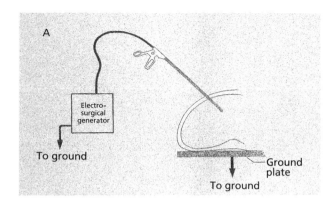

Figure 3.3A The grounded circuit.

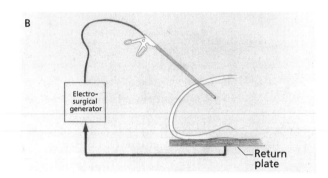

Figure 3.3B The isolated circuit.

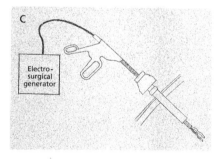

Figure 3.3C The bipolar circuit.

on the patient's thigh and connected to a metallic connector in the operating room, i.e., "earthed" (Figure 3.3A). Once the current is applied to the tissues, electrons flow from the active electrode, through the patient to the ground plate, and then into the ground. An electric circuit is made by also connecting the electrosurgical generator to the ground, which is, therefore, said to be "earthed" or "grounded."

This arrangement is dangerous because if there is a faulty connection between the patient and the ground plate, current will still flow from the electrosurgical generator into the patient, and this current must find its way back to ground to complete the circuit. It will take the path of least resistance, which may be, for example, an EKG lead, and because this has a small contact area with the skin, the current density (see below) in the skin may be high enough to cause a burn.

For this reason, isolated, monopolar circuits have replaced grounded circuits, which are no longer used. The second pole, now called the disperse electrode, is still attached (usually) to the patient's thigh, but it is now connected to the electrosurgical generator rather than being "grounded" (Figure 3.3B). Electrons flow into the patient at the site of the active electrode and are returned to the generator via the disperse electrode. This arrangement is safer because if there is a faulty connection at the site of the disperse electrode and the circuit is broken, current will not flow from the generator to the patient. However, improper placement of the disperse electrode can still reduce the area of contact between it and the skin, without breaking the circuit, in which case the current will continue to flow and may cause a burn where the disperse electrode is attached to the skin if the current density is high enough.

In the bipolar mode, as the name implies, two poles or electrodes are present where the current is applied to the tissues (Figure 3.3C). These are the active and return electrodes that make up the electric circuit, and they are incorporated into the design of bipolar instruments. Consequently, the distance between the two poles is only a few millimeters and current flows only through the tissues between the two poles of the instrument, which is almost always some kind of forceps. The patient is not part of the circuit, and this type of circuitry is, therefore, much safer. It is also, however, less versatile. Because the electric current has to pass through much less tissue to complete the circuit, the impedance of the bipolar circuit is much less than that of a monopolar circuit, and much less power is required. Therefore, the current densities generated with a bipolar circuit are not high enough to allow tissues to be cut, and the bipolar mode is used only for coagulation.

Both an unmodulated and a modulated current can be used with a monopolar circuit depending on the tissue effect desired. However, as Sonderstrom and Levy (5) have elegantly demonstrated, only unmodulated currents should be used with bipolar circuits, and modern electrosurgical units no longer allow the option of choosing a modulated current with the bipolar mode. These authors investigated the reasons for the high failure rate of bipolar sterilization when this was carried out with a Kleppinger forceps attached to a generator other than the one it was designed to be used with (Wolf). What they found was that the Wolf generator used an unmodulated current with a bipolar circuit whereas other generators allowed an option, and gynecologists usually opted for a modulated current, presumably because they associated it with "coagulation." However, the peak voltage of a modulated current of a given wattage is higher than that of an unmodulated current of the same wattage because the current flows for a much shorter period of time. Therefore, if a modulated current is used with a bipolar circuit, the resistance of the surface tissues quickly rises as they are rapidly heated, and sufficient current does not reach the inner part of the tube adequately to coagulate the endosalpinx and occlude the tube.

Biological Effects of Electric Currents

Electric currents, like lasers, produce their clinical effects by the heating of tissues. Heat is generated when an electric current is applied to tissues (ohmic heating) because charged particles are set in motion and collide with each other as well as with uncharged molecules, and these collisions convert the kinetic energy of the particles into heat (thermal energy).

Irreversible damage and cell death occur if tissues are heated to ≥45°C, but the changes and the clinical effects that are produced depend on the rate of heating. If heating occurs slowly, over a period of seconds, first (at 45°–60°C) tissue proteins are denatured, lose their quaternary structure, and solidify; then (at ≥70°C), collagen is converted to glucose; and finally (at ≥90°C), the tissues begin to dry out (desiccation) as tissue water evaporates, but there is no loss of tissue. To the naked eye, these changes first cause tissues to blanch, then swell as tissue water boils away, and, finally, to shrink once they are desiccated. The process is referred to as "coagulation," and it is most commonly used to seal blood vessels.

If heating is very rapid and the temperature in the tissue increases almost instantaneously from 37° to 100°C, tissue water is converted to steam, causing cells to expand rapidly and to explode. This is called vaporization, and it causes loss of solid material, which is dispersed with the plume of smoke. Electrosurgical cutting may be likened to cutting with a saw, which causes some of the material being cut to be lost as sawdust. By contrast, a scalpel, like an axe, cuts by separating tissues without loss of tissue. The electrosurgical effect we call cutting is caused by vaporization of tissue over a small (thin) area; lasers cut tissue by exactly the same mechanism. When vaporization affects a large area, such as an endometriotic implant, we call the tissue effect ablation.

The amount of heat generated by a current and the rate of heating is determined by a number of factors: (1) tissue resistance, (2) the rate of current flow (amps), (3) the type of current (modulated or unmodulated), (4) the time for which the current is applied (dwell time), and (5) the area to which the current is applied (current density). Most of these variables (2–5) are under the control of the operator, and the art of electrosurgery is to select the right conditions for the tissue effect desired.

The amount of heat generated by a current increases with the resistance of the tissue to which it is applied and which is inversely related to its water content. The more resistance the current meets, the more heat is generated. Once all tissue water has been evaporated, tissue resistance becomes extremely high, and continued application of a current causes very high temperatures and charring. Charring indicates that tissues are being incinerated to carbon and that the surface temperature is very high.

The amount of heat generated also increases as the rate of electron flow through the tissues increases.

$$\text{Temperature} = \text{Resistance} \times \text{amps}^2$$

The rate of electron flow increases whenever the setting on the generator is increased because this increases its power output and the current [power (watts) = volts × amps]. For a given power output (wattage), current flow is greater for an unmodulated current than for a modulated current, and heating is more rapid. Modulated currents have higher voltage and lower amperage and cause slower heating.

The total amount of heat generated by a current increases with dwell time, which is the main determinant of the depth of heating and tissue necrosis because it determines the total amount of electric energy delivered to the tissues for a given power output.

$$\text{Energy} = \text{Watts} \times \text{time} \ (\uparrow \text{time} = \uparrow \text{energy})$$

High currents applied for short periods of time cause more rapid heating, because temperature $\propto$ current^2, but less deep tissue heating (because less energy is imparted to the tissues) than low currents of the same wattage applied for a long period of time.

The most important variable determining the tissue effect of a given current is, however, the current density, or the cross sectional area through which the current is flowing. Current density is measured in amps/cm^2, and it is related to the temperature to which the current heats the tissues by,

$$\text{Temperature} = (\text{Current density})^2$$

Current density is increased by either increasing the current or decreasing the area to which the current is applied. Both these variables can be controlled by the operator, and the art of electrosurgery lies in the skillful variation of current density to achieve the tissue effect desired. It would, however, be impractical to constantly change the setting on the generator, and current density is controlled by varying the surface area to which a given current is applied and, to a lesser extent, by the type of current (modulated or unmodulated) selected.

Clinical Applications

Put simply, electrosurgery is used either to cut tissues or to coagulate vessels, and this is achieved by controlling the rate of tissue heating. A high rate of heating is used to cut, and a low rate of heating is used to coagulate. Although the rate of heating can be controlled in several ways, the central strategy used is to vary the current density.

High current densities are required to cut tissues. This can be achieved by applying a modulated (blended) current to a very small area using a needle electrode or by applying a higher, unmodulated current to a somewhat larger surface area using the side of a spatula electrode or the dissecting scissors. Needle electrodes would be used, for example, to ablate endometriotic implants close to the ureter, although we prefer excision to ablation.

We do not like to cut with a modulated current because of its tendency to "spark." To generate a spark, the electric current must "jump" across a small gap between the tissues (usually only a millimeter or so). This requires "force" or high voltage. Watt for watt, a modulated current has up to 10 times the voltage of a cutting current.

It is important to appreciate that during electrosurgical "cutting," the electrode does not actually come into direct contact with the tissues, even if one wishes it to. The very high temperature generated by the high current density instantly vaporizes the tissue water, the cell explodes, some tissue is vaporized along with the steam produced, and the electrode floats in the tissue crater created. Some of the electrical energy is dissipated by heating the air between the electrode and the tissues, rather than the deeper tissue.

Lower current densities are needed for coagulation because the rate of heating must be much lower, otherwise vaporization and tissue loss will occur, and, depending on the size of the contact area, the current will "cut" or "ablate" rather than coagulate the tissues. Coagulation can be achieved in the contact or the noncontact mode, also called "fulguration."

Several strategies can be used to reduce current density and coagulate in the contact mode. First, the area to which the current is applied can be increased. Since we use scissor dissection exclusively, we achieve this by applying the current with the broad, front end of the scissors. Alternatively, the tissue to be coagulated is grasped with grasping forceps, and its end touched with the scissors.

Second, the current is effectively reduced, using one of three strategies: (1) reducing the setting on the generator (although this is rarely done); (2) selecting a modulated current; or (3) using the bipolar mode. The bipolar mode uses much less power, and although the current is unmodulated, this is tantamount to reducing the current. We do not like to use a modulated current for the reasons already stated. If a modulated current is applied to a clamp on a sizeable vessel, e.g., up to the size of the uterine artery, what seems to happen is that after the area between the jaws of the clamp is desiccated (coagulated), the current then "jumps" to a fresh area along the artery, and bleeding can occur (Reich, personal communication).

Coagulation in the noncontact mode is called fulguration. The electrode is held off the tissue, and a modulated (high voltage) current used to create a spark, which causes very superficial heating and necrosis and has a coagulating effect. Fulguration is best used to arrest diffuse capillary oozing rather than bleeding from a discrete vessel. The argon beam coagulator simply consists of a point electrode in a stream of argon (inert) gas, which carries the electrons from the electrode to the tissues. It is a form of assisted fulguration, as it were. I have seen the argon beam coagulator used to good effect, but one cannot help wondering whether the high voltages required may not create new problems.

Electrical Injuries

With the exception of skin burns, which are caused by high current densities at the disperse electrode due to its improper application and contact with the skin, the causes of electrical injuries have been incompletely understood and were often a matter for speculation. The most dreaded of these are bowel injuries, which have caused death from peritonitis. They are thought to result from one of four mechanisms: (1) direct contact between the bowel wall and a "hot" electrosurgical instrument (direct coupling), (2) direct contact between the bowel wall and an insulated instrument whose insulation is faulty (insulation failure), (3) arcing of current from a monopolar instrument to the bowel wall, and (4) capacitative coupling. Adding to the confusion as to causation was the fact that many bowel injuries that were thought to be electrically induced were, in fact, mechanical, as elegantly demonstrated by Sonderstrom and colleagues (6,7).

The first two causes are self-explanatory, and they are almost certainly the most common causes of electrosurgical bowel injuries today. The other two causes have been largely eliminated and are of interest more because they demonstrate important properties of electrosurgery.

▶ **Direct Coupling:** Injury due to direct coupling or contact between bowel and an active electrode occurs either unknowingly or because the surgeon takes what amounts to a calculated risk by working close to bowel. The most treacherous area is the omentum. Bleeding from omental vessels is usually caused by direct injury during insertion of the Veress needle or the first trocar. As the bleeding points are coagulated, the underlying bowel can be injured even if bipolar forceps are used because the bowel may be included in the jaws of the forceps, it may come into contact with the back of the heated instrument, or it may be injured by lateral current spread, which always occurs to some extent. The omentum must always be elevated and checked to ensure that nothing is in contact with its undersurface before any bleeding points are coagulated.

▶ **Insulation Failure:** Injury caused by insulation failure is also straightforward to understand, but it is sobering to note that a freshly opened, disposable instrument that has never been used may have faulty insulation and damage structures it comes into contact with (Indman, personal communications). Even if the insulation around such an instrument is at first sound, it may break down during surgery, especially if the instrument is flimsy and bends easily, like some of the disposable scissors currently available. The author has used such scissors in various circumstances, and has found them to be a liability. On several occasions, these scissors have bent and the insulating coating around them fractured during dissection, particularly during operations on obese patients. The problem is compounded because the valve mechanism on the trocars scrapes and scratches the insulation from around the instrument as it is repeatedly inserted and removed from the abdomen.

This problem is not confined to one product, however. In a recently presented study, Hodgson tested 34 instruments from one hospital for insulation breaks and found defects in all the instruments tested (8). At the same time, it is important not to be alarmist, however, and to remember that it is impossible to completely contain radiofrequency currents within the insulating sheath of an operating instrument, and some current will always leak through its coating. Some circumspection is required before leaping to conclusions about what effects these current leaks are likely to have in vivo.

▶ **Spark Injury (Arcing):** The idea behind this type of injury is that an electric current will travel along paths of least resistance, and when it reaches an area of high resistance, it can "jump" to an area of lower resistance before continuing on its way to the return electrode. The lowest impedance pathway in the vicinity of the high resistance area may be bowel wall, which could sustain an electrical burn at the point of sparking.

For a current to "jump" from one area to another, however, requires electromotive force, i.e., high voltage. For example, it requires an electromotive force of approximately 8000 volts for a current to jump 3 mm, and electrosurgical generators simply do not produce such high voltage currents. For example, the maximum peak voltage of the Valley Lab Force 2 generator is 7000 volts in the "coagulation" mode, and 3000 volts for an unblended current. Thus, the bowel is probably never injured by this mechanism.

▶ **Capacitance Coupling:** As we have said, high voltage radiofrequency currents cannot be completely contained within an instrument (a conductor) by the insulating coat around it, and some current will always leak through the insulating housing. This current usually dissipates through the tissues along low current density pathways. However, if an electrostatic field is created and electrical energy builds up, the energy will eventually be discharged as a spark, which can cause injury to surrounding tissues, such as the bowel wall. Any arrangement that allows electrical energy to build up, i.e., be stored, is called a capacitor, and a capacitor is created whenever two conductors of different charge are separated by insulation.

Precisely this arrangement is created when a unipolar electrode is used down the operating channel of an operating laparoscope, which is a conductor. However,

the electrical energy that builds up around the laparoscope is dissipated into the anterior abdominal wall through its contact with a metallic trocar sleeve. Because this has a large contact area with the tissues, the energy is dispersed along low current density pathways and is harmless. But, if a plastic trocar sleeve is used, or if, as was once done, an insulating tube is placed around the metal trocar sleeve, this harmless exit for the current is cut off, and the energized laparoscope may discharge its energy along high current density pathways and cause a burn if, for example, it makes contact with the bowel wall over a small surface area.

At secondary trocar sites, the metallic sleeve of the trocar itself becomes the capacitor, but the energy is again dissipated into the abdominal wall, and if a plastic sleeve is used, a capacitance effect cannot be created. However, some companies are manufacturing instruments that are a combination of a suction-irrigator and a unipolar spoon electrode. Capacitance coupling is very likely to occur in this type of instrument and it should be used with caution and its design clearly understood.

REFERENCES

1. Sutton C. The role of laparoscopic surgery in the treatment of minimal to moderate endometriosis. Gynaecol Endosc 1993;2:131-133.

2. Luciano AA, Whitman G, Maier DB, et al. A comparison of thermal injury, healing pattern, and postoperative adhesion formation following CO_2 laser and electrosurgery. Fertil Steril 1987;48:1025-1029.

3. Daniell JF, Diamond MP, McLaughlin DS, et al. Clinical results of terminal salpingostomy with use of a CO_2 laser: report of the intra-abdominal laser study group. Fertil Steril 1986;45:175-178.

4. Mage G, Bruhat M. Pregnancy following salpingostomy: comparison between CO_2 laser and electrosurgery procedures. Fertil Steril 1983;40:472-475.

5. Sonderstrom RM, Levy BS. Bipolar systems—do they perform? Obstet Gynecol 1987;69:425–426.

6. Levy BS, Sonderstrom RM, Dail DH. Bowel injuries during laparoscopy: gross anatomy and histology. J Reprod Med 1985;30:168–179.

7. Sonderstrom RM. Bowel injury litigation after laparoscopy. JAAGL 1993;1:74–77.

8. Hodgson JF. Injury from electrosurgery in laparoscopic surgery. (Abstract) World Congress of Gynecologic Endoscopy, 22nd Annual AAGL Meeting, San Francisco, November 10–14, 1993;84.

▼　　▼　　▼　　▼　　▼　　▼　　▼　　▼　　▼

Chapter 4
Techniques for Ligating and Suturing Tissues

If you can describe clearly without a diagram the proper way of making this or that knot, then you are a master of the English tongue.—Belloc

TYING KNOTS

The ability to tie knots is the starting point for suturing, and techniques for knot tying should first be mastered before the surgeon attempts to suture endoscopically. There are two ways to tie knots laparoscopically, *intracorporeally* and *extracorporeally*. The extracorporeal method is the most versatile, and it is the technique we usually use.

Knot tying, like everything else, can only be mastered by practice, and the best way to practice tying knots is to ligate tissues as frequently as possible. The most obvious candidate for ligation is the infundibulopelvic ligament, which should be ligated rather than coagulated whenever ovaries are being removed.

LIGATING THE INFUNDIBULOPELVIC LIGAMENT

To ligate the infundibulopelvic ligament, the ureter is identified as described in Chapter 7, and a small opening ("window") is made in the broad ligament below the infundibulopelvic ligament (Figure 4.1A). A 30″ 2-0 silk thread is then introduced into the abdomen, passed around the infundibulopelvic ligament, and pulled out through a different trocar with grasping forceps (Figure 4.1B). The grasping forceps are then reinserted through this second trocar and the other end of the thread retrieved (Figure 4.1C).

Variations on this scheme are possible depending on how much assistance the surgeon has, but however the suture is passed around the ligament, it is important to avoid "sawing" it with the suture as the suture is pulled out through the trocar. This is achieved by making sure that the suture is not taut as it is being pulled out of the abdomen.

Once the thread has been passed around the infundibulopelvic ligament and both its ends retrieved, an extracorporeal knot is tied. The hitches are made outside the peritoneal cavity exactly the same way as a double-handed square knot is made at laparotomy. Square knots with single hitches ("throws") are used, and they are tied down with the Clarke knot pusher (Marlow Surgical Technologies Inc.) (Figures 4.2A–C).

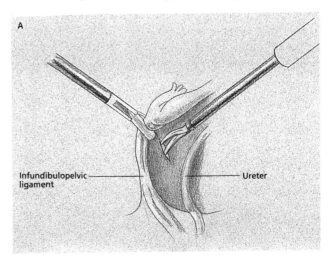

Figure 4.1A An opening is made in the broad ligament below the infundibulopelvic ligament after the ureter has been identified.

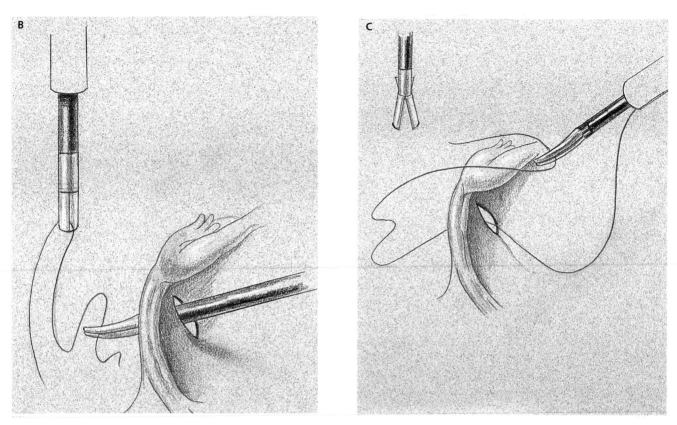

Figures 4.1B,C A silk thread is passed through the opening in the broad ligament and around the infundibulopelvic ligament.

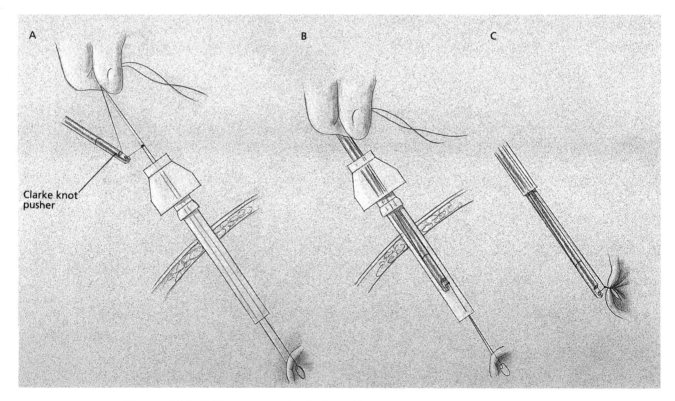

Clarke knot pusher

Figures 4.2A–C Extracorporeal technique of knot tying using the Clarke knot pusher.

There are two tricks to placing knots with the Clarke knot pusher. First, the knot pusher should be placed on one of the strands about half an inch from the knot and not on the knot itself (Figure 4.2A). It is helpful to think of forming a triangle with the suture as the knot is tied down. The ends of the thread are held in the left hand by a right-handed operator, and these make up one corner of the triangle. The other corners are made up by the knot and by where the pusher is placed (Figure 4.2A). The second trick to tying knots with the knot pusher is never to stop halfway. Once knot placement has begun, it has to be completed. Before starting to place the knot, the surgeon should have a clear picture in his mind of the path along which the knot pusher must travel and then follow it in a smooth even thrust (Figures 4.2B,C).

LIGATING WITH PREFORMED LOOPS

Semm popularized the use of the Roeder loop for ligating tissues endoscopically. The Roeder knot is a sliding knot formed by looping one end of the suture back around both strands of suture three and a half times and then bringing the free end under the first loop made (Figure 4.3). Pre-tied loops are commercially available from both the Ethicon (Endoloop) and the Autosuture (Surgiloop) companies. The loops can be used to ligate free pedicles, as for example, in an oophorectomy (see Chapter 14). The loop consists of a lasso with a Roeder knot at its base. The thread then continues through a plastic cannula and is attached to its end (Figure 4.4). Once the loop has been placed around the free pedicle that is to be ligated, the knot is tied down by breaking off the end of the cannula and pushing the cannula over the thread to secure the Roeder knot.

The Endoknot and Surgitie are variations on this concept. They are designed for suturing rather than ligating, but knot tying depends on a Roeder slip knot, which the surgeon has to make. The knot is tied down with a hollow cannula through which the proximal end of the suture has been threaded (Figure 4.5). The distal end of the suture is swaged onto a ski needle. After the needle has been passed through the tissue to be sutured (see below), the thread is brought back out through the same cannula through which it was introduced into the peritoneal cavity. A Roeder knot is made and pushed down into position with the plastic cannula after its distal end has been snapped off.

Unpublished observations by the author have led him to mistrust the Roeder knot. Three operators

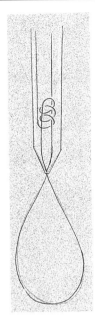

Figure 4.3 The Roeder loop.

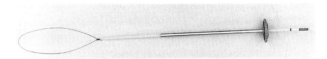

Figure 4.4 The Surgiloop (U.S. Surgical Corp.).

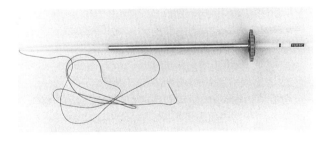

Figure 4.5 The Surgitie (U.S. Surgical Corp.).

were asked to form a single square knot, a surgeon's knot, and a Roeder knot on a tensiometer in vitro. Several braided and monofilament sutures were used, and random numbers were generated to determine the order of knot tying, which was in duplicate for each knot, type of suture, and operator. (The types of suture selected were simply those made available to us by the operating room.) After the knots were tied, the force required to break or unravel the knot was measured on the tensiometer. The operators were the author, Dr. Howard Homesley, head, Division of Gynecologic Oncology, Bowman Gray School of Medicine, and Mr. William Logue, stapling technician, Autosuture Company. Analysis of variance was used to determine the effect of the operator and the type of suture and knot used to tie the knot. There was no difference in knot strength between operators; as expected, the thicker the suture, the stronger the knot, and surgeon's knots were stronger than single knots. The Roeder knot, however, had, at most, only one quarter of the tensile strength of the other knots, and the knots almost always unravelled before the thread broke. Unfortunately, we could not obtain commercially preformed loops from the companies to test.

INTRACORPOREAL TECHNIQUE OF SUTURING

The intracorporeal technique was the first method used for endoscopic suturing. It makes use of a specially designed straight needle, which has a curved tip (so that it resembles a "ski") and a short thread. Knots are made with endoscopic instruments in exactly the same way as an instrument tie is made during conventional surgery (Figures 4.6A–G). The main advantage of the technique is that the needle used is easy to introduce into the peritoneal cavity and to grasp securely with needle holders. However, the technique has many limitations and encumbrances.

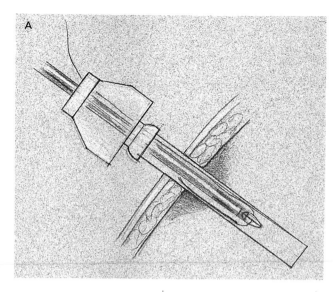

Figure 4.6A The "ski" needle is introduced into the peritoneal cavity.

The main limitation of intracorporeal suturing is that tension cannot be maintained on the suture after the first (double) throw has been placed and the second throw is being prepared. Therefore, the technique cannot be used for certain operations, such as a col-

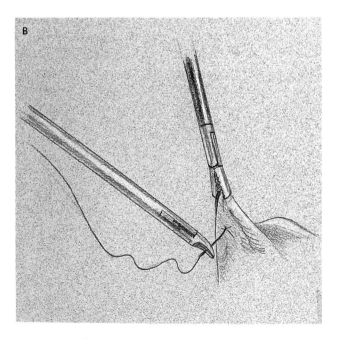

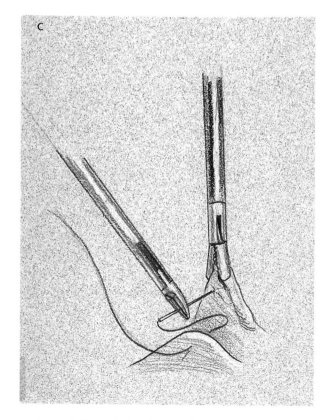

Figures 4.6B,C The needle is grasped with needle holders and passed through the tissue to be sutured.

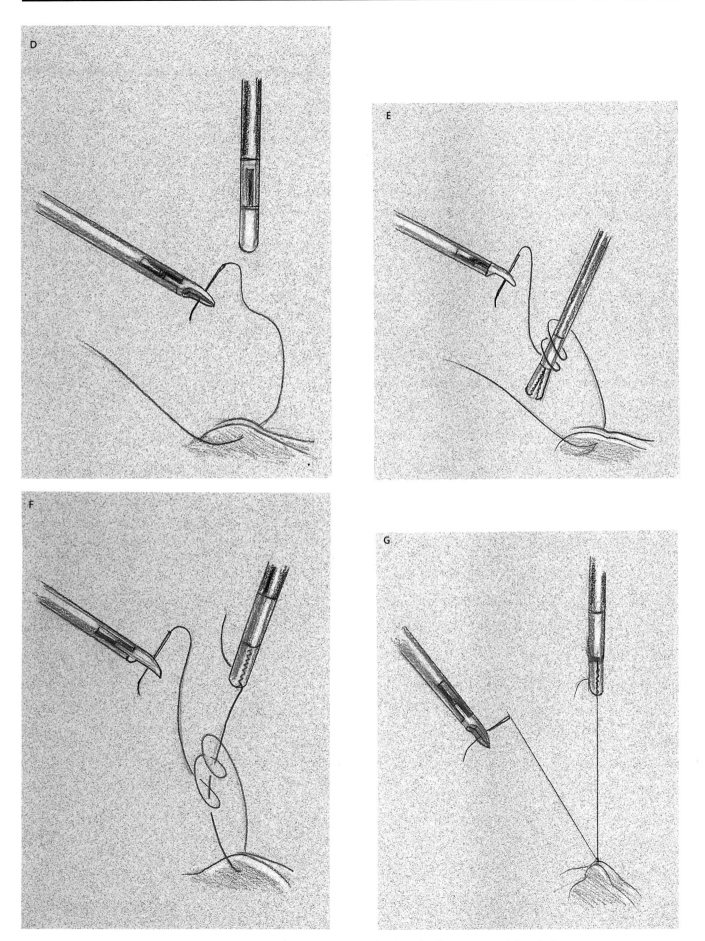

Figures 4.6D–G An intracorporeal knot is tied using the "instrument tie" technique.

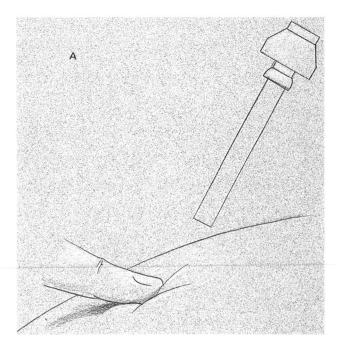

Figure 4.7A The trocar through which the suture is to be placed is removed from the abdominal wall.

posuspension, when tension has to be maintained on the suture after the first and before the second throw has been placed. Intracorporeal suturing techniques are most suited for the placement of fine sutures, as in ureteric or tubal reanastomosis. However, the technique is rather crude for this application as reflected by the poor results obtained with laparoscopic reversal of sterilization (1).

The other difficulty encountered during intracorporeal knot tying is that the suture tends to snag on the hinges of many grasping forceps as the hitches are being tied down. Specially designed graspers have to be used to avoid this problem, and this incurs added expenses.

EXTRACORPOREAL TECHNIQUE OF SUTURING

The extracorporeal technique of suturing was developed by Drs. Courtney Clarke and Harry Reich (2,3). The method consists of introducing a curved needle into the abdominal cavity, picking it up with needle holders, transfixing the tissues to be sutured, tying a knot, cutting the thread, and removing the needle. Originally, straight needles were used as with the intracorporeal method, but use of a curved needle has greatly expanded the scope of the technique without which many operations, such as colposuspension, could never have been carried out laparoscopically.

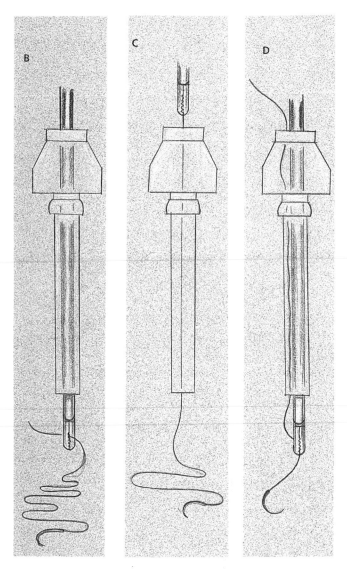

Figures 4.7B,C The thread of the suture is pulled through the trocar. Figure 4.7D The suture is picked up an inch from the needle with a grasper placed through the trocar.

Introducing Curved Needles into the Peritoneal Cavity

▶ **The Reich Technique:** There are two methods of introducing curved needles into the peritoneal cavity. The first method was developed by Reich (3). Essentially, Reich found that any size needle could be introduced into the peritoneal cavity through the tract of a 5-mm trocar by grasping the suture about an inch from the needle with a forceps and then pushing it through the trocar tract. The needle simply follows the instrument.

The trocar through which the suture is to be placed is first removed from the abdomen and the site occluded with a finger (Figure 4.7A). A grasping for-

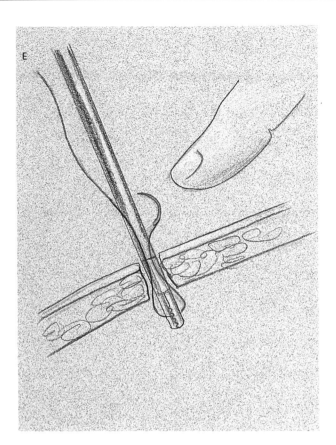

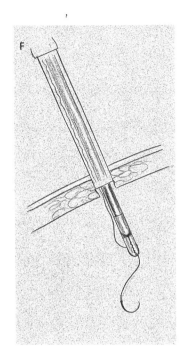

Figures 4.7E,F The grasper is reinserted through the trocar tract, and the trocar cannula slid over it into the peritoneal

ceps is passed through the trocar, the end of a suture picked up and pulled through the trocar (Figures 4.7B,C). The forceps is now passed back through the trocar, the thread of the suture grasped about an inch from the needle (Figure 4.7D), and the forceps and needle inserted into the peritoneal cavity through the trocar tract (Figure 4.7E). The trocar is then pushed back into the peritoneal cavity along the shaft of the grasping forceps (Figure 4.7F).

The forceps are now removed and replaced with a needle holder and the needle picked up (Figure 4.8A). The tissue to be sutured is transfixed (Figure 4.8B), and the distal end of the needle grasped with forceps before the needle holder is released (Figure 4.8C). The needle is then regrasped with the needle holder and pulled through the tissue (Figure 4.8D). The needle is tacked to the peritoneum and cut off, leaving about a 1- to 2-inch tail (Figure 4.8E). The end of the suture is pulled out through the trocar (Figure 4.8F) and an extracorporeal knot tied (Figures 4.2A–C). The needle is then removed by grasping its end with forceps and then simply pulling it through the trocar tract. The trocar is removed ahead of the needle by sliding it along the shaft of the forceps (Figures 4.8G,H).

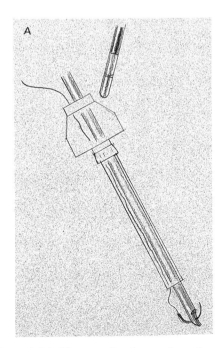

Figure 4.8A The grasping forceps is replaced by needle holders.

Techniques for Ligating and Suturing Tissues   37

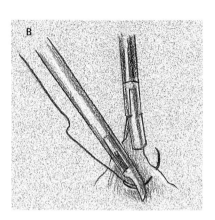

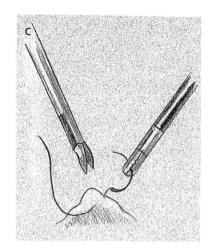

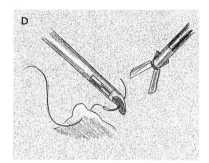

Figures 4.8B–D The tissue to be sutured is transfixed.

We have stopped cutting the needle off inside the peritoneal cavity and simply grasp the thread about an inch from the needle and remove it in exactly the same way as when the suture is cut prior to its removal. This saves a few steps. However, before removing the needle, it is important to pull the suture through the tissues so there is plenty of slack and the tissues will not be pulled or jerked as the needle is being withdrawn (Figures 4.9A–C).

♦ **The Direct Method:** The direct method, as the name implies, consists of passing the needle directly down a 10- or 12-mm trocar without removing the trocar from the abdomen. The thread of the needle is first pulled through a 5-mm reducer with a forceps (Figures 4.10A,B), the forceps passed back through the reducer to grasp the suture about an inch from the needle (Figure 4.10C). The forceps and needle are then inserted into the peritoneal cavity, and the reducer is quickly reattached (Figure 4.10D). A CT2 needle can be introduced through a 10-mm trocar, and a CT1 or V37 needle can be passed down a 12-mm trocar.

The obvious advantage of this method is that the trocar does not have to be removed from the peritoneal

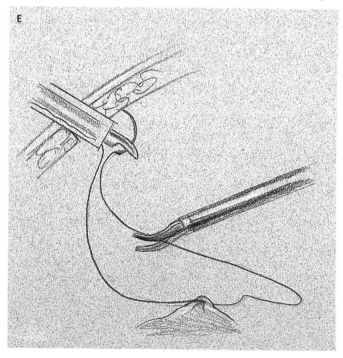

Figure 4.8E The needle is tacked to the peritoneum and cut off leaving a 1- to 2-inch tail.

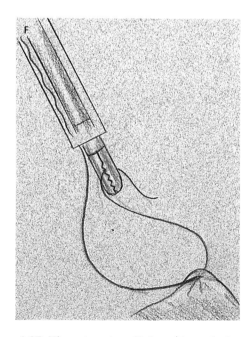

Figure 4.8F The suture is pulled out through the trocar for knot tying.

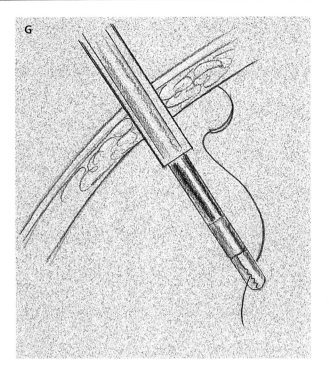
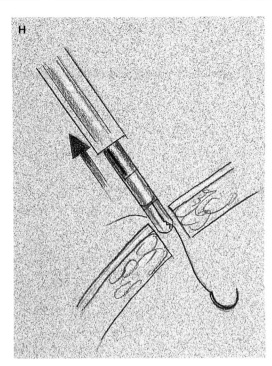

Figures 4.8G,H The needle is removed from the peritoneal cavity.

cavity, but the method is not as satisfactory as it sounds. A great deal of gas escapes when a 5-mm forceps or needle holder is inserted through a 10- or 12-mm trocar. Rapid deflation of the abdomen before the reducer can be snapped back onto the trocar brings tissues closer to the abdominal wall and creates two difficulties. First, the forceps cannot be inserted very far before the reducer is replaced, and frequently there is insufficient length of suture inside the abdomen. Second, the tissues in close proximity to the anterior abdominal wall could theoretically sustain blunt trauma as the forceps is introduced. Another annoying problem is that the reducer frequently traps part of the suture as it is placed back onto the trocar. A 10-mm needle holder may obviate the problems with the reducing valve but not with deflation of the abdomen, but we have not had access to such a needle holder. Also, both the U.S. Surgical and Ethicon companies are now manufacturing reducers with different designs from that shown in Figures 4.10A–D. Although we

have not had the opportunity to test these as yet, it is obvious from the design of these new reducers that the one manufactured by Ethicon will require the same technique of direct needle insertion as shown in Figures 4.10A–D, because these reducers simply clip on to the trocar as did the original Autosuture reducer. However, the new trocars recently developed by the U.S. Surgical Corporation have an entirely new mechanism and should allow the needle to be introduced into the trocar and the 5-mm rubber sleeve to be pulled up over the shaft of the needle holder before the flapper valve is opened and gas escapes (Figures 4.11A,B). The mechanism certainly facilitates the removal of specimens such as lymph nodes. (Unfortunately, surgeons have been barred from using the Autosuture trocars at the Jersey Shore Medical Center by contract even though almost all of them prefer these trocars to the ones they have been constrained to use, a disturbing issue that will be discussed further in Chapter 24.)

COMMENT

Current techniques of endoscopic suturing clearly rely on emulating the method used at laparotomy, but the techniques do not translate well, and even when honed to a fine art, as in the hands of Dr. Harry Reich, they are inherently crude and time-consuming. This is, of course, not said to detract anything from the massive contributions that Reich has made to laparoscopic surgery but rather to underscore that current suturing techniques are *inherently* limited.

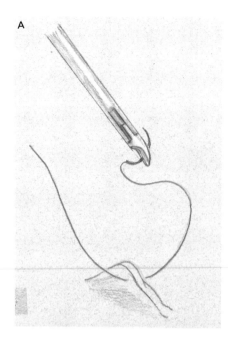

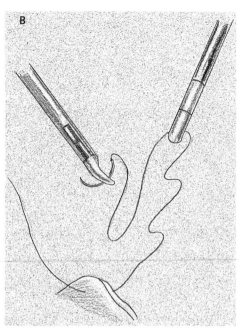

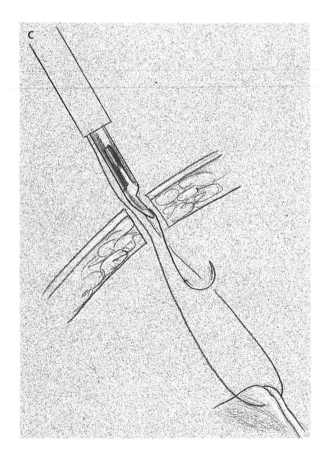

Figures 4.9A–C Modified Reich technique for extracorporeal suturing. The needle is removed from the peritoneal cavity after the suture has been placed, and it is cut off extracorporeally prior to knot tying.

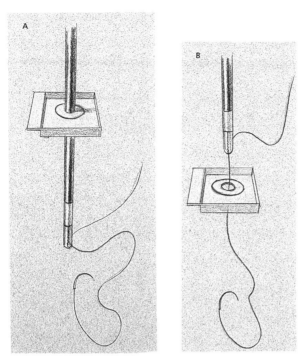

Figures 4.10A,B *The thread of the suture is pulled through a 5-mm reducer.*

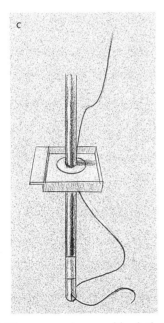

Figure 4.10C *The grasper is passed back through the reducer, and the thread of the suture picked up about an inch from the needle.*

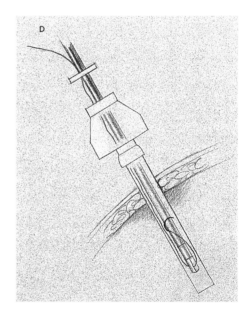

Figure 4.10D *The grasper and needle are inserted into the peritoneal cavity and the reducer reattached.*

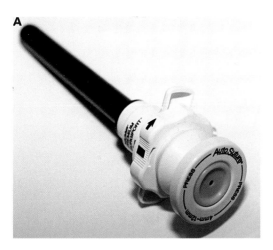

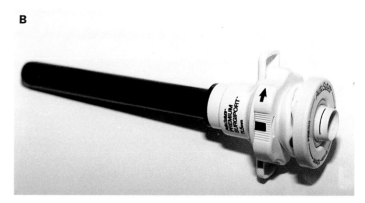

Figure 4.11 Reducer valve mechanism of the new Surgiport trocars (U.S. Surgical Corp.); (A) 5-mm port (B) valve retracted to expose 10-mm port.

COMMENT (*Cont.*)

Available techniques have become somewhat easier to learn and apply with the availability of instruments that are better designed for endoscopic suturing. Manufacturers have finally recognized the need for needle holders to hold needles securely, including curved needles, but many still on the market continue to be woefully inadequate in this respect. Grasping forceps hold needles even less well, and many are even unsatisfactory for pulling the suture through the trocar because the thread slips through their grooved jaws. Despite some improvements in instrumentation, it seems to us that entirely different types of instruments or suturing techniques need to be developed. We are currently working on an Endodrive, which is essentially a needle holder with a needle fixed to it that will pick up a thread after it is driven through the tissues, and we envisage that handheld sewing machines will be developed eventually.

REFERENCES

1. Reich H, McGlynn F, Parente C, Sekel L, Levie M. Laparoscopic tubal anastomosis. J Assoc Gynecol Laparosc 1993;1:16–19.

2. Clarke HC. Laparoscopy—new instruments for suturing and ligation. Fertil Steril 1972;23:274–277.

3. Reich H, Clarke HC, Sekel L. A simple method for ligating with straight and curved needles in operative laparoscopy. Obstet Gynecol 1992;79:143–147.

▼ ▼ ▼ ▼ ▼ ▼ ▼ ▼ ▼

Chapter 5
Complications

Be near me when my light is low,
When the nerves prick and tingle
And the heart is sick,
And all the wheels of being slow.
—In Memoriam, Tennyson

Profound hemodynamic and respiratory changes take place during laparoscopic surgery that are a direct consequence of creating a pneumoperitoneum with carbon dioxide and placing the patient into a head-down (Trendelenburg) position for prolonged periods of time.

The effects of the pneumoperitoneum and postural changes depend largely on how much abdominal pressure increases. Over the recommended range of pressures (10–15 mm/Hg), blood pressure either does not change or rises as venous return is augmented. At higher intra-abdominal pressures, however, cardiac output falls as the vena cava is compressed and venous return impaired. Inadequate muscle relaxation can contribute significantly to a rise in abdominal pressure.

Both the pneumoperitoneum and Trendelenburg position produce cephalad pressure on the diaphragm. The diaphragm is elevated, its excursions restricted, volumetric expansion of the lungs impaired, and overall lung compliance decreased. This is reflected in an increase in airway pressure, which rises by an average of 5–7 cm/H_2O as abdominal pressure increases to 25 cm/H_2O. Lung compliance is further compromised by the increase in pulmonary blood volume that results from redistribution of blood from the abdomen to the thorax as abdominal pressure rises and the patient is tilted head-down. Higher ventilation pressures have to be used to overcome this decrease in lung compliance.

Carbon dioxide is most commonly used for insufflation because it is rapidly absorbed, soluble, and does not support combustion. These properties make it safe to use in conjunction with electrosurgery and reduce the risk of serious embolic phenomena should intravascular injection occur. Carbon dioxide is absorbed continuously into the blood stream during laparoscopic surgery and causes a steady rise in arterial pCO_2. This rise in pCO_2 causes a respiratory acidosis and catecholamine release. Mean blood pressure increases, and there is a positive inotropic effect on the heart, with an increase in stroke volume, heart rate, and cardiac output. There is also a propensity to cardiac arrhythmias, which is compounded by halothane (but not by other halogenated hydrocarbons, such as isoflurane) because it sensitizes the myocardium to catecholamine-induced ventricular ectopy.

It should be evident from the above that the key to minimizing these changes is to keep the increase in pCO_2 and intra-abdominal pressure to a minimum. Hypercapnia can usually be avoided by increasing minute ventilation. This is best accomplished by increasing ventilatory rate rather than tidal volume (although both may need to be increased) because it does not increase airway pressure, whereas an increase in tidal volume does. Abdominal pressure should be kept below 15 cm/H_2O by setting the patient pressure on the insufflator to this level. Good muscle relaxation, avoidance of the lithotomy position, and tilting the patient excessively, unless really necessary, will usually suffice, although in very obese patients, higher intra-abdominal pressures may have to be accepted.

The constant flow of unheated gas through the peritoneal cavity and irrigation with cold fluids lower body temperature, and hypothermia after prolonged laparoscopic operations is the rule rather than the exception. Hypothermia contributes to a decrease in cardiac output by increasing systemic vascular resistance. It predisposes patients to cardiac arrhythmias, and it increases myocardial oxygen demand by causing postoperative shivering. Heating blankets are frequently used intraoperatively to forestall this problem, but they are not very effective in adults because the ability to raise body temperature by this means is determined by the ratio of the body surface area to body weight, which is much lower for adults than for children (in whom surface heating to raise body temperature is much more effective). The patient can be heated much more effectively by warming the inspired air, but the equipment is apparently expensive and, therefore, not frequently used.

COMPLICATIONS AND CONTRAINDICATIONS

The complications of laparoscopy are those of general anesthesia and the specific operation being performed. In addition, there are complications peculiar to laparoscopy, which can result from inserting instruments blindly into the abdomen, maintaining a pneumoperitoneum, and using electrosurgery or other energy source. The value of recognizing these complications early cannot be overemphasized, and the pressures brought to bear on laparoscopic surgeons by the skepticism of their colleagues should not be allowed to influence surgical judgment. Some of these complications are known risks of laparoscopy and can be beyond the control of the surgeon.

MAJOR COMPLICATIONS

Injury to Blood Vessels

Injury to large vessels (aorta, vena cava, or iliac) during trocar insertion is usually avoidable by adhering to the principles described in Chapter 2, but if an injury does occur, it must be recognized promptly and dealt with by immediate laparotomy to avoid a fatal outcome. Precipitous drop in the blood pressure is, relatively speaking, a late event, especially in young women and especially if most of the bleeding is retroperitoneal. If the injury is recognized only at this stage, many patients succumb even if the laceration is repaired and blood volume restored because reperfusion injury frequently causes irreversible hypotension and shock.

Predisposing factors are those that increase the amount of force necessary to insert a trocar. For this reason, thin patients are at much greater risk than obese ones because their great vessels are closer to the skin, and they have much firmer abdominal muscles. Trocars that are dull also place the patient at greater risk for this type of injury. Although Corson (1) has shown that twice the force was necessary to insert conventional reusable trocars than disposable ones, this finding does not apply to all reusable trocars. Some require a great deal of force to insert and are, in this author's opinion, distinctly dangerous and he has been made aware of a number of aortic injuries that have resulted from their use. Careful attention to the details of trocar insertion described in Chapter 2 should avert these tragedies.

Sometimes bleeding from an injured vessel stops from the combined tamponading effect of an increase in intra-abdominal pressure, decreased venous return, and hematoma formation only to resume postoperatively once the pressure gradients return to normal. To avoid this potentially deadly complication, any evidence of hematoma formation must be investigated by opening the overlying peritoneum if this has not been done already, evacuating the hematoma, and inspecting the integrity of any nearby major vessels. Intraoperative injuries to large vessels must be oversewn, no matter how small, even if the bleeding is arrested with pressure.

Injury to the inferior epigastric vessels is the most common type of vascular injury, but it can also be avoided by inserting the trocars in the lower quadrant lateral to the rectus sheath and above a line joining the anterior superior iliac spines (see Chapter 2). The lower part of the epigastric vessels can usually be visualized laparoscopically under the peritoneum below the arcuate line (where the vessels enter the rectus sheath) but not above this point. Only the superficial epigastric vessels can be identified by transilluminating the anterior abdominal wall.

If the epigastric vessels are injured, several maneuvers can be tried to control the bleeding. Sometimes, simply rotating the trocar sleeve 360° or levering it against the abdominal wall will tamponade the bleeding, and if this is successful, the vessels should be tamponaded for five minutes. If the insertion site is below the arcuate line, the parietal peritoneum can be desiccated above and below the trocar sleeve with bipolar forceps, but this will not arrest the bleeding if the vessel is injured within the rectus sheath. Another strategy is to insert a 30-cc balloon Foley catheter through the cannula. The balloon is then inflated, the cannula removed, and the balloon pulled up into the insertion site to tamponade the bleeding. Finally, using a large retention suture, the entire abdominal wall can be sutured through and through at the bleeding site under direct vision. The trocar can be inserted at a different site, the operation completed, and the suture removed later.

Injuries to the GI and GU Tracts

▶ **Bowel Injuries:** Injuries to the bowel are second only to large vessel injuries as potentially life-threatening surgical complications of laparoscopic surgery. At one time, these injuries were believed to be thermal injuries caused by "sparking" of monopolar current from an electrode to the surface of the bowel. Most of these injuries were, however, subsequently shown to be traumatic in origin (see Chapter 3).

Bowel perforation during laparoscopy occurs most commonly during insertion of either the Veress needle or the first trocar. Injuries caused by the Veress needle can be managed expectantly. Usually, they occur where intestinal loops are adherent to the anterior abdominal wall, and the perforation seals off promptly. The emanation of foul-smelling gas or greenish fluid through the Veress needle is a helpful diagnostic sign. Injury to the bowel caused during insertion of the first trocar can be difficult to detect if the injured segment is adherent to the anterior abdominal wall at the trocar insertion site, and the trocar passes through the entire bowel wall. This type of injury will escape detection unless adhesions around the umbilicus are taken down routinely.

Bowel injury during trocar insertion should always be considered whenever multiple attempts at insertion are required or there are dense adhesions around the umbilicus. To make sure that bowel has not been injured, the area of insertion must be inspected, and adhesions to the anterior abdominal wall in the vicinity of the operative field taken down by sharp scissor dissection. It is rarely necessary to move the laparoscope to another site to take down even extensive adhesions around the umbilicus. The laparoscope is withdrawn into the trocar and then the trocar sleeve is retracted slowly until the edges of the peritoneum come into view. If a portion of the bowel has been transfixed, the bowel lumen will come into view as the trocar is withdrawn. The trocar and laparoscope are then advanced back into the peritoneal cavity and the adhesions to the anterior abdominal wall lysed. To divide adhesions at the umbilicus, it will be necessary to pull back the laparoscope and trocar again until they are almost out of the peritoneal cavity.

If a trocar injury is detected, immediate laparotomy should be performed, and on no account should a lap-aroscopic repair be attempted. The bowel wall opposite the entry site has to be inspected for a possible "exit" injury, and the bowel cannot be inspected reliably enough laparoscopically to ensure that this has not occurred, especially if exit injury would involve the mesenteric border of the bowel. However, the site of the abdominal incision can be strategically selected under laparoscopic guidance, and it need not be very large. If the injury is visible before the offending trocar has been moved, it should be left in place to help localize the site of injury at minilaparotomy. A purse-string suture is then placed around the site of injury and the trocar removed. The purse string is tied down and the area reinforced by a second seromuscular layer. Whether segmental bowel resection is necessary is decided on basic surgical principles—the extent of the injury and condition of the surrounding tissue, whether small or large bowel has been injured, and, if the latter, whether the bowel has been prepared.

Bowel injury during surgery can be either mechanical or thermal, but it is usually the former. The most important factor in the management (and prognosis) of these injuries is to recognize them during surgery and, if this is not possible, early in the postoperative period. Simple injuries can be easily repaired with little morbidity; delay in their recognition can result in death.

Momentary, inadvertent contact between the bowel wall and an activated electrosurgical instrument will not injure the bowel. Purse-string sutures do not have to be placed around the area of contact, and expectant management is all that is required. A recognized thermal injury during surgery requires laparotomy and segmental resection with a wide margin around the injury site. If the resection is inadequate, the anastomosis will break down later.

Most intraoperative injuries are, however, mechanical. Small bowel injuries usually occur during lysis of dense adhesions, and they can be managed by simply oversewing the laceration. This can be done laparoscopically if the surgeon is sufficiently proficient at endoscopic suturing. Two layers of interrupted sutures are placed and sterile milk instilled into the bowel lumen to check the site of repair for leakage (2).

Large bowel injuries may also occur during lysis of adhesion, but the most common site of injury is probably the rectum during the resection of endometriosis. Large bowel injuries can only be repaired laparoscopically in well-prepared bowel. Lacerations can be either sutured or stapled with an Endo-GIA stapler placed transversely to the bowel lumen. Occasionally, very low rectal injuries can be repaired vaginally through a colpotomy incision.

Reich's (3) technique for laparoscopic repair of bowel laceration is to place stay sutures at the transverse edges of the laceration, which are then brought out through the lateral ports, the ports removed and reinserted so that the stay sutures are outside the trocar sleeve (Figure 5.1). He uses a two-layered closure, although the success of one-layered anastomoses with monofilament sutures after conventional large bowel resection suggests that a similar technique could be used laparoscopically.

The reader would be well-advised to take a cautious approach to laparoscopic repair of bowel lacerations. The laparoscopic approach takes longer, even in the most experienced hands, providing greater opportunity for peritoneal soiling. It is best reserved initially for small lacerations involving the rectum in prepared bowel when soiling is minimal or nonexistent and where the integrity of the repair can be properly tested by instilling betadine solution into the rectum through a Foley catheter and then checking the site for leakage, with the pelvis filled with water, as after a conventional, stapled rectal anastomosis. Before undertaking the endoscopic repair of bowel lacerations, the surgeon must have had considerable experience repairing such injuries at conventional surgery and have fully mastered at least one technique for endoscopic suturing and used it under different circumstances, such as a colposuspension or the repair of lacerations in more forgiving organs, such as the bladder (4).

Delayed bowel injury can result from unrecognized traumatic perforation or from electrosurgical thermal damage. Although there is much overlap, as a rule, bowel perforation following electrosurgical injury presents 4 to 10 days after surgery, whereas traumatic perforations present within 24–48 hours. The gross appearances of traumatic and electrical injuries are the same; a perforation surrounded by a white area of necrosis. Microscopically, however, the lesions are distinct (5). Thermal injuries cause coagulation necrosis, and the leucocytic infiltrate typical of healing tissues is absent. The site of traumatic injury, by contrast, has all the histological characteristics of healing tissue: abundant capillary ingrowth, white cell infiltration, and fibrin deposition.

The presentation depends on whether there is diffuse peritonitis or a localized pelvic abscess. Usually, there is increasing abdominal pain, fever, and malaise, but the more dramatic picture of septic shock can also be seen. Examination will reveal an acute abdomen if generalized peritonitis is present or more localized tenderness if the perforation has been walled off in the pelvis. Ancillary tests are helpful when positive, but they are frequently negative. Leucocytosis may be absent, but there is usually a left shift. A flat plate of the

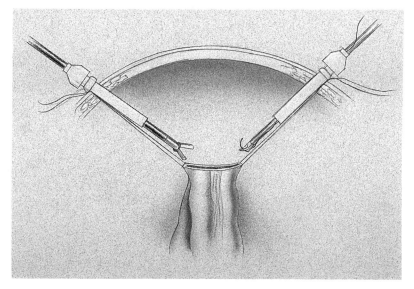

Figure 5.1 Reich's endoscopic technique for suturing bowel lacerrations.

abdomen will show subdiaphragmatic air in only about a third of the patients, and ultrasound can miss up to a third of pelvic abscesses (6).

If the cause of the original injury was traumatic, it may be possible to carry out a wedge resection of the area and then oversew it, especially if small bowel is involved. Large bowel injuries more often require resection and sometimes a colostomy. The decision is made on the traditional surgical criteria already discussed. Thermal injuries always require segmental bowel resection, the margins of which should clear the injured tissue by at least 5 cm. If there is any doubt as to the cause of the original injury, frozen section of the resected segment may be helpful and suggests a wider margin of resection.

▶ Injuries to the Stomach:

Injuries to the stomach are caused exclusively by trocar insertions, and the routine use of a nasogastric tube should make this a rare event. If the stomach is injured, the laceration should be repaired in two layers via a laparoscopically directed minilaparotomy incision and nasogastric suction continued postoperatively.

▶ Incisional Hernias:

Failure to close the fascia at extraumbilical trocar sites larger than 5 mm can result in an incisional hernia (7). These present within the first two postoperative weeks with pain over the insertion site and partial small bowel obstruction. In cases of doubt, the diagnosis can be made by a CT scan of the anterior abdominal wall, which will show a loop of bowel herniating through the fascia (Figure 5.2). In many cases, the hernia can be reduced laparoscopically or under local anesthetic.

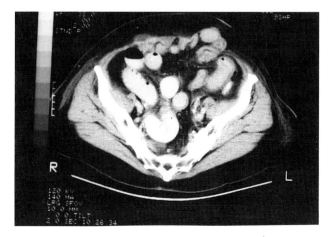

Figure 5.2 Incisional hernia through a 12-mm trocar site in the left lower quadrant (used for the Endo-GIA stapler).

▶ Bladder Injuries:

The bladder can be injured by a secondary trocar placed suprapubically, but this kind of injury can be prevented by placing secondary trocars under direct laparoscopic vision. The bladder may also be injured as it is dissected off the vagina during laparoscopic hysterectomy and during vaginal closure of the cuff following laparoscopic bladder dissection (8). A reliable sign of a bladder laceration is the appearance of gas in the Foley catheter drainage bag (4). Repair is with laparoscopically placed figure-of-eight sutures in the bladder muscularis and postoperative bladder drainage for seven days.

▶ Ureteric Injuries:

Thermal injury to the ureter, which occurs most commonly after fulguration or laser vaporization of endometriosis involving the utero-sacral ligaments, will usually cause a stricture, hydroureter, and hydronephrosis, and can ultimately lead to the loss of the affected kidney. Delayed necrosis with extravasation of urine can also occur although it is more commonly seen after lacerations of the ureter. The ureter can also be inadvertently stapled if an endoscopic stapler is used to divide the pedicles (especially the cardinal ligaments) during laparoscopic hysterectomy (9).

Injuries that occlude the ureter usually cause flank or lower abdominal pain with or without fever early in the postoperative period. It is said that these injuries can be "silent," although this can never be proven and is rather doubtful.

Injuries that cause extravasation of urine can present in a variety of ways. Leakage of urine into the peritoneal cavity will result in reabsorption of the waste products of metabolism by dialysis. This presents as nausea, general malaise, rising creatinine, and, eventually, sepsis. If the urine is walled off, a urinoma will form, which will usually cause an ileus. The urine will eventually find its ways to the surface through an incision, either the trocar site or the vaginal wall, and present as a fistula.

The integrity of the ureter can be checked intraoperatively by injecting 5–10 cc of indigo carmine intravenously, but failure to see extravasation is not an infallible sign of ureteric integrity. Dye may not leak through small holes, excretion of the dye may be very slow due to the position the patient is in and/or some degree of hypovolemia, and even a severed ureter can go into spasm and not leak dye, although this must surely be rare.

Flank or pelvic pain after adnexal surgery or hysterectomy should be investigated with an intravenous pyelogram and so should prolonged postoperative ileus or a "ground glass" appearance on a plain abdominal film, which is indicative of a fluid collection. Injuries that are detected early can frequently be managed by placing a ureteric stent for one to three months.

Laparoscopic repair of ureteric injuries is being reported with increasing frequency, but experience is still limited, and laparoscopic repair cannot be recommended as a routine at this time, except for the repair of small lacerations that only require a single stitch and a stent, until more experience is gained with laparoscopic ureteric reconstruction and the results, particularly long-term follow up, can be assessed (10). The ureter, like the bile duct, is not a very forgiving structure. The results obtained with laparoscopic reversal of sterilization (11) give one sufficient grounds to pause and reflect on whether currently available methods of suturing allow as satisfactory a repair as can be achieved with conventional surgery. Partial injuries can be managed by stenting alone or with a single interrupted suture (12,13). The repair of full thickness injuries by anastomosis after ureteric excisions needs to be thought out and carefully planned. Of particular concern to this author is the use of end-to-end anastomosis without spatulation of the severed ends of the ureter.

OTHER LIFE-THREATENING COMPLICATIONS

Pneumothorax

The presence of an unrecognized congenital defect in the diaphragm will result in the development of a tension pneumothorax shortly after a pneumoperitoneum is established. Under anesthesia, this will present with a rise in airway pressure, engorgement of the neck veins, and cyanosis; breath sounds on the affected side will be absent and the chest will be resonant. The pneumoperitoneum obviously has to be released immediately and a thoracostomy tube quickly placed, preceded by placement of a large angiocath if the pneumothorax needs to be promptly relieved.

Gas Embolus

A very rare but potentially life-threatening complication of laparoscopy is venous gas embolus (13). The cause is usually direct gas insufflation into a large vein. The gas becomes trapped in the right heart and causes right heart outflow obstruction. There is circulatory collapse associated with a "millwheel" murmur, cyanosis, raised CVP, decreased end tidal CO_2 (because the pulmonary circulation is effectively oc-

cluded), and very high arterial pCO_2. Treatment consists of prompt recognition and stopping the insufflation. The patient is given 100% oxygen to breathe and cardiovascular support. A central line is placed to aspirate gas from the ventricle, and the patient is rolled on her left side to facilitate expulsion of gas from the ventricle.

MINOR COMPLICATIONS

Fluid Overload

The use of large amounts of fluid for irrigation can result in fluid overload, especially after long operations. Once it is recognized, it can be easily treated with a small amount of diuretics.

Subcutaneous Emphysema and Edema

Manipulation of instruments during surgery often loosens the parietal peritoneum around the trocars where they enter the peritoneal cavity. Carbon dioxide can escape from the peritoneal cavity at these sites and infiltrate the loose areolar tissue of the body, causing subcutaneous emphysema. This is usually benign and resolves within a day, often within hours. If subcutaneous emphysema is noted in the anterior abdominal wall at the end of an operation, the trapped CO_2 should be "massaged" toward the nearest trocar site and expressed. Swelling of the vulva can be reduced in the same way.

Facial and orbital swelling is a positional phenomenon caused by having the patient in a Trendelenburg position for prolonged periods. It is harmless and resolves within a few hours.

Infection

Infection is uncommon after laparoscopic procedures. It is a closed procedure, there is little dead tissue to serve as a culture medium, blood clots are usually removed at the end of the procedure, and copious irrigation is used, which dilutes the bacterial inoculum introduced into the peritoneal cavity during trocar insertion.

Wound infection in the trocar sites is also uncommon. When it occurs, it is treated in the usual way with drainage, irrigation ± debridement, and packing of the wound. Antibiotics are not used.

Shoulder Pain

Shoulder pain can be the most significant source of discomfort for the patient. It is caused by residual CO_2 in the peritoneum and can be prevented by making sure that all the gas is removed at the conclusion of the operation. To ensure this, *it is important not to take the patient out of Trendelenburg position until the pneumoperitoneum has been completely released,* otherwise, CO_2 can be trapped under the diaphragm as these may be at a higher position than the trocars once the patient is placed flat.

ABSOLUTE CONTRAINDICATIONS TO LAPAROSCOPY

The contraindications to laparoscopic surgery are the same as the contraindications to surgery in general. There are, however, a few situations in which operations, which could otherwise be carried out laparoscopically, should be performed via a laparotomy. These are: (1)hypovolemic shock, (2) severe cardiopulmonary disease, (3) previous abdominopelvic radiation, and (4) multiple operations for: (i) ruptured abscesses, (ii) inflammatory bowel disease with fistula, and (iii) tuberculosis.

REFERENCES

1. Corson SL, Batzer FR, Gocial B, Maislin G. Measurement of force necessary for laparoscopic trocar entry. J Reprod Med 1989;34:282–284.

2. Reich H, McGlynn F, Budin R. Laparoscopic repair of full-thickness bowel injury. J Laparoendosc Surg 1991; 1:119–122.

3. Reich H. Laparoscopic bowel injury. Surg Laparosc Endosc 1992;2:74–78.

4. Reich H, McGlynn F. Laparoscopic repair of bladder injury. Obstet Gynecol 1990;76:909–910.

5. Levy BS, Sonderstrom RM, Dail DH. Bowel injuries during laparoscopy: gross anatomy and histology. J Reprod Med 1985;30:168–179.

6. Sonderstrom RM. Bowel injury ligation after laparoscopy. J Am Assoc Gynecol Laparosc 1993;1:74–77.

7. Kadar N, Reich H, Liu CY, Manco GF, Gimpleson R. Incisional hernias following major laparoscopic gynecological procedures. Am J Obstet Gynecol 1993;168: 1493–1495.

8. Kadar N, Lemmerling L. Urinary tract injuries during laparoscopically assisted hysterectomy: causes and prevention. Am J Obstet Gynecol 1994;170:47–48.

9. Woodland MB. Ureter injury during laparoscopy-assisted vaginal hysterectomy with endoscopic lineal stapler. Am J Obstet Gynecol 1992;167:756–757.

10. Nezhat C, Nezhat F, Nezhat C, Bess O. Laparoscopic management of intentional and unintentional urologic injury. (Abstract) World Congress of Gynecologic Endoscopy, 22nd Annual AAGL Meeting, San Francisco, November 10–14, 1993;79.

11. Reich H. McGlynn F, Parente C, Sekel L. Levie M. Laparoscopic tubal anastomosis. J Am Assoc Gynecol Laparosc 1993;1:16–19.

12. Gomel V, James C. Intra-operative management of ureteral injury during operative laparoscopy. Fertil Steril 1991;55:416–419.

13. Neven P, Vandeusen H, Baert L, Koninckx PR. Ureteric injury at laparoscopic surgery: the endoscopic management. Gynaecol Endosc 1993;2:45–46.

14. Yacoub OF, Cardona I, Coveler LA, Dodson MG. Carbon dioxide embolism during laparoscopy. Anesthesiology 1982;57:533–535.

Chapter 6
Laparoscopic Anatomy of the Pelvis and Dissection of the Retroperitoneum

Over again I feel thy finger and find thee.
—Wreck of the Deutschland,
Gerard Manley Hopkins

The laparoscope affords a much more panoramic and anatomic view of the pelvis than is obtained at laparotomy. The uterus does not need to be displaced to the same extent to expose the pelvic structures, and a number of landmarks can be identified that are simply not visible at laparotomy (Figure 6.1).

LAPAROSCOPIC PELVIC LANDMARKS

The Anterior Pelvis

A prominent peritoneal fold is always visible in front of the uterus. It is the *transverse vesical fold,* which lies over the dome of the bladder and runs horizontally across the anterior pelvis from one superior pubic ramus to the other, crossing each obliterated hypogastric artery about an inch above where they are crossed by the round ligaments.

Prominent peritoneal folds can also be seen hanging from the anterior abdominal wall on either side of the mid-line. These are the *obliterated hypogastric arteries,* or *lateral umbilical ligaments.* They are a continuation of the hypogastric arteries that cross the pelvic brim and run underneath the peritoneum to the umbilicus. The round ligaments cross in front of the obliterated hypogastric arteries about an inch medial to where they enter the internal inguinal ring. The *inferior epigastric artery,* the last branch of the external iliac artery just proximal to the inguinal ligament, winds around the medial edge of the internal inguinal ring and can also be seen running upwards and medially underneath the parietal peritoneum to enter the rectus sheath at the arcuate line. It lies lateral to the obliterated hypogastric artery on the anterior abdominal wall (Figure 6.1).

As the obliterated hypogastric arteries are traced retrogradely into the depths of the pelvis, their first important anatomical relationship is with the external iliac vessels, which lie just lateral to the obliterated hypogastric artery at the level of the pelvic inlet attached to the medial border of the psoas muscle (Figure 6.2). The external iliac vein lies directly below the artery, but the relationship becomes more inferomedial closer to the inguinal ligament. The obturator fossa is situated immediately below and somewhat lateral to the vein, a relationship that is difficult to understand if one envisages the pelvic sidewall as following a vertical course below the psoas muscle. In fact, the obturator fossa is a shallow lateral recess that lies below the iliac vessels and resembles the hollow of a cupped hand. The hollow of the recess is filled out, as it were, with fatty nodal tissue through which runs the obturator nerve and, below it, the obturator artery and vein, which lie just lateral to the obliterated hypogastric artery. Slightly more proximally, the obliterated hypogastric artery meets the uterine to form the internal iliac or hypogastric artery proper (Figure 6.2). Strictly speaking, the superior vesical artery is the next branch encountered as the obliterated artery is traced proximally to the origin of the uterine artery. However, this branch of the obliterated hypogastric artery arises from its posterolateral aspect and runs forward and upward to the bladder in the paravesical space. It cannot be seen before the paravesical is opened medial to the obliterated hypogastric artery, the anterior

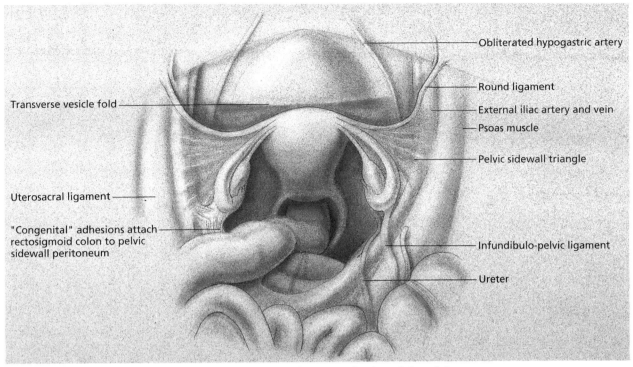

Figure 6.1 Panoramic laparoscopic view of the pelvis.

Labels for Figure 6.1:
- Obliterated hypogastric artery
- Round ligament
- External iliac artery and vein
- Psoas muscle
- Pelvic sidewall triangle
- Transverse vesicle fold
- Uterosacral ligament
- "Congenital" adhesions attach rectosigmoid colon to pelvic sidewall peritoneum
- Infundibulo-pelvic ligament
- Ureter

surface of the uterine artery and cardinal ligament is dissected free of areolar tissue, and the obliterated hypogastric artery deviated laterally. Throughout its pelvic course, the medial border of the obliterated hypogastric artery is related to the lateral wall of the dome of the bladder, but an avascular plane can be developed between these structures.

The Pelvic Sidewall

If the pelvic sidewall peritoneum is put on tension by deviating the uterus to the contralateral side, the triangle of the pelvic sidewall will become evident. The base of this triangle is formed by the round ligament, the lateral border by the external iliac artery, the medial border by the infundibulopelvic ligament,

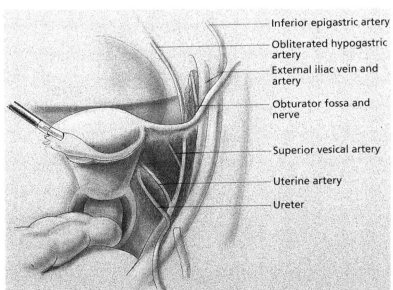

Labels for Figure 6.2:
- Inferior epigastric artery
- Obliterated hypogastric artery
- External iliac vein and artery
- Obturator fossa and nerve
- Superior vesical artery
- Uterine artery
- Ureter

Figure 6.2 Anatomy of the obliterated hypogastric artery and its relationships.

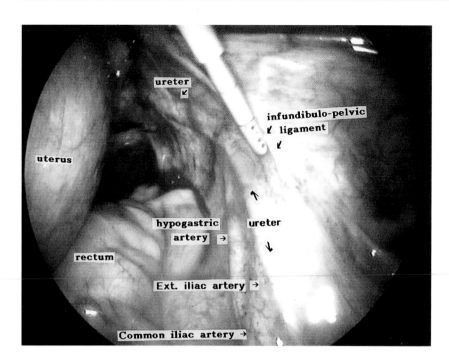

Figure 6.3 Pelvic course of the ureter.

and the apex by where the infundibulopelvic ligament crosses the common iliac artery. On the left side, so-called congenital adhesions attach the rectosigmoid to the pelvic sidewall peritoneum at or just above the pelvic brim, and these usually cover the apex of the pelvic triangle (Figure 6.1). The retroperitoneum is entered lap-aroscopically by incising the peritoneum of the pelvic triangle rather than by dividing the round ligament to preserve the natural tension in the tissues and allow blunt dissection of the retroperitoneal tissue planes .

The Posterior Pelvis

If the uterus is anteverted to expose the posterior pelvis and cul-de-sac, the uterosacral ligaments will be easily seen at the base of the broad ligament on either side of the rectum, running forward and slightly upwards to insert into the back of the cervix (Figure 6.1). The right ureter can usually be seen through the medial leaf of the broad ligament above the uterosacral ligament and, higher up, below the inferior border of the ovarian fossa, but the left ureter is often not visible. The right ureter can usually be traced along the pelvic sidewall, where it lies just above the internal iliac artery, to the pelvic inlet. Here it lies medial to the infundibulopelvic ligament, and crosses the external iliac artery to enter the pelvis (Figure 6.3). The left ureter cannot be seen at the pelvic brim because it is covered by the sigmoid mesentery. If the sigmoid colon is retracted toward the left, the right common iliac artery can often be seen under the posterior parietal peritoneum, especially in thin patients, and the promontory of the sacrum can be "felt" with a probe.

RETROPERITONEAL BLOOD VESSELS

Aorta and Vena Cava

The aorta enters the abdominal cavity through the aortic hiatus in the posterior diaphragm and runs along the front of the lumbar vertebrae to terminate at the lower border of L4 by dividing into the left and right common iliac arteries. The *middle sacral artery* arises just above the aortic bifurcation, crosses the promontory, and runs down the front of the sacrum to terminate by anastomosing with the lateral sacral arteries (Figure 6.4A). Its only surgical significance is that it may be injured during presacral neurectomy. It can be ligated with impunity.

If one proceeds cephalad along the aorta, the first branch encountered is the *inferior mesenteric artery,* which arises from the front of the aorta on the left side about 4 cm above the aortic bifurcation. It runs downward and to the left in the mesentery of the descending colon, gives off the left colic artery, and continues into the pelvis in the mesentery of the rectosigmoid as the *superior rectal* or *hemorrhoidal artery,* which lies medial to the left ureter at the pelvic brim. The superior rectal artery splits into two branches behind the rectum and pierces the fascia of Denonvilliers, where it ends in terminal branches that supply the rectum.

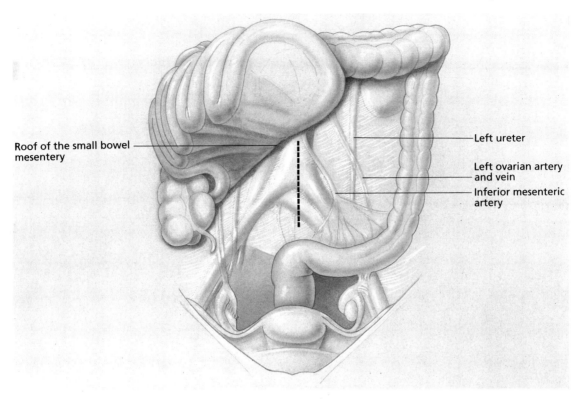

Roof of the small bowel mesentery

Left ureter

Left ovarian artery and vein

Inferior mesenteric artery

Figure 6.4A Anatomy of the posterior peritoneum and retroperitoneum.

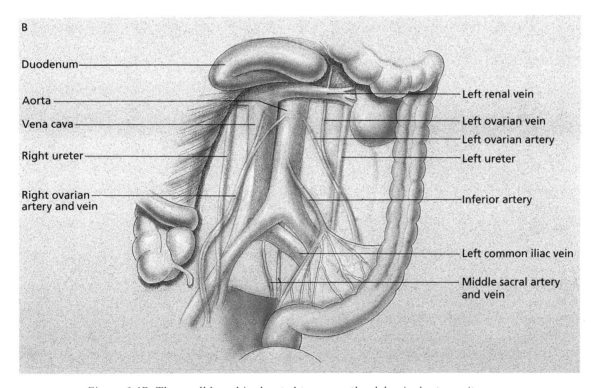

B

Duodenum

Aorta

Vena cava

Right ureter

Right ovarian artery and vein

Left renal vein

Left ovarian vein

Left ovarian artery

Left ureter

Inferior artery

Left common iliac vein

Middle sacral artery and vein

Figure 6.4B The small bowel is elevated to expose the abdominal retroperitoneum.

Laparoscopic Anatomy of the Pelvis and Dissection of the Retroperitoneum   53

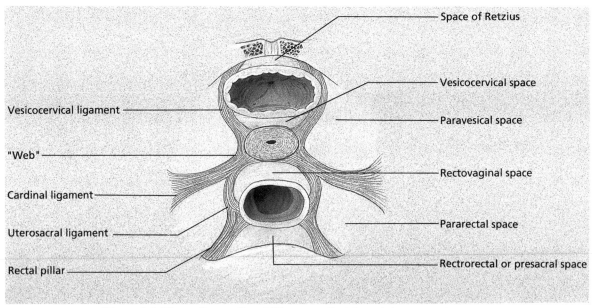

Figure 6.5 Tissue "spaces" and "ligaments" of the pelvic retroperitoneum.

The *ovarian arteries* also arise laterally from the front of the aorta a little more than halfway between the origin of the inferior mesenteric and the renal arteries. (Figure 6.4B). They run obliquely downwards and outwards medial to the ovarian veins, cross in front of the ureters about halfway between the pelvic inlet and the renal pelvis, to lie lateral to the ureters at the pelvic brim. Further cephalad, at the level of L2, lies the *left renal vein* crossing in front of the aorta to join the inferior vena cava, which lies just to the right of the aorta. It covers the *left renal artery,* which is, therefore, usually not seen during aortic lymphadenectomy. The *right renal artery* crosses under the vena cava, and is also not seen during aortic lymphadenectomy.

The *common iliac veins* join to form the *inferior vena cava* on the right side of the aorta, just below and slightly behind the bifurcation. The left common iliac vein crosses the midline below the bifurcation of the aorta just above the sacral promontory and crosses underneath the right common iliac artery to reach the inferior vena cava. It can be injured during presacral neurectomy and resection of sacral nodes during pelvic lymphadenectomy. Except for the lumbar veins posteriorly, there are no branches of the vena cava below the renal veins except for the *right ovarian vein,* which drains into the front of the vena cava on the right side at the level of the origin of the right ovarian artery. The *left ovarian vein* joins the inferior wall of the

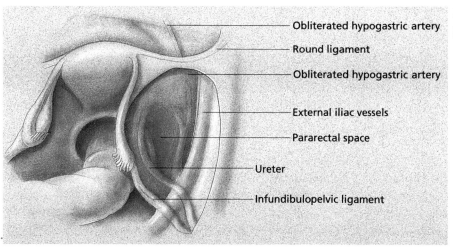

Figure 6.6 Anatomy of the (lateral) pararectal space.

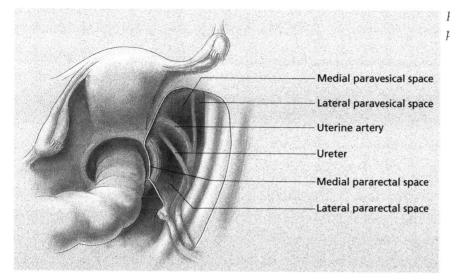

Figure 6.7 The medial and lateral pararectal and paravesical spaces.

left renal vein, and it lies medial to the ureter. The *left adrenal vein* drains into the superior border of the left renal vein opposite the left ovarian vein (Figure 6.4B). The *right renal vein* is extremely short and not exposed during aortic lymphadenectomy; the left renal vein is long, crosses in front of the aorta, and marks the upper limit of aortic lymphadenectomy for gynecological malignancies.

Pelvic Blood Vessels

The common iliac artery ends at the pelvic inlet in front of the sacroiliac joint by dividing into the external and internal iliac arteries. The *external iliac artery* runs along the pelvic brim attached to the medial border of the psoas muscle, and passes under the inguinal ligament to become the femoral artery. It gives off only two branches close to the inguinal ligament, the inferior epigastric and the deep circumflex iliac arteries, both of which supply the anterior abdominal wall (Figure 6.2).

The anatomy of the *internal iliac artery* is complicated, but its surgical anatomy is straightforward because most of its branches are not encountered during pelvic surgery and dissection of the retroperitoneum. The internal iliac artery descends quite steeply into the pelvis along the pelvic sidewalls to where the uterine

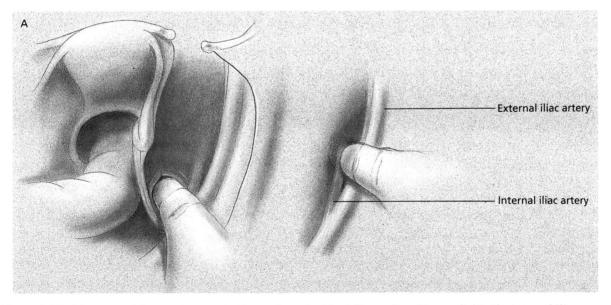

Figure 6.8A The pararectal space is opened at laparotomy by blunt finger dissection medial to the internal iliac artery in the direction of the patient's contralateral femoral head (left). Incorrect dissection between the external and internal iliac arteries may damage the external iliac vein (right).

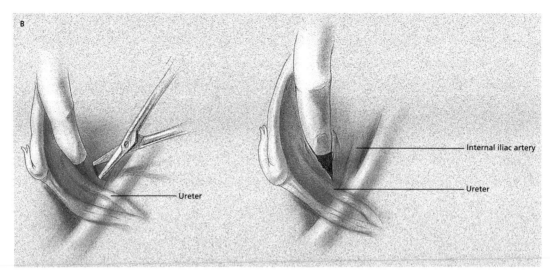

Figure 6.8B Dense areolar tissue covering the pararectal space must be first incised (left) before the space can be opened bluntly by finger dissection.

arteries are given off at the lateral attachments of the cardinal ligaments (Figure 6.3). They then sweep sharply upwards on either side of the bladder as the obliterated hypogastric arteries, which give off the superior vesicle arteries to the bladder, cross the superior pubic rami, and run beneath the peritoneum of the anterior abdominal wall to the umbilicus.

RETROPERITONEAL SPACES OF THE PELVIS

The peritoneum is draped like a cape over the pelvic organs. Between the peritoneum above, the pelvic di-

aphragm below, and the pelvic sidewall laterally, loosely packed fibrous tissue and fat surrounds the pelvic organs, allowing them to distend as necessary. Condensations of this retroperitoneal tissue, referred to as "ligaments," divide the subperitoneal space into compartments or "spaces" (Figure 6.5). These spaces or tissue planes are only potential spaces, and a cavity or "hole" is not encountered within the tissues on opening the peritoneum. However, by blunt dissection in the correct plane, large, avascular, cavernous areas can be exposed within the retroperitoneal tissues. It is impossible to exaggerate the importance to laparo-

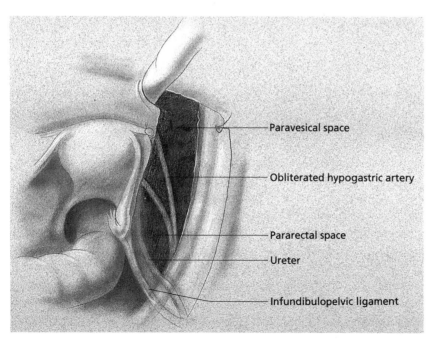

Figure 6.9 The paravesical space is opened by blunt finger dissection in a medial direction against the obliterated hypogastric artery.

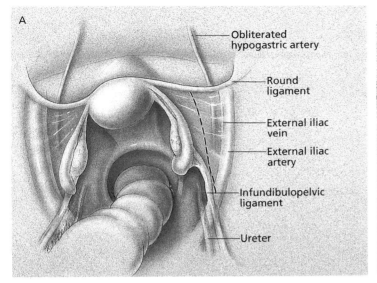

A

Obliterated hypogastric artery

Round ligament

External iliac vein

External iliac artery

Infundibulopelvic ligament

Ureter

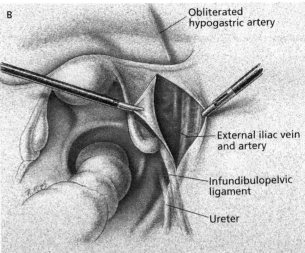

B

Obliterated hypogastric artery

External iliac vein and artery

Infundibulopelvic ligament

Ureter

Figures 6.10A–C The pelvic sidewall triangles are opened to gain access to the retroperitoneum.

C

External iliac artery and vein

Infundibulopelvic ligament

Ureter

Congenital adhesions

Sigmoid colon

scopic surgery of knowing the anatomy of these tissue planes and how to open them correctly.

It is helpful to divide the pelvic spaces into two groups, the central and lateral spaces, and to think of the central spaces as those through which specific operations are carried out and the lateral spaces as being used to identify vital retroperitoneal structures.

The central spaces will be familiar to gynecologists and lie along an imaginary line connecting the symphysis pubis and the sacrum. The space of Retzius lies between the back of the pubic bone and the bladder and must be opened to perform retropubic operations for incontinence, such as a colposuspension. The vesicovaginal space lies between the bladder and vagina and is opened during anterior colporrhaphy whereas the rectovaginal space lies between the rectum and vagina and is opened during posterior colporrhaphy. The retrorectal or presacral space is opened during presacral neurectomy (as well as to resect the rectosigmoid colon). As these spaces, with

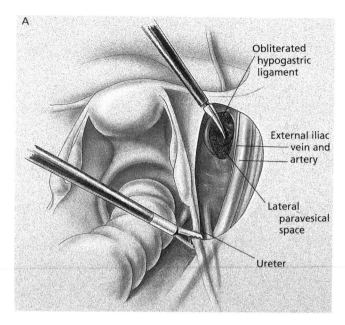

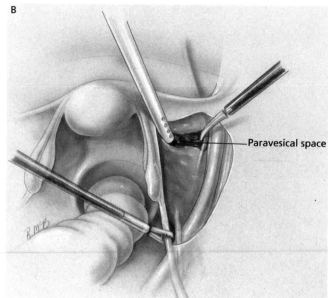

Figures 6.11A,B The paravesical space is opened on either side of the obliterated hypogastric artery.

the possible exception of the retrorectal space, are familiar to all gynecologists, they will not be discussed further. The anatomy of the retrorectal space is discussed in Chapter 19.

The lateral spaces separate the pelvic viscera from the pelvic sidewall. They are the paravesical and pararectal spaces. Although the paravesical space must be opened during pelvic lymphadenectomy and the pararectal space during sacrospinous ligament fixation, these spaces are usually developed to identify vital structures in the retroperitoneum, such as the ureter, uterine artery, and hypogastric artery.

THE LATERAL PELVIC SPACES

Anatomy

If an imaginary line is drawn vertically along the medial leaf of the broad ligament all the way down to the levator floor, the line will successively cross the infundibulopelvic ligament, the ureter, the uterosacral ligament, and, finally, the rectal pillars. The *pararectal spaces* that are used for pelvic surgery are bounded laterally by the internal iliac arteries, medially by the ureters, and below them, the uterosacral ligaments and rectal pillars (Figure 6.6). The cardinal ligament forms the distal boundary of the pararectal space and separates it from the paravesical space, which lies in front of the pararectal space. The uterine artery runs on top of the cardinal ligament from the hypogastric artery to the uterus.

Prior to the development of these tissue spaces, the ureters lie just above the internal iliac arteries on the pelvic sidewall (Figure 6.3); after the pararectal spaces are developed, the ureters mark their medial borders. Therefore, the development of the pararectal spaces always provides a reliable method of identifying the pelvic course of the ureters as well as exposing the iliac vessels, the uterine artery, and the cardinal and uterosacral ligaments.

Another avascular tissue plane can be developed medial to each ureter and uterosacral ligament, but lateral to the peritoneum, which forms the medial portion of the broad ligament and its inferior extension into the cul-de-sac. It is this plane that the general surgeon calls the pararectal space and he/she uses for carrying out either anterior or abdominoperineal resection of the rectum for carcinoma. In other words, our colleagues in general surgery never work laterally to the ureter when performing their pelvic operations but leave it attached in its natural position on the lateral pelvic sidewall. This medial pararectal space is also developed by pelvic surgeons during radical hysterectomy to mobilize the ureter and prepare the uterosacral ligament for division but only after the pararectal space proper has been opened (Figure 6.7).

The *paravesical spaces* are bordered distally or caudad by the pubic bone, proximally or cephalad by the cardinal ligament, medially by the obliterated umbilical artery, laterally by the external iliac vessels and obturator fossa, and inferiorly by the levator floor. Just as

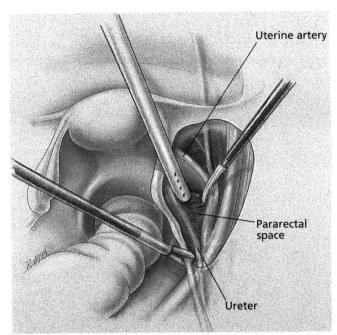

Figure 6.12 The obliterated hypogastric artery is traced retrogradely to the origin of the uterine artery, and the pararectal space opened by blunt dissection proximal and medial to the uterine artery.

a space can be developed medial to the ureter and uterosacral ligament, each being part of the same pararectal space, so a tissue plane can be developed on both sides of the obliterated hypogastric artery (Figure 6.7). The lateral portion of the space lies between the artery and the pelvic sidewall and is the paravesical space proper, but a plane can also be developed medially between the obliterated hypogastric artery and the bladder. It is usually advantageous to open the tissue space on both sides of the obliterated hypogastric artery to obtain good exposure of the anterior aspect of the cardinal ligament and the uterine artery above it.

DEVELOPMENT OF THE LATERAL PELVIC SPACES

Laparotomy

Those who are not accustomed to dissecting the retroperitoneum should first become familiar with how to open the lateral pelvic spaces at laparotomy rather than try to familiarize themselves with the anatomy and learn laparoscopic surgery at the same time. To open the lateral pelvic spaces at laparotomy, the retroperitoneum is first entered by dividing the round ligament and incising the peritoneum in a cephalad direction parallel and lateral to the in-

fundibulopelvic ligament up to the pelvic brim. The broad ligament is next opened by placing a hand against its medial leaf and gently pulling in a medial direction. This maneuver will separate the loose areolar tissue between the leaves of the broad ligament, but an impasse will eventually be reached at about the level of the ureter and internal iliac artery, where the areolar tissue is more condensed and will not separate any further. This point lies at the base of the broad ligament and marks the roof of the pararectal space. This is as far as many gynecologists take the retroperitoneal dissection.

▶ **Pararectal Space:** To open the pararectal space, the external iliac artery is palpated and traced proximally to the bifurcation of the common iliac artery. Both the external and common iliac arteries lie against the medial border of the psoas muscle and are easy to identify by palpation. Once the common iliac artery has been identified at its bifurcation, the index finger of the dissecting hand is placed just medial to the internal iliac artery, and traction is applied with the finger to the tissues medial to the internal iliac artery in the direction of the patient's contralateral femoral head. A bloodless space will start to develop, and as it does, the plane of dissection should follow the curve of the pelvis, which, with the patient in a Trendelenburg position, is at first downward and forward, but then curves in an upward direction (Figure 6.8A). The surgeon will find the ureter lying against the dissecting finger, still attached to the medial leaf of the broad ligament, for the ureter marks the medial border of the pararectal space, and its lateral border is formed by the internal iliac artery.

It is critical to identify the bifurcation of the common iliac artery before starting to dissect the pararectal space to ensure that the plane of dissection will be medial to the internal and not the external iliac artery. The internal iliac artery does not usually lie vertically below the external but below and, to varying degrees, medial to it (Figure 6.8A). Inadvertent dissection medial to the external iliac artery will risk injury to the external iliac vein, which lies between the internal and external iliac arteries.

Quite frequently, especially in thin, young patients, the dense connective tissue forming the roof of the pararectal space cannot be disrupted bluntly, and a small opening must first be made in it with the point of a tonsil clamp or dissecting scissors as the tissue is held taut by medial traction (Figure 6.8B). Once a small nick has been made, the index finger is insinuated into

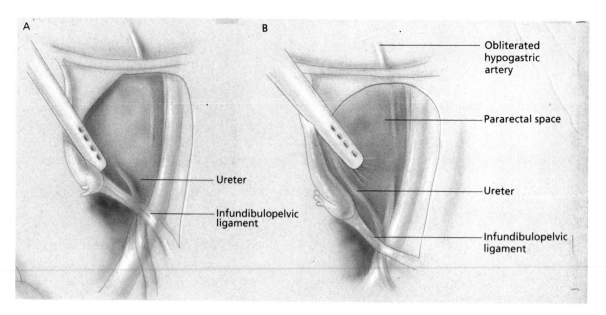

Figures 6.13A,B The pararectal space can often be opened without developing the paravesical space, by identifying the ureter at the pelvic brim (A) and then bluntly dissecting against the ureter in a medial direction (B).

the pararectal space, which will readily open if its medial wall is retracted in a medial direction as previously described. The dense areolar tissue at the base of the broad ligament may be likened to Saran Wrap (cellophane) covering a lunch box. It is difficult to disrupt the Saran Wrap by simply pushing down on it, but once a small nick is made, the Saran Wrap can be separated effortlessly.

▶ **Paravesical Space:** The peritoneal fold containing the obliterated hypogastric arteries is usually not visible at laparotomy, but the paravesical space can be easily opened by blunt dissection. After the broad ligament has been opened, the external iliac artery is again identified by palpation. The index finger of the dissecting hand is placed against the medial edge of the artery and follows it down distally as far as the pubic ramus. On reaching the pubic bone, the direction of the dissection changes abruptly through a 90° angle and is again directed medially towards the patient's contralateral femoral head (Figure 6.9). A large bloodless plane, which is the paravesical space, will again open and a cord-like structure will be found by the dissecting finger, which is the lateral umbilical ligament or obliterated hypogastric artery.

Laparoscopy

The pararectal spaces cannot be easily developed laparoscopically in the same way as during laparotomy. First, with each successive step of the dissection,

that is, division of the round ligament, opening of the broad ligament, and separation of the areolar tissues, the tissues become progressively more slack, and blunt dissection becomes increasingly more difficult and usually eventually impossible because the tissues cannot be maintained on tension. Second, the internal iliac artery is buried in areolar tissues and cannot be at first visualized after the broad ligament is opened, and, obviously, it cannot be palpated. The precise level (in a cephalad-caudad sense) at which to begin dissection of the pararectal space is, therefore, not at first obvious, and troublesome bleeding can occur if the dissection is begun over the cardinal ligament rather than proximal to it or too close to the sacrum. To overcome these difficulties, the technique of entering the retroperitoneum must be altered, and a different strategy is used to find the pararectal space.

▶ **Opening the Pelvic Peritoneum:** To enter the retroperitoneum, the pelvic sidewall triangle (see above) is first delineated by deviating the uterus to the contralateral side. The peritoneum in the middle of the triangle is then desiccated with bipolar forceps, incised with dissecting scissors, and the incision extended to the round ligament, but round ligament is not divided (Figure 6.10A). The broad ligament is opened by bluntly separating the extraperitoneal areolar tissues, usually with the tip of the suction irrigator. Even tiny vessels are coagulated because the slightest amount of bleeding can stain the extraperitoneal areo-

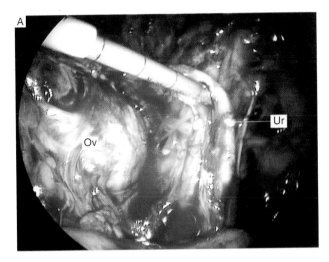

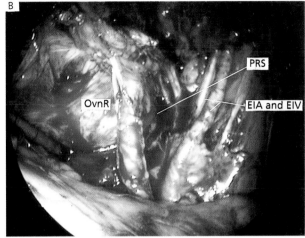

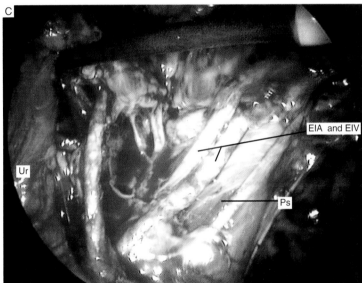

Figures 6.14A–C Resection of a residual ovary after identifying the ureter and freeing it from the ovary.

lar tissues and obscure view of the underlying structures (Figure 6.10B).

On the left side, so-called congenital adhesions attach the rectosigmoid to the peritoneum laterally at or just above the pelvic brim. These usually cover the apex of the pelvic triangle. The dissection on the left side is begun by separating these adhesions from the underlying peritoneum, and the pelvic sidewall triangle is opened at or near its apex (Figure 6.10C). The peritoneal incision is then carried distally to the round ligament, which is not divided at this time.

▶ **Dissection of the Retroperitoneum:** The secret to dissecting the retroperitoneum laparoscopically is not to compartmentalize one's thinking about the dissection. The laparoscopic surgeon is already placed at a disadvantage by not being able to palpate retroperi-

toneal structures, and this is compounded by the absence of reliable retroperitoneal landmarks below the peritoneum. If a technique for pelvic dissection is to be reproducible, however, reliable laparoscopic landmarks must be found, even if it means making use of structures not in the immediate vicinity of where the surgeon wants to be.

The most useful and reliable laparoscopic landmark in the pelvis is the obliterated hypogastric artery; from its anatomy, it is easy to understand why it truly serves as a laparoscopic gateway to the retroperitoneum.

First, the obliterated hypogastric artery is nearly always identifiable, even in obese patients. In perhaps 10% of women, it is not very prominent, but it can still be located by making use of its anatomic relationship to the round ligament and transverse vesical fold (Figures 6.1, 6.2).

Second, because the obliterated hypogastric artery lies within the paravesical space it can be easily dissected free of the surrounding tissues by developing the avascular tissue planes on either side of the artery using blunt dissection (Figures 6.11A,B).

Third, the obliterated hypogastric artery is a continuation of the hypogastric artery after it gives off the uterine artery. Therefore, once it is dissected free of the surrounding tissues in the paravesical space, the artery can be traced retrogradely to identify the uterine arteries at their origin from the internal iliac artery (Figure 6.2).

Fourth, the uterine arteries run along the cardinal ligament, which separates the paravesical and pararectal spaces. Once the uterine arteries have been identified, the paravesical spaces developed, and the anterior aspect of the cardinal ligament delineated, the dissection of the pararectal space can be started accurately proximal and medial to the cardinal ligament and uterine artery (Figure 6.12).

Thus, although at laparotomy, the pararectal space can be and usually is opened without developing the paravesical space, at laparoscopy, it is helpful to open the paravesical space first because this allows the pararectal space to be opened much more accurately with less risk of annoying, diffuse bleeding.

The pararectal space can be opened without developing the paravesical space by using the ureter, which forms the medial border of the pararectal space, as the landmark. As we shall discuss more fully in the next chapter, the key to this approach is to identify the ureter at the pelvic brim, where it lies medial to the infundibulopelvic ligament, and then trace it into the pelvis along the broad ligament, gently pushing it medially with the tip of the suction irrigator or a probe, whereupon the pararectal space will open lateral to the ureter (Figures 6.13A,B). This approach works best in thin patients who have little extraperitoneal fat, and the ureter and internal iliac artery are easily identified.

This is the overall strategy we use to dissect the lateral pelvic spaces laparoscopically whether we are performing a simple laparoscopic hysterectomy, pelvic lymphadenectomy, or resecting a symptomatic, enlarged residual ovary (Figures 6.14A–C). A more detailed account of each step will be found in Chapter 11, which describes and discusses laparoscopic hysterectomy, and a more detailed discussion of laparoscopic dissection of the ureter can be found in the next chapter.

Chapter 7
The Ureter

It is new no matter how long we have known it. Its values crowd each other, its symbols are inexhaustible.—Susan Langer

The gynecologist's relationship to the ureter has been the butt of many surgical jokes, and Symmonds maintained that "... surgeons who do not have sufficient knowledge of the pelvic anatomy to practice routine and constant identification of the ureter should not operate in the pelvis" (1). However understandable this rather harsh edict may be, the truth of the matter is that most gynecological operations can be carried out perfectly safely, indeed impeccably, without identification of the ureter. This is true for almost every vaginal operation, operations on the fallopian tube and ovary, and operations for incontinence, and it is even true for most hysterectomies, the core operation of gynecology. Thus, if many gynecologists feel uneasy at the prospect of having to identify the ureter, not to say dissect it free, it is only because they are rarely called upon to do this in their daily work and not because they do not have the necessary surgical skill to do so or because the ureter is particularly difficult to identify and dissect.

By contrast, identification of the ureter is required to perform a number of laparoscopic operations safely. In addition to radical pelvic operations, such as pelvic lymphadenectomy, these include laparoscopic hysterectomy, transection of the uterosacral ligaments, presacral neurectomy, resection of residual ovaries, and operations for advanced endometriosis. Anyone tempted to question the truth of this statement needs only to study the frequency with which ureteric injuries have occurred during laparoscopic hysterectomy in the hands of both expert laparoscopists and pelvic surgeons (1–8).

ROLE OF URETERIC STENT

Ureteric stents serve three useful functions, and we now pass them routinely for all major laparoscopic operations. First, they make the ureters much more prominent and easier to see. Second, by making the ureters more rigid, the stents not only make it easier to dissect the ureters free of surrounding tissues, but once they have been freed, the stents prevent the ureters from falling into the depths of the pelvis and out of view. Third, should the ureter be inadvertently tied or divided, the injury is much more likely to be recognized intraoperatively if stents are in place. Published accounts of ureteric injuries during laparoscopic surgery clearly indicate that, with rare exceptions (3,4), these injuries are usually not recognized intraoperatively unless stents have been used. Compared with delayed recognition, the intraoperative recognition and repair of a ureteric injury spares the patient a great deal of morbidity. That is not to say that advanced laparoscopic operations cannot be performed without stents, and, in fact, approximately half of the laparoscopic hysterectomies performed by the author were done without them. Nonetheless, stents assist considerably in identifying the ureter.

We cannot stress strongly enough that the purpose of the stent is not to help "palpate" the ureter endoscopically with instruments, and their use does not absolve the gynecologist from the need to identify the ureters properly and to dissect them free when necessary. We are frankly alarmed by suggestions that illuminated stents (or any other gadgets for that matter) can circumvent the need to identify the ureter (9). Indeed, in an instructive letter to the editor, Alderman (10) clearly describes that even the ability to move a ureteric stent back and forth is no guarantee that the ureter has not been clamped.

PASSING URETERIC STENTS

The insertion of ureteric stents is extremely straightforward provided the surgeon knows how to perform cystoscopy. We use #6 whistle-tip catheters and insert them through a 30°-angled cystoscope with perforated rubber nipples placed over the working channels. After introducing the cystoscope into the bladder, any urine present is drained, and approximately 200 cc saline are instilled into the bladder. It is important not to overfill the bladder as this will make the ureteric orifices harder, not easier to locate.

To locate the ureteric orifices, the cystoscope is withdrawn until the urethrovesical junction becomes visible and then slowly advanced back into the bladder until the triangular-shaped trigone is identified at its base. We usually look for the right ureteric orifice first by rotating the cystoscope on its long axis through an angle of about 30° from the midline toward the surgeon's left until the right ureteric orifice at the right upper corner of the trigone is identified. (The cystoscope is not moved from side to side in the horizontal plane.) The left ureteric orifice is identified by rotating the cystoscope in the opposite direction through an angle of about 60°. The ureteric orifice is a slit-like opening, which may be flush with the bladder mucosa (especially if the bladder is overfilled), the "moon crater" appearance, or it may lie on top of a small heaped-up mound of mucosa, the "golf-tee" appearance. Once the ureteric orifice has been located, the whistle-tip catheter is threaded through the working channel of the cystoscope on the side opposite to the ureteric orifice. The catheter should be threaded with a light touch so that the slightest resistance to its advancement can be appreciated, which, with a normal ureter, signifies that the tip of the stent is in the renal pelvis. If the catheter is advanced too roughly, the renal parenchyma can be perforated, and this will cause bleeding and even clot colic postoperatively.

Once the stents have been passed, a Foley catheter is inserted into the bladder, and the distal end of the stents threaded into the tubing of the draining bag through two holes made in the end of the Foley catheter with a No. 11 blade. (We make small stab incisions before we pass the stents.) The stents are then tied to the shaft of the catheter with silk thread. The catheters are removed when the operation is finished before the patient leaves the operating room.

RELEVANT ANATOMY

The ureters vary between 25 and 30 cm in length depending on the height of the individual, and their abdominal and pelvic components are approximately equal in length. The ureters follow a straight, almost perpendicular line from the renal pelvis to the pelvic brim. They lie on the anterior surface of the psoas muscles but are attached to the undersurface of the posterior parietal peritoneum and move with the peritoneum when this is elevated. In their abdominal course, the right and left ureters are located approximately 4–5 cm lateral to the inferior vena cava and aorta, respectively (Figure 7.1).

Approximately halfway between the pelvic inlet and the renal pelvis, the ovarian vessels cross the abdominal ureters (the left one at a higher level than the right) to lie lateral to them at the pelvic brim (Figure 7.1). Here, the ovarian vessels enter the infundibulopelvic ligament and cross the ureters again to lie at first above and then medial to them, as the vessels runs medially in the roof of the broad ligament from the pelvic brim to the ovaries. The surgical significance of this relationship is that (1) the ureter cannot be damaged if the pelvic sidewall peritoneum is incised lateral to the anatomic position of the infundibulopelvic ligament and (2) the infundibulopelvic ligament must be retracted medially to expose the ureter at the pelvic brim and on the medial leaf of the broad ligament.

The Pelvic Ureter

The ureters cross the iliac vessels to enter the pelvic brim. The right ureter almost always crosses the external iliac artery whereas the left ureter lies closer to the midline and crosses the common iliac artery. Throughout their pelvic course, the ureters lie in a connective tissue sheath attached to the medial leaf of the broad ligament. Upon crossing the pelvic brim, the ureters descend quite abruptly and follow the contours of the pelvis between the iliac arteries and lie lateral to the infundibulopelvic ligament. In other words, on crossing the pelvis, the ureters actually bend laterally to run along the pelvic sidewalls just above the internal iliac arteries (Figure 7.2A). This is not appreciated surgically, however, because once the broad ligament is opened, the ureters are displaced medially from their natural position on the pelvic sidewall and are seen as

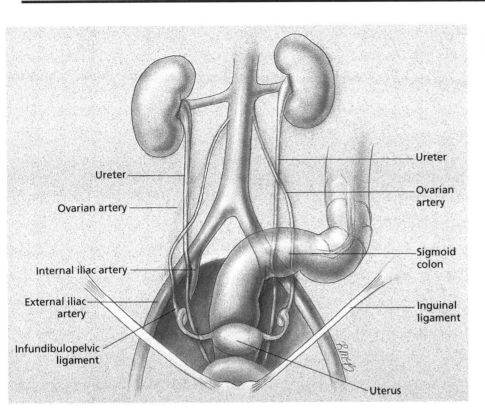

Figure 7.1 Retroperitoneal relationships of the ureter.

Ureter

Ovarian artery

Internal iliac artery

External iliac artery

Infundibulopelvic ligament

Ureter

Ovarian artery

Sigmoid colon

Inguinal ligament

Uterus

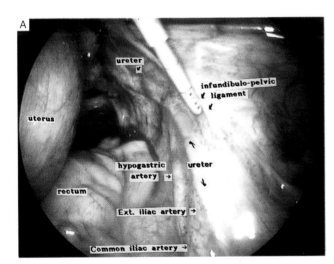

Figure 7.2A Anatomic position of the ureter in the pelvis, where it lies lateral to the infundibulopelvic ligament.

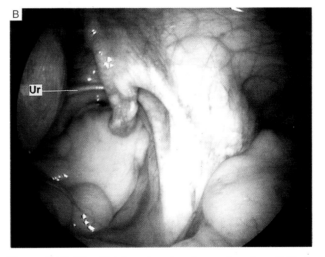

Figure 7.2B The distal ureter runs forward and medially in the base of the broad ligament.

following a more or less straight course from the renal pelvis to the bladder, turning medially to join the bladder only after they have entered the ureteric tunnel in the vesicocervical ligaments or bladder pillars.

In the undisturbed state, at about the level of the ischial spines, the ureters run forward and medially in the base of the broad ligament (Figure 7.2B) to pass under the uterine arteries approximately 1.5 cm lateral to the internal cervical os. (The left ureter is usually closer to the cervix than the right.) The ureters then turn abruptly medially to enter the bladder, passing over the anterior vaginal fornices as they do so. The terminal 1–2 cm of the ureter is called the *genu* or knee of the ureter. It lies in the vesicocervical ligament (also called the vesicouterine ligament or bladder pillar), the surgical anatomy of which can only be fully appreciated during radical vaginal hysterectomy or the Schauta-Amreich operation (see Chapter 23).

Surgical Injuries to the Ureter

From its anatomy, it should be evident that the ureter is particularly vulnerable to injury at three points during pelvic surgery: (1) at the pelvic brim as the infundibulopelvic ligament is being divided, and the closer this is divided to the pelvic brim, the greater the vulnerability of the ureter; (2) at the ovarian fossa, especially during resection of ovaries or ovarian remnants that are bound by adhesions to the pelvic sidewall; and (3) lateral to the cervix during division or coagulation of the uterine artery, the uterosacral ligament, or the cardinal ligament, especially in the presence of endometriosis or pelvic inflammatory disease.

Laparoscopic Identification of the Ureter

The ureter can be identified using three quite different approaches, which may be called medial, superior, and lateral.

▶ **The Medial Approach:** The medial approach to the ureter is the most simple and least useful but, unfortunately, still the most, if not the only, method of laparoscopic ureteric identification taught. If the uterus is anteflexed, the ureter can usually be visualized in its natural position on the medial leaf of the broad ligament (at least on the right side) provided there is no significant cul-de-sac or adnexal pathology. This allows the peritoneum immediately above the ureter to be incised to create a "window" in the peritoneum, which makes for safe division of the infundibulopelvic ligament or adnexal pedicle (Figure 7.3). The peritoneal incision must be very superficial, however; otherwise, the iliac vessels, which lie just lateral, out of view, can be injured. This approach is obviously very limited for a number of reasons.

First, the distal ureter often cannot be seen through the broad ligament. The medial approach, therefore, is usually not helpful in identifying the ureter over the distal part of the uterosacral ligaments, the area divided during a LUNA operation.

Second, the left ureter frequently cannot be visualized at all because the sigmoid mesentery obscures the view of its proximal portion. Thus, if it can be seen at all, the left ureter is visible only for a short distance in the region of the ovarian fossa.

Third, the technique obviously cannot be applied when there is significant pathology in the cul-de-sac or adnexa.

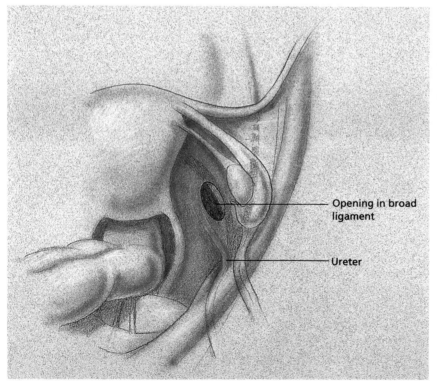

Opening in broad ligament

Ureter

Figure 7.3 An opening is made in the medial leaf of the broad ligament above the ureter to allow the infundibulopelvic ligament or adnexal pedicle to be safely divided.

Fourth, it does not allow proper access to the retroperitoneum and development of the pararectal space.

▶ The Superior Approach:

The superior approach to identifying the ureter is used during laparotomy when the retroperitoneal spaces have been obliterated by prior retroperitoneal surgery. The idea is to identify the ureter outside the pelvis, where its anatomy has not been distorted by prior surgery or disease. The ureters are identified at the pelvic brim, or higher if need be (but then the ascending and descending colon covering them have to be mobilized medially by incising the white line of Toldt in the paracolic gutters), and traced into the pelvis along the medial leaf of the broad ligament. When this approach has been used laparoscopically, the ureter is separated from the infundibulopelvic ligament and dissected progres-sively off the broad ligament, but this is both time-consuming and not very helpful. Reflection of the ureter off the proximal part of the broad ligament in no way facilitates subsequent division of the uterine arteries or uterosacral or cardinal ligaments; only reflection of the distal ureter just proximal to the cardinal ligament does.

A superior approach can be used laparoscopically, and it is useful when only an ovary or ovarian remnant is being removed and the pelvic sidewall is distorted (Figures 7.4A–C). The pelvic sidewall peritoneum is incised in the middle of the pelvic triangle and the incision extended proximally at least to the pelvic brim, but usually beyond, and often to the cecum on the right or the descending colon on the left (Figure 7.4A). The infundibulopelvic ligament is then pulled medially with a suitable grasping forceps and the ureter identi-

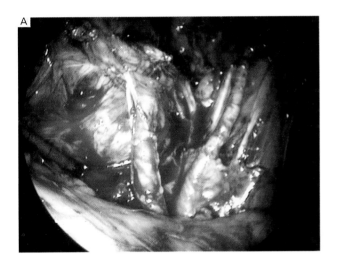

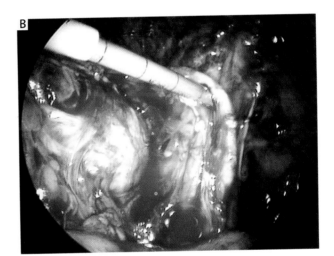

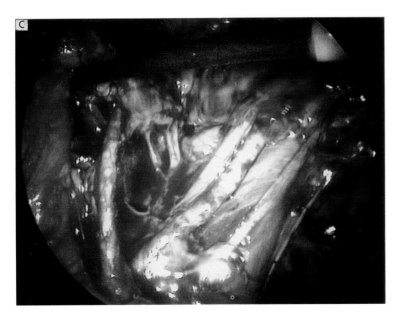

Figures 7.4A–C The right pararectal space has been developed and the ureter identified and dissected off the residual ovary, which is then removed.

fied at the pelvic brim (Figure 7.4B). We emphasize again that failure to find the ureter at the pelvic brim always means that the infundibulopelvic ligament has not been displaced medially enough, and this, in turn, is always due to the fact that the peritoneal incision has not been extended sufficiently proximally.

Once the ureter is identified, it is pushed gently medially with the tip of the suction irrigator or dissecting forceps at successively more distal points, whereupon the pararectal space will open lateral to the ureter (Figure 7.4C). The ureter should not be dissected off the whole length of the broad ligament as this serves no purpose (other than in a radical hysterectomy).

▸ **The Lateral Approach:** The lateral approach is the laparoscopic equivalent of the open technique for it makes use of the pararectal space to identify the ureter, and the ureter does not have to be peeled off the broad ligament for its entire pelvic course to be visible (11). The technique makes use of three basic strategies. First, the sidewall peritoneum is incised without dividing the round ligament, and the infundibulopelvic or adnexal pedicles are only divided after the retroperitoneal dissection is complete. Second, the ureter is identified at the pelvic brim, before it dives deep into the pelvis; the infundibulopelvic ligament must be adequately mobilized to make this possible. Third, the obliterated hypogastric artery, which is easily identified and dissected free laparoscopically, is traced retrogradely to the origin of the uterine artery. The uterine artery, which runs on top of the cardinal ligament and, in turn, marks the caudal (distal) border of the pararectal space, is used as a landmark for the pararectal space.

▸ *STEP 1. The pelvic sidewall triangles are opened.* The triangle of the pelvic sidewall is delineated by displacing the uterus to the contralateral side. The base of this triangle is formed by the round ligament, the lateral border by the external iliac artery, the medial border by the infundibulopelvic ligament, and the apex by where the infundibulopelvic ligament crosses the common iliac artery (Figures 7.5A–C). The peritoneum in the middle of the triangle is desiccated with a bipolar current and incised with dissecting scissors, and the broad ligament is opened by bluntly separating the extraperitoneal areolar tissues (Figure 7.6). Even tiny vessels should be coagulated because the slightest amount of bleeding can stain the extraperitoneal areolar tissues and obscure view of the underlying structures.

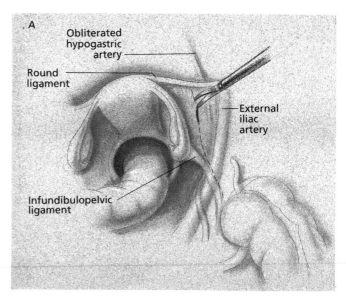

Figure 7.5A *The peritoneum of the pelvic sidewall triangle is opened to gain access to the retroperitoneum.*

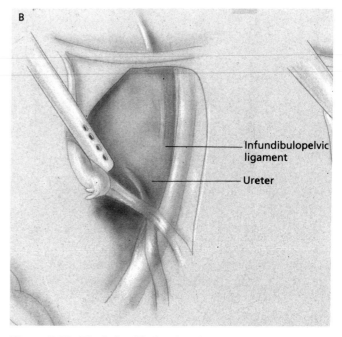

Figure 7.5B *The infundibulopelvic ligament is mobilized and pulled medially to expose the ureter at the pelvic brim.*

The peritoneal incision is extended first to the round ligament, which is not divided at this time, and then to the apex of the triangle lateral to the infundibulopelvic ligament. It is important not to displace the infundibulopelvic ligament from its anatomic position before the peritoneal incision is completed; otherwise, the natural anatomic relationship between the ureter and the infundibulopelvic ligament, which serves to

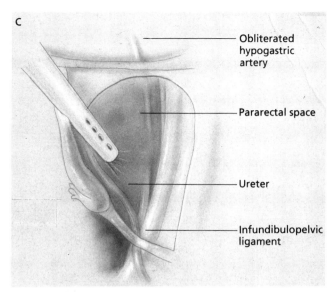

C

Obliterated hypogastric artery

Pararectal space

Ureter

Infundibulopelvic ligament

Figure 7.5C The pararectal space is opened by blunt dissection against the ureter in a medial direction.

protect the ureter from injury as it lies medial to the infundibulopelvic ligament, will be lost.

On the left side, so-called congenital adhesions attach the recto-sigmoid to the peritoneum laterally at or just above the pelvic brim. These usually cover the apex of the pelvic triangle. The dissection on the left side is begun by separating these adhesions from the underlying peritoneum, and the pelvic sidewall tri-

angle is opened at or near its apex (Figure 7.7). (The external iliac artery will be below the plane of dissection.) The peritoneal incision is then carried distally to the round ligament, which is, again, not divided at this time.

▶ *STEP 2.* **The ureter is identified at the apex of the pelvic triangle.** The infundibulopelvic ligament is pulled medially with grasping forceps to expose the ureter at the pelvic brim where it crosses the common or external iliac artery (Figure 7.5B). This is a crucial step. It may be necessary to reflect the ureter off the medial leaf of the broad ligament for a short distance to aid in its identification, although this is rarely required.

It is important to mobilize the infundibulopelvic ligament adequately; otherwise it will not be possible to retract its proximal end sufficiently medially to expose the ureter at the pelvic brim. Failure to achieve adequate mobilization of the infundibulopelvic ligament is the most common error in carrying out the dissection. The operator then searches for the ureter distal to the pelvic brim and lateral to the infundibulopelvic ligament but frequently fails to find it, for the ureter is at that point covered by fatty areolar tissue, or, more distally, by the infundibulopelvic ligament itself and cannot be seen except in the thinnest of patients. The error stems from the fact that the peritoneal incision has to be extended much further proximally than is re-

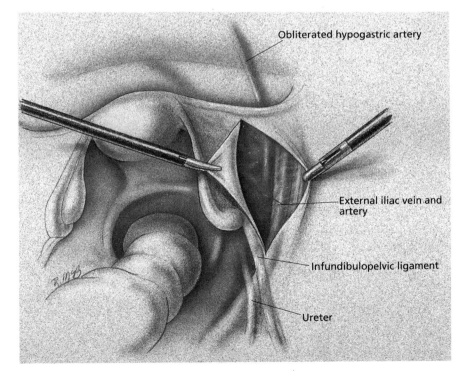

Obliterated hypogastric artery

External iliac vein and artery

Infundibulopelvic ligament

Ureter

Figure 7.6 The broad ligament is opened.

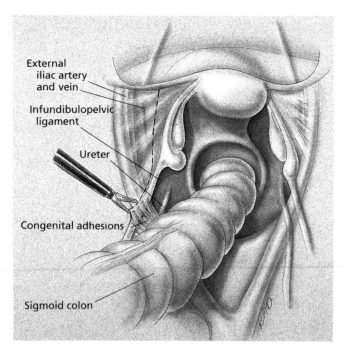

External
iliac artery
and vein

Infundibulopelvic
ligament

Ureter

Congenital adhesions

Sigmoid colon

Figure 7.7 The attachments of the sigmoid colon are divided and the incision on the left is started at the apex of the pelvic sidewall triangle.

quired in an open case, frequently to the cecum on the right and the descending colon in the paracolic gutter on the left.

The dissection of the apex is more difficult on the left side partly because the ureter is covered by the mesentery of the sigmoid colon but mainly because it crosses the iliac vessels higher (more proximally) and, consequently, lies more medial than the right ureter. As a result, it is more difficult to expose the left ureter by retracting the infundibulopelvic ligament medially. The peritoneal incision frequently has to be extended to the white line in the paracolic gutter to mobilize the sigmoid colon and, with it, the infundibulopelvic ligament, which, at this point, lies extraperitoneally under the mesentery (Figure 7.8). It is also sometimes necessary to mobilize the medial leaf of the broad ligament from the pelvic brim and sacrum. To do this, the operator has to dissect bluntly in a medial direction under the infundibulopelvic ligament, taking care not to perforate the medial leaf of the broad ligament or the right plane of dissection will be lost. Finally, the operator needs to be aware that the external iliac artery will be below the plane of dissection much of the time.

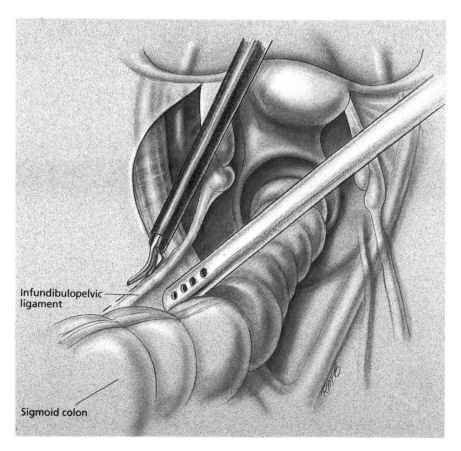

Figure 7.8 The peritoneal incision is extended into the paracolic gutter to mobilize the left infundibulopelvic ligament.

Infundibulopelvic
ligament

Sigmoid colon

STEP 3. *The obliterated hypogastric arteries are identified extraperitoneally.* The dissection is carried out bluntly underneath and caudad to the round ligament, until the obliterated hypogastric artery is identified extraperitoneally (Figure 7.9). Although the anatomy will be unfamiliar to most general gynecologists, this step is, in fact, the most straightforward part of the dissection. If any difficulty is encountered, the artery should be first identified intraperitoneally where it hangs from the anterior abdominal wall, traced proximally to where it passes behind the round ligament, and then with both its intraperitoneal portion and the dissected space under the round ligament in view, the intraperitoneal part of the ligament should be moved back and forth. It will almost always be possible to detect corresponding movements in the extraperitoneal portion of the ligament.

STEP 4. *The paravesical spaces are developed.* Once the obliterated hypogastric arteries have been identified extraperitoneally, it is a simple matter to develop the paravesical space by bluntly separating the areolar tissue on either side of the artery. The dissection is started lateral to the artery, mindful that the external iliac vein is just lateral to it. The tips of the closed dissecting scissors are placed against the lateral edge of the artery and the artery is simply pulled medially, whereupon a bloodless plane will open lateral to it (Figure 7.10). The medial border of the artery is then freed in an identical manner, but working in the opposite direction. During this maneuver, the operator must take care not to press on the external iliac vein as the artery is displaced laterally (Figure 7.11). It is better, in fact, to dissect mostly medially, against the bladder, while the umbilical ligament is held fixed and deviated slightly laterally.

STEP 5. *The pararectal spaces are developed.* The obliterated hypogastric arteries are next traced proximally to where they are joined by the uterine arteries and the pararectal spaces opened by blunt dissection proximal and medial to the uterine vessels, which lie on top of the cardinal ligaments. Once the pararectal spaces have been opened, the ureter on the ipsilateral side is easily identified on the medial leaf of the broad ligament, which forms the medial border of the pararectal space. The uterine artery and cardinal ligament at the distal (caudal) border of the space and the internal iliac artery on its lateral border also become clearly visible at this stage (Figure 7.12).

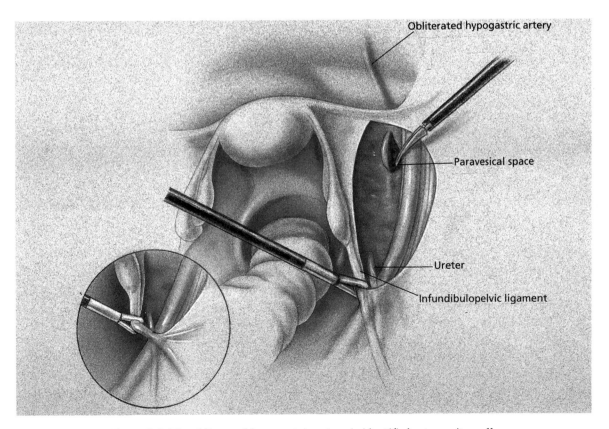

Figure 7.9 The obliterated hypogastric artery is identified extraperitoneally.

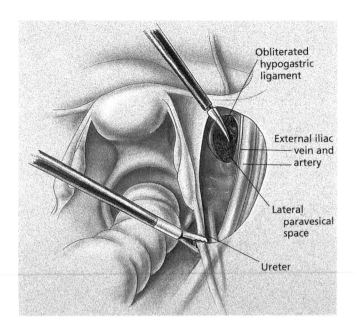

Figure 7.10 *The lateral paravesical space is opened.*

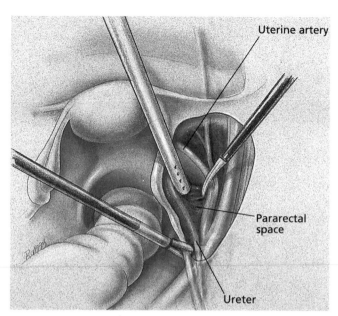

Figure 7.12 *The pararectal space is developed.*

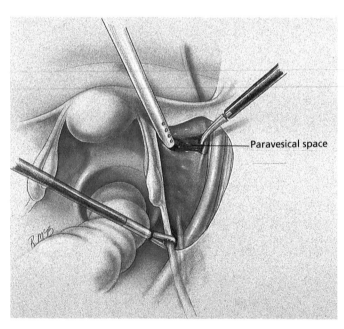

Figure 7.11 *The medial paravesical space is opened.*

REFERENCES

1. Hourcabie JA, Bruhat M-A. One hundred and three cases of laparoscopic hysterectomy using endo-GIA staples and a device for presenting the vaginal fornices. Gynaecol Endosc 1993;2:65–72.

2. Grainger DA, Sonderstrom RM, Schiff SF, Glickman MG, DeCherney AH, Diamond MP. Ureteral injuries at laparoscopy: insights into diagnosis, management and prevention. Obstet Gynecol 1990;75:839–843.

3. Gomel V, James C. Intraoperative management of ureteral injury during operative laparoscopy. Fertil Steril 1991;55:416–419.

4. Neven P, Vandeusen H, Baert L, Koninckx PR. Ureteric injury at laparoscopic surgery: the endoscopic management. Gynaecol Endosc 1993;2:45–46.

5. Kadar N, Lemmerling L. Urinary tract injuries during laparoscopically assisted hysterectomy: causes and prevention. Am J Obstet Gynecol 1994;170:47-48.

6. Hunter RW, McCartney AJ. Can laparoscopic assisted hysterectomy safely replace abdominal hysterectomy? Br J Obstet Gynaecol 1993;100:932–934.

7. Childers JA, Brzechffa PR, Hatch KD, Surwit EA. Laparoscopically assisted surgical staging (LASS) of endometrial cancer. Gynecol Oncol 1993;51:33–38.

8. Blecharz A, Rzempoluch J, Zamlynski J. Laparoscopic hysterectomy; review of 33 cases (Abstract). Presented at the 2nd European Congress in Gynaecologic Endoscopy and New Surgical Techniques, Heidelberg, October 21–23, 1993. Gynaecol Endosc 1994;3:21.

9. Phipps JH, John M, Hassanaien M, Saeed M. Laparoscopic- and laparoscopically assisted vaginal hysterectomy: a series of 114 cases. Gynaecol Endosc 1993;2:7–12.

10. Alderman B. Ureteric injury (letter). Gynaecol Endosc 1993;2:186.

11. Kadar N. A laparoscopic technique for dissecting the pelvic retroperitoneum and identifying the ureter. J Reprod Med (in press).

Chapter 8
Basic Laparoscopic Surgical Techniques and Instrumentation

Mechanical excellence is the only vehicle of genius.
—Blake

The prerequisites of any operation are a thorough understanding of anatomy and the pathology being treated; its goals are to remove diseased tissues and restore normal anatomy; and its execution requires proper exposure of the operative field, separation of tissues, control of bleeding, and, sometimes but not always, the approximation or reapproximation of tissues. The prerequisites and goals of surgery do not alter when an operation is carried out laparoscopically, and its execution changes much less than one might at first imagine.

EXPOSURE

Adequate exposure during laparoscopic surgery requires maintenance of the pneumoperitoneum, a good quality laparoscope, light source, and video camera-monitor system, and the ability to clear the operative field of blood and to retract structures that might otherwise obscure the operative field. Exposure is the *sine qua non* of surgery, and, not surprisingly, the technical innovations that made advanced laparoscopic operations possible all had to do with providing the surgeon with continuous exposure during endoscopic surgery.

The pressure-regulated high-flow insufflator and the high-pressure suction irrigation device were pivotal innovations introduced by Professor Kurt Semm in the 1970s. They allowed the surgeon rapidly to clear the operative field of blood and other debris and to maintain or quickly reestablish the pneumoperitoneum during instrument exchanges and suctioning. High-flow insufflators should have a maximal flow

rate of at least 9 L/min. The flow rate, preset pressure, and patient pressure should be displayed digitally and be easy to read from the operating table (Figure 8.1).

The suction irrigator is the edoscopist's surgical sponge, and the irrigation cannula can be used simultaneously for blunt dissection. The Nezhat-Dorsey system we use has a disposable trumpet valve attached to a reusable cannula (Figure 8.2). The original, completely reusable handle was much too small and forced the hand to work almost closed, at a considerable mechanical disadvantage. The trumpet valve was an important addition to the system for it allowed the surgeon to switch rapidly between suction and irrigation unaided using one hand. We prefer to use a cannula that has perforations on its side to facilitate

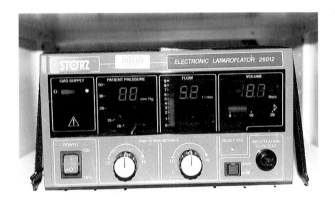

Figure 8.1 Insufflator with a digital read out that can be clearly seen by the surgeon.

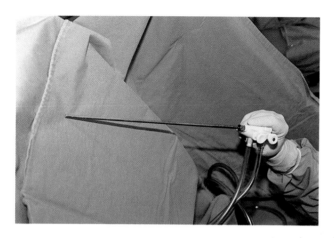

Figure 8.2 *The Nezhat-Dorsey trumpet valve suction irrigator.*

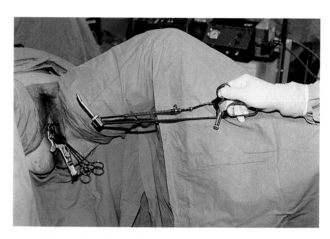

Figure 8.3 *The Pelosi hinged uterine mobilizer.*

suctioning, but because these perforations are small, they do not interfere with the direction of the irrigating jet when the instrument is being used for irrigation.

The ability to display the operative field on a video monitor was a very significant development that freed the surgeon's eye from the laparoscope, allowed two-handed operative techniques to be applied, and provided a view of the operative field for surgical assistants. To make this possible, however, required many improvements and innovations in light sources, laparoscopes, and, of course, the silicon microchip camera. Different manufacturers frequently use the same type of light source and identical chips in their cameras, so differences in quality only become apparent with extended use of the equipment. Presumably adverse features, such as glare or color bleeds, can be as much a function of the design of the iris system and of how the camera's computer processes the analogue images as of the quality of the basic components (see Chapter 2).

The design of mechanical devices, such as retractors and traditional surgical instruments, has lagged far behind optics and lasers. Most endoscopic retractors and grasping instruments serve more as objects of curiosity than as effective means of retracting, and the pelvic surgeon still has to rely largely on gravity and a good uterine manipulator to expose pelvic structure. The availability of a hinged uterine manipulator, which allows the uterus to be moved in any direction independently of the shaft of the instrument, cannot be overemphasized. There are only two available, the original Valtchev (Conkin Surgical Instruments) and the Pelosi Mobilizer (Nova, Endoscopy), which, in our view, is far superior (Figure 8.3).

DISSECTION

Surgical dissection involves separating tissues and controlling bleeding. In conventional surgery, tissues are separated by cutting them with scissors or, less frequently, with a scalpel and then bluntly separating natural tissue planes. Precisely the same technique of dissection is used endoscopically. However, technology has been slow to provide the laparoscopic surgeon with instruments that can serve as counterparts to the dissecting scissors and tissue forceps used in open surgery. Endoscopic dissecting scissors were originally crude, hook-shaped instruments, or had straight blades (Figure 8.4). It is an astonishing fact that for all the breathtaking technological advances that have occurred in recent years, a good pair of dissecting scissors with a rotating, insulated shaft is hard to find, and the original Endoshears (U.S. Surgical) are still unsur-

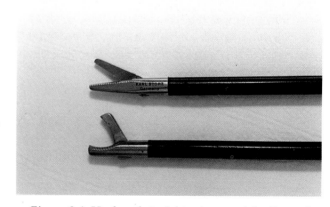

Figure 8.4 *Hook and straight scissors originally used for endoscopic dissection.*

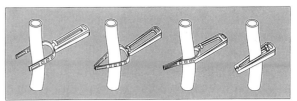

Closure sequence of lapro-clip ligating clip

Figure 8.6 The locking mechanism of the new 12-mm resorbable Laproclip (Davis & Geck).

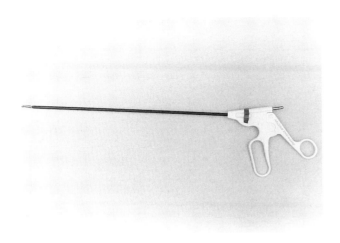

Figure 8.5 The Endoshears.

passed (Figure 8.5). Nondisposable scissors have been available for only about one year, but they are heavy, and many are poorly balanced and cannot match the original Endoshears in performance.

In conventional surgery, hemostasis is achieved by ligating, suturing, clipping, or coagulating bleeding points or vessels. The same techniques are used for hemostasis during laparoscopic surgery, although much less reliance is placed on suturing because, as we have observed (see Chapter 4), presently available techniques, even in the best of hands, are clumsy, crude, and time-consuming. Electrosurgical coagulation of tissues remains the mainstay of hemostasis. Small vessels can be coagulated with a unipolar, modulated, or unmodulated current, larger vessels with the bipolar mode, and diffuse oozing in the noncontact mode (fulguration) using a monopolar, high-voltage modulated current (see Chapter 3). Endoscopic clips and clip appliers have matched those used at laparotomy, but the application of clips has limited usefulness as a surgical technique. The uterine artery is larger than the cystic artery and cannot be clipped with metal clips, although we have recently used a resorbable 12-mm clip (Laproclip, Davis & Geck, Danbury CT) successfully to ligate both the uterine artery and the infundibulopelvic ligament (Figure 8.6). The Laproclip has become our preferred method of occluding the uterine and ovarian vessels prior to division.

In summary, then, our approach to laparoscopic dissection is straightforward and follows as much as possible the techniques used at laparotomy. We use a two-handed approach with dissecting scissors held in the right hand and tissue-type grasping forceps in the

left. When dissecting retroperitoneal tissue planes, the grasping forceps are replaced by the suction irrigator, which is held in the left hand, and the cannula used for blunt dissection as well as suctioning and irrigation as the need arises. The dissecting scissors are attached to a unipolar circuit, and an unmodulated current is used exclusively except when fulgurating in the noncontact mode, in which case a modulated ("coagulation") current is used. When tiny, hair-like vessels are encountered, the current is momentarily activated as the blades of the scissors are transecting the vessel. If slightly larger bleeders are encountered, the scissors are rotated front end on to decrease the current density, and the vessels are coagulated with an unmodulated current. The side or tip of the scissors can also be used as a knife electrode to cut peritoneum, the posterior vaginal wall, or structures, such as the uterosacral and round ligaments. Larger vessels or bleeding points need to be coagulated with bipolar forceps using a low-voltage unmodulated current. We use the Kleppinger forceps with a modified grip for bipolar coagulation because this allows a fuller range of rotation (Figure 8.7).

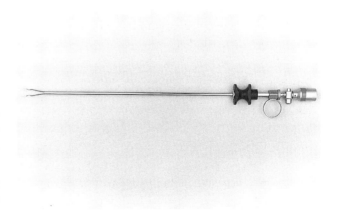

Figure 8.7 Kleppinger bipolar forceps with a syringe-type handle.

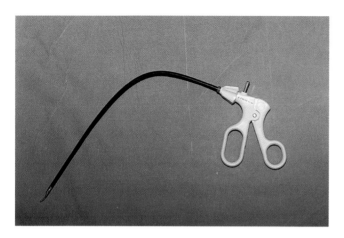

Figure 8.8 The Ethicon scissors and forceps have a much too flexible shaft.

INSTRUMENTATION

It is helpful to consider operating instruments as falling into three different categories. Let us call them scissors, forceps, and graspers.

Scissors

For reasons that are not clear to this author, the original endoscopic dissecting scissors were medieval-looking implements, which, even more surprisingly, were devised by infertility surgeons, who generally need small and delicate tools for their work (Figure 8.4). The straight scissors, both the 5-mm and 3-mm, are a design that is also difficult to understand. After all, who would imagine dissecting the pelvis with straight suture scissors? Nonetheless, master surgeons who use classical techniques of dissection, such as Drs. Harry Reich and David Redwine, have been able to bring sharp-scissor dissection to a fine art with these instruments. The scissors do have the advantage of having rounded ends, the hallmark of the dissecting scissor, making them useful for simultaneously spreading and cutting extraperitoneal areolar tissue by a sweeping motion with jaws half open.

Not until the U.S. Surgical Corporation developed the Endoshears did endoscopic scissors with properties similar to those used at laparotomy become available (Figure 8.5). This scissor set a standard yet to be surpassed. It has curved blades and rounded tips, and its shaft can be rotated with a single finger. After a long time, the Ethicon Company managed to develop its own version of this scissor, but, in my opinion, this instrument is frankly dangerous. It is much too flimsy, the tips are too sharp, the shaft bends much too easily (Figure 8.8), and I have known its insulating coating to fracture as the shaft of the scissor bends, which is usual during operations on obese patients.

It is, perhaps, surprising that in this space age, it took a very long time for reusable scissors incorporating all the features of the original Endoshears, including the rotatable shaft, to be developed. The reusable scissors I have used, however, have been much too heavy or poorly balanced, and, like the Ethicon disposable scissor, their blades tended to scrape on each other as the jaws were opened and closed. Very recently, Microsurge introduced a scissor that is semireusable and promising. They come in 5-mm and 3-mm sizes (Fig-

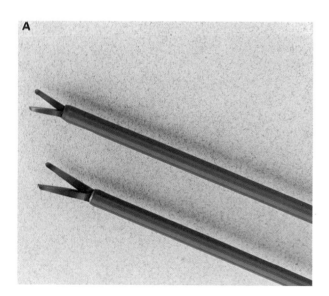

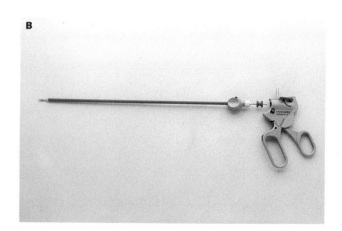

Figures 8.9A,B New semireusable (resposable) dissecting scissors.

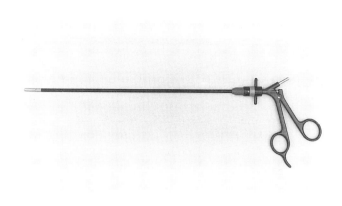

Figure 8.10 The Aesculap "alligator"-type grasping forceps used in the manner of dissecting forceps at laparotomy (PL-146).

ure 8.9A). The handle is reusable (Figure 8.9B), and the tip can be used up to about 10 times. My personal recommendation at the present time would be to use the U.S. Surgical Endoshears for sharp-scissor dissection (Figure 8.5). Although reusable instruments are preferred to disposable ones on economic grounds, proper cost comparisons must take into account the cost of sharpening scissors as well as their overall lifespan. Reusable or semireusable scissors may not have as great an economic advantage as is generally supposed, especially if the manufacturers of disposable instruments reduce their prices in the future.

Forceps

Although the term forceps is not applied to endoscopic grasping instruments, if one is to use the classic two-handed approach to dissection, there is a need for an endoscopic instrument to take the place of the dissecting forceps that are used in conventional surgery. Candidates for the job all go under the heading of grasping forceps in instrument catalogs. It should be noted that the term dissecting forceps, when applied to endoscopic instruments, does not have the usual connotation of an instrument that is used to pick up tissues, but rather, of one used to spread tissues apart, and that is, in fact, quite useless for picking them up. The surgeon will, therefore, have to seek a pair of endoscopic dissecting forceps from instruments listed as grasping forceps.

To be useful during sharp-scissor dissection, the instrument must have several features that enable it to pick up small amounts of tissue, hold tissue securely, and pick up and release tissues easily, repeatedly, and at different angles. Few available grasping forceps are, in fact, ideal for this purpose. Many do not have rotating shafts, which is extremely useful, even if not absolutely essential. Many others have jaws that are unsuitable because they either have teeth or do not grasp tissues well. Most dissecting forceps that have slightly curved ends are like this. To determine whether an instrument will hold tissue adequately, its closed jaws should be help up to the light. If the middle portion of the jaws do not meet tightly, the instrument will not function well as dissecting forceps. Others still have unsuitable locking, ratcheted handles. Although this is not absolutely ideal, the most suitable pair of dissecting forceps this author has found is made by Aesculap (catalogue no. PL-146) (Figure 8.10).

Grasping Instruments

The laparoscopic pelvic surgeon will need essentially three different types of grasping instruments.

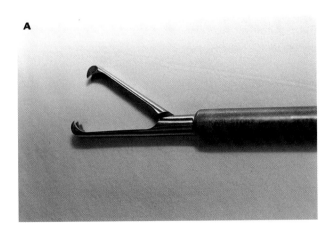

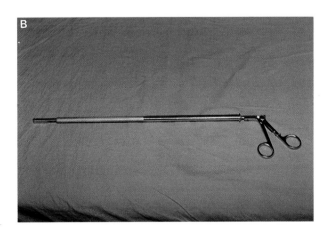

Figures 8.11A,B 10-mm Claw tooth grasping forceps (available in 5 mm as well).

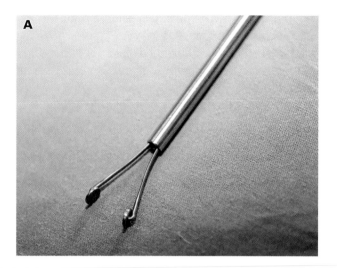

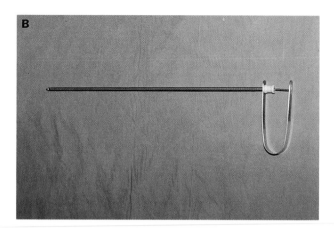

Figures 8.12A,B Bowel-grasping forceps.

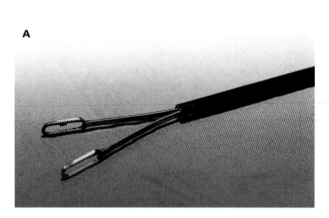

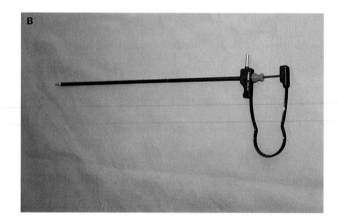

Figures 8.13A,B All-purpose, nontraumatic grasping forceps (Wolf 8383.141).

First, he or she will need a rather crude but firm instrument to pick up or stabilize structures that are to be removed and can, therefore, be traumatized, such as a fibroid or an ovary. The best type of instrument for this purpose is the clawtooth grasper, which comes in 5-mm and 10-mm sizes and is available from all the instrument manufacturers (Figures 8.11A,B).

Second, the surgeon will need an instrument that can be used to grasp bowel. I have tried many different types of nontraumatic grasping instruments for this purpose and have found that only one design works well under all circumstances, and that is the bowel grasper originally made by WISAP (Figures 8.12A,B). The instrument has a spring-loaded grip and two small discs for jaws mounted at right angles onto the shaft. Grasping forceps with this design are now available from most manufacturers (e.g., Wolf 8383.43), but they should be tried out before they are

purchased to ensure that they are functionally as effective as the original.

Third, the surgeon will need what, for want of a better word, may be called a stabilizing instrument. This is an all-purpose, nontraumatic grasping instrument that is used, for example, to retract the peritoneum during aortic lymphadenectomy or the infundibulopelvic ligament during retroperitoneal dissection and ureteric identification, or to grasp the ovarian ligament and stabilize the ovary during ovarian cystectomy. To find a grasper like this is, in fact, surprisingly difficult. Many of the forceps that one might think will do the job, in fact, either do not hold tissues well or traumatize them. Paradoxically, forceps that hold tissues the least well are sometimes the most traumatic. The author recently found an ideal instrument for this purpose, which, ironically enough, was not even designed as a grasping forceps

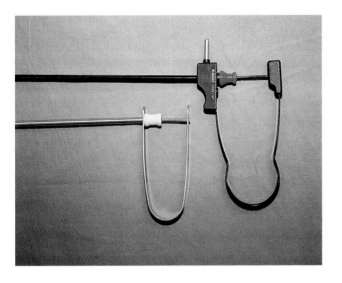

Figure 8.14 Spring-loaded handles; the larger handle is mechanically easier to use.

(Wolf 8383.141, Figures 8.13A,B). This is the best grasping instrument I have yet had the opportunity to use.

Spreading Instruments

There are circumstances in which a fine-pointed instrument with jaws that can open widely is useful for opening up tissue planes. An obvious example would be dissection of the ureteric tunnel under the uterine artery. There are a number of instruments designed for this purpose, and they are referred to as dissecting forceps. I have found most of these to be disappointing. Either the instrument does not rotate, making it awkward to use, or, as with the Maryland dissector, the

tips are far too thick, and an area that is big enough to accommodate their jaws can be easily opened under direct vision by blunt dissection with the irrigating cannula. A major disadvantage of this type of instrument is that for its jaws to open widely enough for the instrument to be useful, the instrument has to be at least 10 mm in diameter. Many dissecting forceps that have a 60° angle frequently do not fit down a 5-mm trocar, even though the shaft of the instrument is only 5 mm. At one time I used the Jarit right angle forceps to insert under the uterine artery and free it from the underlying ureter, but the same effect can be achieved just as easily by dividing the uterine artery more laterally, elevating it, and dissecting the tissue underneath with scissors.

Handles

There are essentially two types of handles, those that lock or maintain the tips of the instrument closed, and those that do not. Nonlocking handles have the traditional ring design, and the important thing to check is that the two rings are not close together and that the hand does not impinge on any electrosurgical attachment as the handles are opened and closed. A number of instruments with ring handles are designed with the rings much too close together, particularly those manufactured by Marlowe, and this places the hand at a mechanical disadvantage.

As regards locking handles, the original pistol handle design by Wolf is, in my opinion, preferable to ratcheted handles because grasping instruments frequently have to be replaced and are rarely kept in the same position for very long periods of time. The pistol

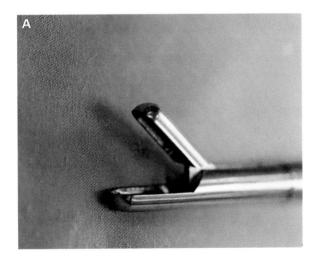

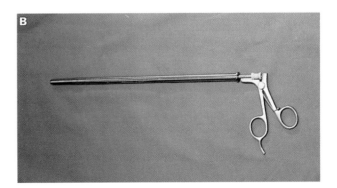

Figures 8.15A,B Spoon forceps used for pelvic and aortic lymphadenectomy.

Basic Laparoscopic Surgical Techniques and Instrumentation 79

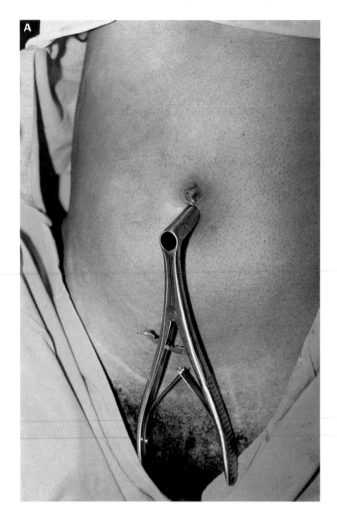

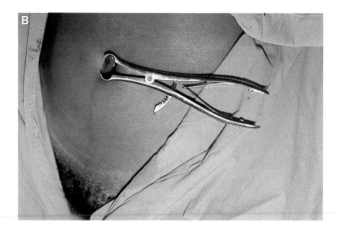

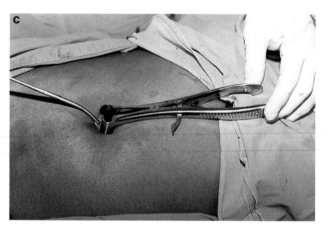

Figures 8.16A–C The gall bladder extractor used to enlarge the umbilical trocar tract (Davis & Geck).

grip is much easier to open and close than ratcheted handles, but it allows tissues to be held just as securely. The width of the handle is again important because if the two loops of the U-shaped pistol grip are too close together, the hand will be working at a mechanical disadvantage (Figure 8.14).

To summarize, there is a very large variety of instruments available, but many of these are not needed for a traditional, two-handed approach to sharp-scissor dissection. Some instruments are, however, vital, and these are more difficult to obtain than one might imagine from the variety available. Grasping forceps are needed that will fulfill the role of the classic dissecting forceps used at laparotomy. They should have a rotating shaft and jaws that can be easily opened and closed and that will hold tissues without traumatizing them. Dissecting scissors with a rotating shaft are required that are at the same time light and stable and whose blades glide smoothly over each

other without rasping. A bowel grasper and an atraumatic grasper are needed for retraction, and strong, toothed forceps are required to grasp and hold solid tissue that will be removed, such as fibroids and ovarian masses.

SPECIMEN REMOVAL

The question of how to remove a surgical specimen from the peritoneal cavity is unique to endoscopic surgery and, for obvious reasons, does not arise during a laparotomy. If total hysterectomy is being carried out, the vaginal vault will be opened and the specimen can almost always be removed through the vagina after prior morcellation, inside an impermeable bag, if need be (see Chapter 13). However, if an operation is being performed on the adnexa (oophorectomy, ovarian cystectomy, salpingectomy, or salpingostomy), or a myomectomy or subtotal hysterectomy is being car-

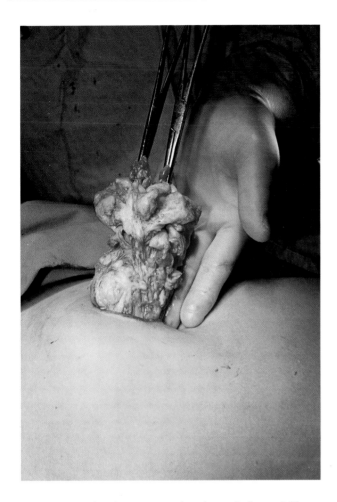

Figure 8.17 Specimen extraction through the umbilicus.

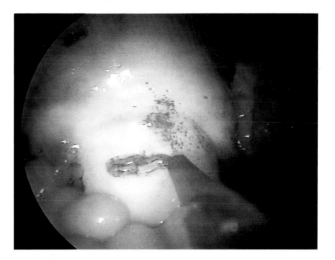

Figure 8.18 Culdotomy incision made against the hub of the Pelosi uterine mobilizer.

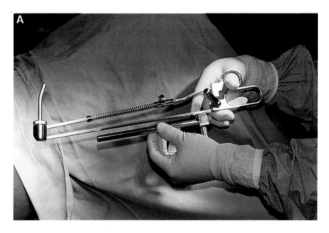

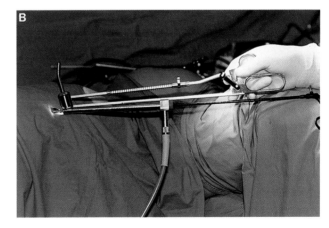

Figures 8.19A,B Illuminator attachment of the Pelosi uterine mobilizer.

ried out, a decision must be made about how to remove the excised specimen.

Small specimens, such as lymph nodes, can be removed with spoon forceps (Figures 8.15A,B), which compress the tissue into the hollow of their jaws. Specimens that are too large to be removed in this way can often be removed through the umbilical trocar site after the trocar tract is bluntly spread with a gall bladder extractor (Davis & Geck) (Figures 8.16A–C). To remove larger specimens, the umbilical incision has to be formally enlarged with a scalpel and the incision in the deeper layers extended under direct vision using the operating laparoscope if necessary. After the skin incision has been extended, the skin edges are reapproximated with Allis clamps, and the pneumoperitoneum (which will have been lost as the incision is extended) is reestablished. The operating laparoscope is reinserted into the peritoneal cavity, and the specimen grasped with grasping forceps passed down the operating channel of

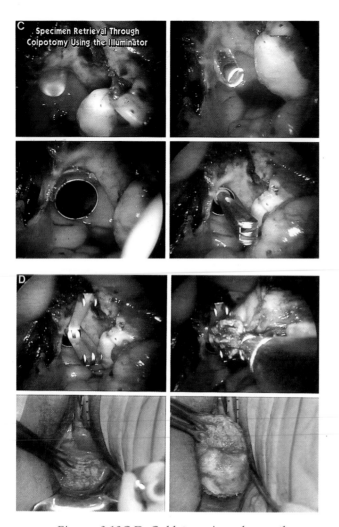

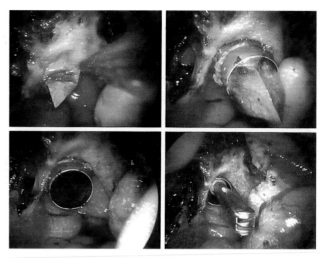

Figure 8.20 Colpotomy made by directly inserting a trocar and cannula into the cul-de-sac under direct laparoscopic guidance.

Figures 8.19C,D Culdotomy is made over the illuminated posterior vaginal wall, and 10-mm grasping forceps are inserted into the cul-de-sac through the lumen of the illuminator.

the laparoscope. The laparoscope is then slowly withdrawn until the specimen is pulled up into the trocar sleeve. The laparoscope, trocar sleeve, and the biopsy forceps are then all withdrawn together, which will bring the specimen into the umbilical incision, where it is grasped with a Kocker clamp. The specimen is then teased out through the umbilical incision (Figure 8.17), or, if it is a large fibroid or the uterine fundus, it will need to be morcellated (see Chapters 13 and 17).

Laparoscopic Culdotomy

Large fibroids and large ovarian masses or cysts are best removed through the vagina by making a culdotomy incision, i.e., incising the vagina transabdominally through the cul-de-sac rather than through

vagina (colpotomy). Culdotomy is greatly facilitated by the Pelosi mobilizer. This instrument allows the uterus to be sharply anteflexed, whereupon the hub of the instrument on which the cervix sits will be seen bulging into the posterior vaginal fornix between the uterosacral ligaments. The vagina is incised against the hub of the mobilizer using the closed tips of the dissecting scissors and an unmodulated monopolar current (Figure 8.18). Contact between the dissecting scissors and the metal hub of the mobilizer is of no consequence because its surface area is large and any current that flows down the instrument will be dissipated along low current density pathways (see Chapter 3). If there is any difficulty in identifying the posterior vaginal wall, culdotomy is facilitated by the illuminator attachment of the uterine mobilizer, which attaches and slides down the grooved lower border of its shaft (Figures 8.19A,B). The illuminator not only lights up the posterior vaginal wall, but by having a hollow cannula, 10-mm grasping forceps can be inserted down its operating channel and pushed against the cul-de-sac. An incision can then be made laparoscopically over the prominence created in the cul-de-sac by the open jaws of the grasping forceps using a needle electrode or the closed tips of the dissecting scissors and an unmodulated monopolar current. The specimen can then be removed through the vagina but may need morcellation (Figures 8.19C,D). Finally, a trocar can be inserted directly into the cul-de-sac under laparoscopic guidance, just as it is inserted through the anterior abdominal wall. Grasping forceps can then be introduced into the peritoneal cavity through the trocar sleeve (Figure 8.20).

Once the culdotomy incision is made, the pneumoperitoneum will be lost, but by pulling the uterus downwards, the culdotomy site can usually be sealed off to allow the specimen to be manipulated into the cul-de-sac, whereupon it will seal the culdotomy site. Large fibroids will need to be morcellated transvaginally after stabilization with a tenaculum or corkscrew. Ovarian masses are best placed in an endoscopic bag and pulled out intact or, if need be, morcellated inside the sac (see Chapter 14).

▼ ▼ ▼ ▼ ▼ ▼ ▼ ▼ ▼

Chapter 9
Single-Puncture Techniques

Marco Pelosi

How can I tell what I think until I see what I say?
—Foster

It is impossible to understand the evolution and rationale of single-puncture laparoscopic techniques if they are taken out of historical context. First of all, single-puncture techniques are not new. The operating laparoscope, on which single-puncture techniques depend, was developed by Ruddock in 1934 (1), and Power and Barnes (2) reported their experience of using Ruddock's operative laparoscope for sterilization in 1941. Single-puncture sterilization techniques gained popularity but were ultimately replaced by multiple-puncture techniques because the operative laparoscope was felt to provide a limited field of vision and compromise the ability to place tissues on tension. Advanced single-puncture techniques, like their multiple-puncture counterparts, are relatively recent developments, made possible by technological advances such as high flow, pressure regulated CO_2 insufflators, high-pressure suction irrigating pumps, and bipolar coagulation.

The author began to develop single-puncture techniques in the early 1970s, when minor endoscopic operations, such as adhesiolysis and ovarian cystectomy, were being performed with increased frequency. The pioneering work of Bruhat and colleagues, in France, and Semm, in Germany, extended the range of operations that could be performed endoscopically to include salpingostomy for ectopic pregnancies, the resection of endometriosis, and the treatment of benign ovarian tumors. However, when these operations were first performed, the videoscopic display of laparoscopic images (video laparoscopy) had not yet been developed, and multiple-puncture tech-

niques offered no very great advantages over their single-puncture counterparts. Multiple-puncture techniques were cumbersome and frustrating because the surgeon worked with his eye to the laparoscope, which left only one hand free with which to operate, and assistants could not help him very much because they could not see the operative field. It was disappointment with these multiple-puncture techniques that led the author to continue to use and develop single-puncture approaches to more complicated operations.

The introduction of video laparoscopy in the mid 1980s eliminated the drawback of blind assistance and the difficulties of coordinating multiple instruments, and multiple-puncture techniques gained ascendancy. At this time, the author also began to use multiple-puncture video laparoscopic techniques in conjunction with single-puncture laparoscopy without video camera for the same type of operations. To his surprise, single-puncture techniques proved to be as effective as the multiple-puncture modality, at least for benign gynecological operations.

BASIC TECHNICAL CONSIDERATIONS: SINGLE- VERSUS MULTIPLE-PUNCTURE TECHNIQUES

The ability to maintain a pneumoperitoneum, to clear the operative field of blood and other debris, and to maintain hemostasis are essential prerequisites for the successful performance of advanced laparoscopic operations by whatever means they are to be carried out. These prerequisites were met with the introduction of high flow, pressure regulated insufflators, high-pressure suction irrigation pumps, and bipolar forceps with an appropriate (unmodulated, low wattage) electric circuit.

Another feature common to both single- and multiple-puncture techniques is the need to extract surgical specimens from the peritoneum, be it an ectopic pregnancy, an ovarian cyst, a fibroid, or the uterine fundus. Two basic techniques are used to extract specimens that are too large to fit through one of the trocar cannulas. The specimen may be removed through the vagina (culdotomy) or through an enlarged trocar insertion site (microceliotomy). These techniques are, again, common to both single- and multiple-puncture techniques, and the sole difference between these two techniques is the method used to expose tissues and to place them on proper tension to allow them to be desiccated and divided. This is the greatest challenge to single-puncture techniques.

ADEQUATE EXPOSURE

The female pelvic organs have the unique feature of being attached to a large central mobile organ, the uterus, which can be accessed and manipulated externally through the vagina. It became clear to the author that use of a uterine manipulator that allowed the uterus to be moved in any direction would allow the surgeon optimum laparoscopic visualization and exposure of the pelvic structures, and exposure could be maintained at will by simply holding the manipulator in the required position. The ability to retrovert the uterus is particularly helpful for exposing and stabilizing the tube and ovary, for it allows the tube and ovary to be "flipped" anteriorly, in front of the broad ligament, and then to be stabilized by pressing them against the pelvic sidewall with the uterine mobilizer (Figure 9.1).

TRACTION–COUNTERTRACTION

Many structures, such as the round or infundibulopelvic ligament, can be placed on adequate tension for coagulation and division by appropriate manipulation of the uterus with a hinged uterine manipulator. If tension is still insufficient, it can be created with proper use of the endoscopic instruments. For example, if the infundibulopelvic ligament to be coagulated is not on sufficient tension, the ligament can be placed on tension after it is grasped with a bipolar forceps and before it is coagulated. Also, before the ligament is divided, one blade of the scissors is placed under the ligament and traction is applied before the ligament is divided. The same technique is used to divide the anterior cul-de-sac peritoneum, or "bladder flap." One blade of the dissecting scissors is placed under the cut edge of the peritoneum, the peritoneum is elevated, placed on tension, and then divided.

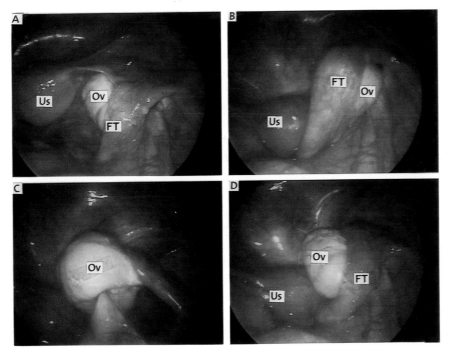

Figure 9.1 (A) Uterus and adnexa are shown in their anatomic position, (B) uterus is retroverted with the uterine mobilizer, (C) the adnexa is "flipped" in front of the broad ligament, and (D) the tube and ovary are stabilized by pressing them against the pelvic sidewall with the fundus of the uterus.

ADVANTAGES OF SINGLE-PUNCTURE LAPAROSCOPY

Single-puncture techniques have several inherent advantages. First, they are much easier to learn than multiple-puncture techniques because the instrumentation is simpler, there is no need to use a video camera, and even if a camera is used, problems with hand-eye coordination (triangulation) do not arise. Single-puncture laparoscopy is performed with an operative laparoscope placed through an intraumbilical cannula (Figure 9.2A) and three basic instruments: bipolar forceps for hemostasis, unipolar scissors for tissue dissection, coagulation, and cutting, and a high-pressure suction irrigation probe for hydrodissection, lavage, and aspiration (Figure 9.2B). Frequent instrument exchanges are necessary during an operation, but this minor disadvantage is likely to be minimized in the future by the availability of multiple purpose

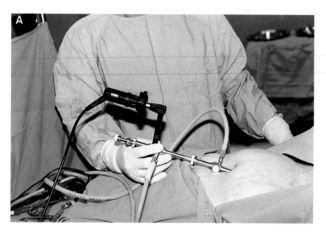

Figure 9.2A The operative laparoscope inserted through an umbilical cannula.

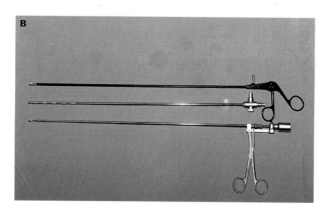

Figure 9.2B The basic instruments needed for single-puncture laparoscopic operations.

instruments that combine, for example, a knife or spoon electrode with a suction-irrigation cannula. Lack of absolute dependence on a video camera obviates the difficulties that can arise from camera malfunction, which has, on occasions, necessitated conversion of an otherwise uncomplicated laparoscopic procedure to a laparotomy.

Second, single-puncture techniques circumvent the complications that can arise from the use of auxiliary trocars. The most common of these are hemorrhage from injury to the inferior epigastric artery and herniation at the trocar site. Although, in principle, these complications can be avoided by using the technique of trocar insertion described in Chapter 2 and closing the fascia below trocar sites ≥10 mm (3), respectively, they cannot be entirely eliminated.

Third, single-puncture techniques are less costly than multiple-puncture ones, although the difference can be minimized by using reusable instruments for multiple-puncture operations. A single intraumbilical scar is also cosmetically more appealing than multiple scars. Although the scars from auxiliary puncture sites may be small and inconspicuous, this is by no means always the case, especially if keloids form in the scars.

Finally, single-puncture techniques are very versatile. Although in experienced hands, additional trocars for ancillary instruments are seldom required, auxiliary trocars can be placed if considered necessary. Moreover, in the presence of dense abdominal adhesions, adhesiolysis can be performed through the operating laparoscope to create a safe area for the placement of additional trocars. Single-puncture techniques are particularly useful if combined operations, such as hysterectomy plus cholecystectomy, have to be performed because they avoid the need to use an undesirable total number of abdominal punctures (4).

CLINICAL EXPERIENCE WITH SINGLE-PUNCTURE TECHNIQUES

The author has performed over 4,000 single-puncture operative laparoscopic procedures, excluding tubal sterilizations. Operations on the uterus included myomectomies (Chapter 17), total and subtotal hysterectomies, and, recently, a case of laparoscopically assisted vaginal metroplasty (5,6). Recently, the author successfully performed a hysterectomy for a 910-gram fibroid uterus using Kadar's extraperitoneal technique (Figures 9.3A,B). Operations on the fallopian tube have included conservative and extirpative operations for ectopic pregnancy (Figures 9.4A–E), ter-

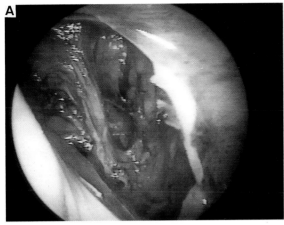

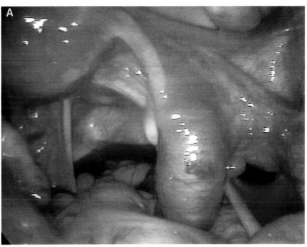

Figure 9.4A Right unruptured ampullary pregnancy.

Figure 9.4A Right unruptured ampullary pregnancy.

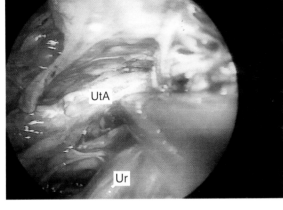

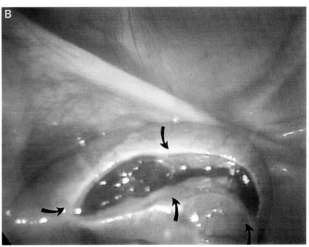

Figures 9.3 A,B Extraperitoneal hysterectomy technique performed using a single umbilical puncture. (A) the paravesical spaces have been developed (Step 4—see Chapter 11), (B) the pararectal space is developed and ureter and uterine artery identified (Step 5).

Figure 9.4B Linear salpingostomy made with a needle electrode.

minal neosalpingostomy for hydrosalpinx (Figures 9.5A,B), and the treatment of pelvic inflammatory and adhesive disease, benign tumors, and endometriosis. Operations on the ovary have included oophorectomy and ovarian cystectomy (Figures 9.6A-C). Urogynecologic procedures have included the performance of single-puncture Burch and MMK colposuspension, vaginal needle suspension of the bladder neck, and single-puncture sling procedure (Chapter 18). The single-puncture treatment of endometriosis includes excision/fulguration of endometrial implants, LUNA, presacral neurectomy, and surgery for endometriosis obliterating the cul-de-sac/rectovaginal septum, re-

moval of endometriomas ranging from small to very large (>20 cm), and appendectomies (7).

The overall conversion rate to laparotomy was 2%. Average hospital stay was 22 hours, and patients returned to work, on average, after 12 days. The overall mortality among these 4,000 single-puncture operative laparoscopic procedures was zero, and serious complications requiring laparotomy occurred in six (0.15%) patients. This is far lower than that reported for multiple-puncture techniques from other centers (8).

Two patients with advanced endometriosis required laparotomy and transfusion two and four days postoperatively to control bleeding from areas where endometriotic nodules had been resected. Both patients recovered without further complications.

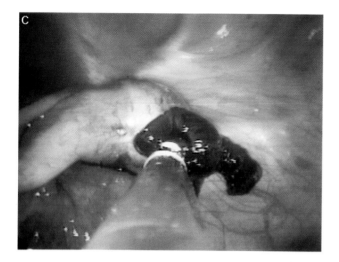

Figure 9.4C *The products of conception are removed.*

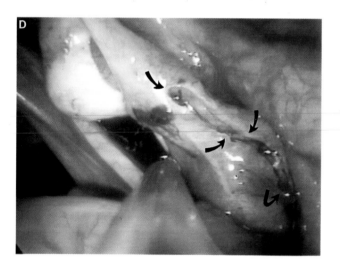

Figure 9.4D *The final appearance of the tube.*

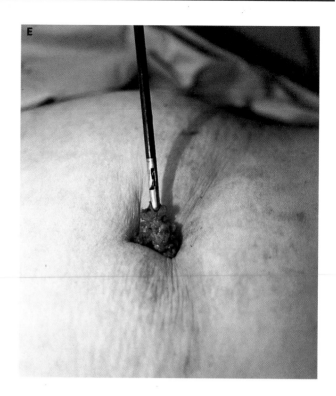

Figure 9.4E *The specimen is removed through the umbilicus.*

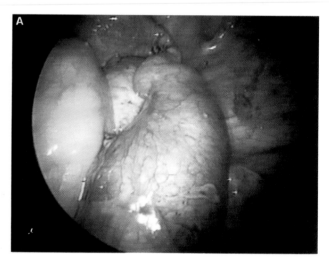

Figure 9.5A *Right hydrosalpinx.*

Two other patients required laparotomy and partial bowel resection three and six days after surgery because of unrecognized bowel injuries. In one instance, the bowel injury probably occurred during extensive sharp and blunt dissection of dense adhesions associated with advanced pelvic inflammatory disease. The other patient developed a button-hole injury of the rectum as a result of resection of deep endometriosis involving the full thickness of the right uterosacral ligament. Both patients had uneventful recoveries. Finally, 2 of 180 patients undergoing laparoscopically assisted hysterectomy suffered complications related to the use of an endoscopic stapler (with a multiple-puncture approach). The right ureter was divided in one patient as the stapler was used to divide the right uterine artery. The ureter was subse-

quently reimplanted, and the patient recovered without sequelae. The other patient required emergency repeat laparoscopy for intra-abdominal bleeding several hours after an uneventful laparoscopic hysterectomy during which an endoscopic stapler was again used to divide the uterine arteries and cervical ligaments. At repeat laparoscopy, a small bleeding artery was found in the middle of the stapled cardinal ligament. The bleeding was arrested by the application of

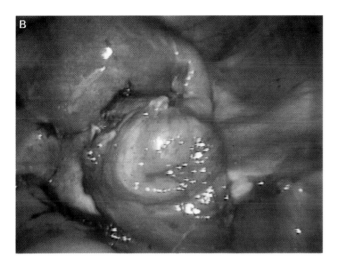

Figure 9.5B Single-puncture terminal neosalpingostomy.

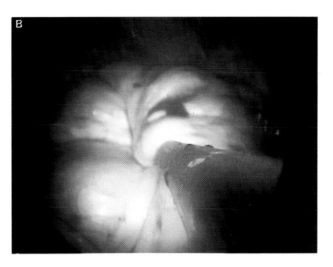

Figure 9.6B The collapsed cyst is grasped, "rolled" on itself with grasping forceps, and exteriorized through the umbilical puncture site.

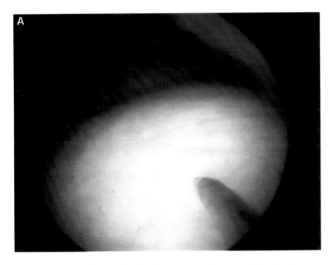

Figure 9.6A The wall of a large ovarian cyst that is about to be aspirated.

an endoclip. The patient required four units of blood, but recovered without further complications.

DISCUSSION

None of the textbooks of laparoscopic surgery published within the last 10 years describe or discuss single-puncture laparoscopic techniques. Some do comment on the operative laparoscope, but only to dismiss it as an instrument that provides a limited view of the operative field, and the instruments that are placed down the operative channel, as having limited maneuverability and not allowing tissues to be placed on proper tension. The exception is Friedrich's editorial comment in Semm's textbook (9),

where he states, "I have a more positive attitude regarding the use of operating endoscopes. Since monocular vision and, consequently, inadequate depth perception are handicaps inherent in the use of all endoscopes, every endoscopic surgeon must first learn to compensate for these handicaps and, with increasing experience, will become quite proficient. With the experience of several thousand cases, I am convinced that the advantages of an operating endoscope far outweigh the disadvantages."

Needless to say, we agree with his point of view. Any operating endoscope that has an operating channel will have a blind spot, but the area obscured while the operating channel is in use will have been inspected during the exploratory-diagnostic phase of the laparoscopic operation. There is, of course, a limit to what can be exposed with the use of a uterine manipulator and proper use of the instruments placed down the operating channel of the laparoscope. For example, the oncological operations described in Section D of this atlas could not be performed using only a single umbilical puncture. However, our experience with single-puncture techniques clearly demonstrates that more than adequate exposure can be achieved by means of a uterine manipulator, proper use of the operating laparoscope, and correct technique of dissection with the endoscopic instruments.

Although we use it exclusively for benign gynecological operations, we do not regard the single-puncture approach to be a competitor of the widely used multiple-puncture techniques but as comple-

COMMENT

I asked Dr. Pelosi to describe his single-puncture techniques for this atlas for two reasons. First, I wanted to cover all the laparoscopic techniques that made use of traditional approaches to surgery. Second, these techniques have been so successful in his hands that I felt there must be some lessons we could all learn from studying them.

The first thing that strikes me about these surgical techniques is that the term "single puncture" fails to capture or convey their essential technical underpinnings, which are the use of an operative laparoscope and a hinged uterine manipulator, and the close communion between the endoscopic operative field and the outside world, either via the umbilicus or the vagina. These serve not merely as sites for specimen removal but as conduits to the pelvic structures that allow endoscopic procedures to be assisted and enhanced by conventional surgical techniques. The constraint, then, is not the single puncture for one could easily use another 5-mm suprapubic puncture site without losing any of the advantages of Dr. Pelosi's techniques. Rather, it is the use of the operative laparoscope.

The use of an operative laparoscope for dissection does bring with it certain advantages, the most important of which is easier coordination of endo-scopic instruments in the new spatial environment of the endoscopic visual world. There is also greater simplicity of instrumentation, less reliance on a camera, and fewer potential problems with instrumentation of the abdomen. Clearly, this makes for rapid and efficient surgery once one becomes adept at these techniques. However, these advantages are bought at a price. For me, the greatest of these is not that securing adequate exposure or stabilizing structures is more difficult, for these problems can be solved with a little ingenuity. Rather, it is the inability to use the classic two-handed approach to dissection, which would make it impossible to perform a proper pelvic lymphadenectomy, for example, using a single umbilical puncture. One could envisage being able to do the operation with a supplementary suprapubic puncture, but even if it were to be feasible, it would not be, at least in my view, the optimal approach.

However, these are rather parochial concerns, and almost all gynecologic operations can be expeditiously performed with these techniques. Even if the techniques are not used exclusively in the way that Dr. Pelosi uses them, we should all certainly become adept at dissecting through the operating laparoscope.

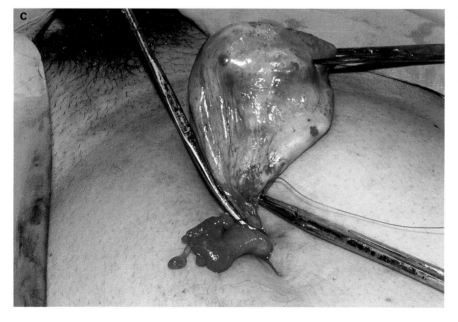

Figure 9.6C The uterus and adnexa are held in place at the umbilicus with the uterine mobilizer, and a traditional extracorporeal ovarian cystectomy is performed.

mentary to them. The purpose of describing these techniques is also not to demonstrate that they can be done. Single-puncture techniques have genuine inherent advantages over multiple-puncture techniques, and they can be learned relatively easily and quickly by any experienced pelvic surgeon. Whether these inherent advantages are considered sufficient to avoid multiple-puncture techniques altogether as we do or to use single-puncture techniques only in some situations or, indeed, not at all, is a decision that each gynecologist must make for himself or herself.

REFERENCES

1. Ruddock JC. Peritoneoscopy. West J Surg 1934; 42:392–405.

2. Power FH, Barnes AC. Sterilization by means of peritoneoscopic fulguration: a preliminary report. Am J Obstet Gynecol 1941;41:1038–1042.

3. Kadar N, Reich H, Liu CY, Manco GF, Gimpleson R. Incisional hernias following major laparoscopic gynecological procedures. Am J Obstet Gynecol 1993;168: 1493–1495.

4. Pelosi MA, Villalona E. Laparoscopic hysterectomy, appendectomy, and cholecystectomy. NEJM 1993;90: 207–212.

5. Pelosi MA, Pelosi MA III. Laparoscopic hysterectomy with bilateral salpingo-oophorectomy using a single umbilical puncture. NEJM 1991;88:721–726.

6. Pelosi MA, Pelosi, MA III. Laparoscopic supracervical hysterectomy using a single umbilical puncture (minilaparoscopy). J Reprod Med 1992;37:777–784.

7. Pelosi MA, Pelosi MA III. Laparoscopic appendectomy using a single umbilical puncture (minilaparoscopy). J Reprod Med 1992;37:588–594.

8. Querleu D, Chevallier L, Chapron C, Bruhat MA. Complications of gynecological laparoscopic surgery. A French multicenter collaborative study. Gynaecol Endosc 1993;2:3–6.

9. Friedrich ER. In Semm K: Operative manual for endoscopic abdominal surgery. Translated and edited by Friedrich ER. Chicago: Yearbook Medical Publishers, 1987;54–55.

Part B
Laparoscopic Hysterectomy

Chapter 10
Laparoscopic Hysterectomy: Controversies, Indications, Classification

Seek simplicity and distrust it.
—Whitehead

The term laparoscopic hysterectomy means different things to different people. The technique of laparoscopic hysterectomy has not been standardized, a uniform nomenclature for the procedure has not been adopted, and its indications remain undefined and in question. In short, laparoscopic hysterectomy is an operation mired in controversy.

CONTROVERSIES

It is generally accepted that laparoscopic hysterectomy is intended to replace abdominal hysterectomy and not vaginal hysterectomy, and its advantages over abdominal hysterectomy stem from the elimination of a laparotomy incision. Laparoscopic hysterectomy, of course, involves the same operative steps as an abdominal hysterectomy but postoperative discomfort and recovery time seem to be much more influenced by the size and site of an abdominal incision than by what is done under the incision or how long an operation takes.

In principle, therefore, the indications for laparoscopic hysterectomy should be the same as those for an abdominal hysterectomy. However, exponents of vaginal hysterectomy argue that what endoscopists seek to achieve with a laparoscopic approach can be accomplished by the vaginal route, and, if it cannot be, a laparoscopic hysterectomy becomes technically so time-consuming and demanding that very little, if any, reduction in morbidity results. What seems to be at issue, therefore, is (1) whether laparoscopic hysterectomy is required to replace abdominal hysterectomies or if this can be achieved by a vaginal hysterectomy and (2) whether laparoscopic hysterectomy is feasible and reduces morbidity in the subset of women who are not suitable candidates for a vaginal hysterectomy.

We attempted to settle these questions by analyzing our laparoscopic hysterectomies in a subset of women who were difficult surgical candidates and in whom no one would have attempted a vaginal hysterectomy. We chose women who were obese ($\geq$200 lbs) and those who had uteri weighing more than 500 grams (1,2). Historically, these women have a high wound infection rate, stay in hospital for at least five days, and often require midline incisions. Laparoscopically assisted hysterectomies could be carried out in 90% of women with uteri weighing $\geq$500 grams (mean, 837 grams), and the only complication was a single case of hemorrhage from a uterine injury during trocar insertion, which we believe can be avoided in the future (2). There were no failures or significant complications among 24 obese (mean weight, 237 pounds) women undergoing laparoscopic hysterectomy, 30% of whom also had either pelvic lymphadenectomy for endometrial cancer or bladder-neck suspension for incontinence and many of whom were nulliparous (1). Average hospital stay for both groups was three days. Despite the fact that we were unable to find any reported series in which similar patients had successfully undergone vaginal hysterectomies, the referees for *Obstetrics and Gynecology* and the *American Journal of Obstetrics and Gynecology* demanded proof from randomized trials before accepting that vaginal hysterectomy was not possible in these women.

Because objective criteria for the feasibility of vaginal hysterectomy do not exist and strong biases for and against laparoscopic hysterectomy have already developed, it will never be possible to prove that vaginal hysterectomies could not have been carried out in women subjected to laparoscopic hysterectomy. The only scientifically rigorous way to demonstrate this would be to conduct a trial involving a random selection of surgeons favoring laparoscopic and vaginal surgery and randomly assign to them patients requiring hysterectomy without regard to the feasibility of a vaginal or laparoscopic approach. Such a trial could never be conducted, would be arguably unethical, and, in the end, may still only show that surgeons with prior biases obtained the best results with the operation they preferred.

History is, in fact, on the side of the laparoscopists, and there is little a priori reason to believe that most women undergoing laparoscopic hysterectomy could have been treated by a vaginal hysterectomy for they have not been so treated in the past. With few exceptions (3), only 30% of hysterectomies, at most, are carried out vaginally in most centers, and if women with significant uterine prolapse are excluded, the figure drops to about 5% (4). At St. Peter's Medical Center, New Brunswick, New Jersey, for example, 470 hysterectomies were performed during the 18-month period from January 1990 to June 1991. Of these, 75 (16%) were vaginal and all but 7 (1.5%) were carried out for prolapse. Only 3 of 68 (4.4%) women undergoing vaginal hysterectomy for prolapse had an oophorectomy (Kadar, unpublished observations).

There is quite good circumstantial evidence that uteri can be removed laparoscopically even if vaginal hysterectomy was deemed impossible by experienced pelvic surgeons. In a prospective study involving 149 women who required a simple hysterectomy for benign disease other than prolapse, Querleu and colleagues attempted to remove the uterus vaginally whenever possible and reserved laparoscopically assisted procedures for those who had adnexal disease, significant adhesions, or a very narrow vagina and an enlarged uterus (5). Abdominal hysterectomy was only carried out if neither vaginal nor laparoscopic hysterectomy was possible. Vaginal hysterectomy was attempted in 116 of 149 (78%) women and it was successful in 114 (98%). However, four women sustained intraoperative bladder and rectal lacerations, which were repaired without sequelae. A total of 9 laparotomies and 26 (17%) laparoscopic hysterectomies were carried out without any complications (5).

The reasoning behind good faith objections to laparoscopic hysterectomy seems to be that because the uterosacral and cardinal ligaments are the main supports of the uterus, the ability to divide these structures vaginally, as is done in a laparoscopic or laparoscopically assisted hysterectomy, must signify that the entire uterus could have been removed by that route. This reasoning is faulty, however, for it assumes that the only barrier to removing a uterus vaginally are its supports, which is simply untrue. In fact, many factors concatenate to render vaginal hysterectomy feasible or impossible, and these include adnexal or cul-de-sac pathology, the size of the uterus, the patient and her buttocks, the caliber of the vaginal canal, and the angle subtended by the subpubic arch. Even when these factors render vaginal hysterectomy impossible, however, it is usually possible to take at least one extraperitoneal "bite" of the uterosacral or cardinal ligaments vaginally. Indeed, at one time this was not infrequently done at the start of a really difficult abdominal hysterectomy if it was felt that abdominal access to these structures was going to be particularly difficult because they could usually be accessed from the vagina, and even partial division of these ligaments could increase the mobility of an otherwise fixed uterus. The same, of course, applies in the reverse direction.

SUMMARY OF INDICATIONS

To summarize, there is very strong presumptive evidence to suggest that laparoscopic hysterectomy can eliminate most abdominal hysterectomies in women who are not suitable candidates for a vaginal hysterectomy. It follows immediately that the indications for laparoscopic hysterectomy should be the same as they are for an abdominal hysterectomy and include persistent menorrhagia, symptomatic fibroids, pain ± abnormal bleeding secondary to pelvic inflammatory disease or endometriosis, endometrial carcinoma, and so on. Although the indications for vaginal hysterectomy can and, in some centers, have been extended to encompass most of these conditions, historically, this has not been a widespread practice, nor has it been shown to be safe.

It might be argued that the same fate awaits laparoscopic hysterectomy and that the operation will only have wide applicability in some hands. However, by its very nature, laparoscopic hysterectomy is a more versatile operation and potentially increases the surgeon's ability to circumvent abdominal hysterectomy, however adept he or she is at vaginal surgery. Average figures are meaningless in this context. Laparoscopic hysterectomy may allow one surgeon to reduce his or her frequency of abdominal hysterectomies from 30% to 10%, and another to reduce it from 70% to 30%, but the operation will have served them both well.

Some may argue that the second surgeon would be better served by extending his or her indications for vaginal surgery, but this is to take us back to the rhetorical question of how one can know that a laparoscopic hysterectomy could not have been carried out vaginally. The implication that most could have been is pure speculation that finds no support in historical data. The suggestion that most should have been is an expression of personal preference that finds no support in published data either and certainly not in the kind of studies now being demanded for laparoscopic surgery. Indeed, to the extent that any data speak to the feasibility of achieving with a vaginal hysterectomy what it has not been possible to achieve up to now, they are grounds for reminding ourselves that just because a uterus can be removed vaginally it does not follow that it should be so removed. Of the 143 vaginal hysterectomies performed as part of prospective studies involving laparoscopic hysterectomy, 5 (4%) women sustained injuries to the bladder and rectum, and in one case, this resulted in a fistula (5,6).

CLASSIFICATION

A standard nomenclature for hysterectomies involving laparoscopy is desirable to enable the indications for and the results obtained with different techniques to be evaluated and compared. It is also made necessary by the fact that the laparoscopic component of laparoscopic hysterectomies varies enormously in complexity and has not been standardized. Several classifications have already been proposed (7). Each makes use of an ordinal scale on which operations are assigned progressively higher numerical values as the laparoscopic contribution to the operation increases in complexity. The classifications proposed by Johns and Diamond, Bruhat, and Reich, are shown in Table 10.1 (7), and that of Munro and Parker in Table 10.2 (8).

To be useful, a classification system must be above all simple, and the nomenclature, so far as possible, self-explanatory. This is the great merit of Reich's classification, and it is the weakness of that proposed by

Table 10.1 Classification schemes for laparoscopic hysterectomy

Classification of Johns and Diamond

Stage 0: diagnostic laparoscopy + VH

Stage 1: laparoscopic adhesiolysis or excision of endometriosis + VH

Stage 2: adnexectomy + VH

Stage 3: Stage 2 + laparoscopic dissection of bladder flap

Stage 4: Stage 3 + laparoscopic division of the uterine arteries

Stage 5: entire uterus is freed laparoscopically

Classification of Bruhat

Type 1: laparoscopic surgery confined to the adnexa

Type 2: laparoscopic division of uterine arteries

Type 3: entire hysterectomy is carried out laparoscopically

Reich's Classification

1. diagnostic laparoscopy + VH

2. laparoscopic vault suspension after vaginal hysterectomy

3. laparoscopically assisted vaginal hysterectomy (LAVH)

4. laparoscopic hysterectomy (LH)

5. total laparoscopic hysterectomy (TLH)

6. laparoscopic supracervical hysterectomy

7. laparoscopic hysterectomy with lymphadenectomy

8. laparoscopic hysterectomy with lymphadenectomy and omentectomy

9. radical laparoscopic hysterectomy

VH = vaginal hysterectomy

Munro and Parker, which, exhaustive and thoughtful though it is, is, in our view, far too complex to be clinically useful (Table 10.2). Reich's term, "total laparoscopic hysterectomy" is, for example, much preferable to their "type IVE laparoscopic hysterectomy."

A classification system must also be clinically relevant, however, and focus on procedures that are in danger of being confused. For all its attractions, there-

Table 10.2 Classification system for laparoscopically directed and assisted total hysterectomy

Type 0		Laparoscopically directed preparation for vaginal hysterectomy
Type I*		Dissection up to but not including uterine arteries
	Type IA	Ovarian artery pedicle(s) only
	Type IB[†]	A + anterior structures
	Type IC	A + posterior culdotomy
	Type ID[†]	A + anterior structures and posterior culdotomy
Type II*		Type I + uterine artery and vein occlusion, unilateral or bilateral
	Type IIA	Ovarian artery pedicle(s) plus unilateral or bilateral uterine artery and vein occlusion only
	Type IIB[†]	A + anterior structures
	Type IIC	A + posterior culdotomy
	Type IID[†]	A + anterior structures and posterior culdotomy
Type III*		Type II + portion of cardinal-uterosacral ligament complex; unilateral or bilateral, plus:
	Type IIIA	Uterine and ovarian artery pedicles with unilateral or bilateral portion of the cardinal-uterosacral complex only
	Type IIIB[†]	A + anterior structures
	Type IIIC	A + posterior culdotomy
	Type IIID[†]	A + anterior structures and posterior culdotomy
Type IV*		Type II + total cardinal-uterosacral ligament complex; unilateral or bilateral, plus:
	Type IVA	Uterine and ovarian artery pedicles with unilateral or bilateral detachment of the total cardinal-uterosacral ligament complex only
	Type IVB[†]	A + anterior structures
	Type IVC	A + posterior culdotomy
	Type IVD[†]	A + anterior structures and posterior culdotomy
	Type IVE	Laparoscopically directed removal of entire uterus

The system describes the portion of the procedure completed laparoscopically.

*A suffix "o" may be added if unilateral or bilateral oophorectomy is performed concomitantly, e.g., type IoA.

[†]The B and D subgroups may be further subclassified according to the degree of dissection involving the bladder and whether an anterior culdotomy is created: (1) incision of vesicouterine peritoneum only, (2) dissection of any portion of bladder from cervix, (3) creation of an anterior culdotomy.

fore, Reich's classification seems to us to be more an inventory of what can be accomplished laparoscopically than a classification of laparoscopic hysterectomy. Clearly, for example, "laparoscopic hysterectomy with lymphadenectomy" is not a type of hysterectomy, and the term is unsatisfactory for it fails to define either the type of hysterectomy or the type of lymphadenectomy to be performed. Similarly, the term "radical laparoscopic hysterectomy" refers to a completely different class of operations, and, however ambiguous the connotations of the term "laparoscopic hysterectomy," they do not encompass radical operations for cancer. Indeed, laparoscopic techniques for radical hysterectomy are as variable as those for simple hysterectomy, and a separate classification for laparoscopic radical hysterectomy may be necessary (see Chapter 23).

At the other extreme are procedures that are a combination of diagnostic laparoscopy, laparoscopic adnexectomy, adhesiolysis, or excision of endometriosis and vaginal hysterectomy. Their names are self-explanatory, and it is difficult to see why these procedures need to be included in a classification of laparoscopic hysterectomy at all, much less what the perceived advantages of a term like "stage 0 laparoscopic hysterectomy" are over "diagnostic laparoscopy plus vaginal hysterectomy."

It is worth noting the similarity between this kind of nomenclature and the rather contrived classification Piver (9) proposed for radical hysterectomy, in which a simple hysterectomy for in situ cancer was rechristened "class I radical hysterectomy," a term that no one adopted. To carry the analogy further, Piver's classification was useful because it distinguished between two operations that had the same name but different indications and complication rates (class II and class III radical hysterectomy). The other three categories, however, were never used for they were either not clinically meaningful, e.g., type V radical hysterectomy, or already had perfectly adequate names, e.g., type I radical hysterectomy.

It seems to us that the same fate awaits overly elaborate classifications of laparoscopic hysterectomy. If a classification is to be successful, it must be simple and effective, and result in a clarification of terms that are ambiguous, rather than that create artificial categories, however "academically" or nosologically appealing. Reich coined three terms: "total laparoscopic hysterectomy" (TLH), "laparoscopic hysterectomy" (LH), and "laparoscopically assisted vaginal hysterectomy" (LAVH), of which only LAVH and LH need clarification. TLH is self-explanatory; the entire operation is carried out laparoscopically, and the vagina is sutured laparoscopically as well.

Table 10.1 shows that a general consensus has developed that the distinguishing feature between LAVH and LH should be whether the uterine arteries are divided laparoscopically or vaginally, as originally proposed by Reich. The rationale for this is not entirely clear, but the division is clearly inequitable. From the perspective of technical difficulty, LAVH refers to a fairly uniform group of procedures that consist essentially of laparoscopic adnexectomy plus a vaginal hysterectomy but can include laparoscopic adhesiolysis, excision of endometriosis, and dissection of the bladder flap. By contrast, LH refers to a much more diverse group of procedures that have in common some or all of the steps allowed in a LAVH and laparoscopic division of the uterine vessels but differ considerably with respect to what is done laparoscopically thereafter. We regard this as highly unsatisfactory because the technical difficulties encountered during laparoscopic dissection of the pelvis escalate after the uterine vessels are divided and not with their division. After all, the uterine vessels are divided in a subtotal hysterectomy, and the main advantages of this operation are its simplicity and lower complication rate (see Chapter 11). Moreover, if nothing further is done laparoscopically, division of the uterine arteries per se does not facilitate the hysterectomy, except in the case of very large uteri (see Chapter 13). It is, therefore, difficult to see the rationale for laparoscopic division of the uterine arteries if nothing further is to be done laparoscopically.

RECOMMENDATION

It seems both unnecessary and undesirable to incorporate every conceivable permutation of laparoscopically and vaginally performed operative steps into a classification of laparoscopic hysterectomy (Table 10.2) just as it is unnecessary to classify abdominal hysterectomies, for example, according to whether or not the vaginal cuff is closed. The basis for grouping and separating procedures should be operative steps that significantly alter the technical difficulty, scope, and/or complication rate of the procedure. We would argue that the only operative steps that meet these criteria are division of the uterosacral and/or cardinal ligaments, which require identification of the ureter at the level of the cardinal ligament, and reflection of the ureter off the broad ligament. Thus, we suggest adopting the modified Reich classification shown in Table 10.3

The adnexal pedicles can be safely divided, the uterine artery can be safely coagulated high on the fundus, and the posterior (or anterior) vaginal wall can be safely incised laparoscopically without identifying the ureter deep in the pelvis. The technical difficulty of adnexectomy, adhesiolysis, dissection of the bladder flap, and excision of endometriosis does not vary significantly if like cases are compared. Therefore, subdivision of these cases into different types of LAVH seems unnecessary. We would also consider an operation that consists of laparoscopic adnexectomy, dissection of the bladder flap, and coagulation and division of the uterine vessels high on the fundal wall a LAVH, not

Table 10.3 Modified Reich classification of laparoscopic hysterectomy

Laparoscopically Assisted Vaginal Hysterectomy (LAVH)

vaginal hysterectomy + laparoscopic adnexectomy and/or adhesiolysis and/or excision of endometriosis (dissection of bladder flap and coagulation of uterine arteries allowed but not recommended)

Laparoscopic Hysterectomy (LH)

Any hysterectomy procedure in which the uterosacral or cardinal ligaments are divided, and the vagina opened laparoscopically

(both anterior and posterior dissections allowed, but posterior dissection is recommended)

Total Laparoscopic Hysterectomy (LC)

The entire procedure is carried out laparoscopically (indications presently unclear)

a LH, although we would question the need to divide the uterine arteries unless the uterus is very large and will require morcellation. Ideally, self-explanatory terms should be used to describe these various laparoscopic additions to a vaginal hysterectomy, but the term LAVH is already so widely used that it is probably unrealistic to believe that its use can be successfully discouraged.

Neither the uterosacral nor the cardinal ligaments can be safely divided without first developing the pararectal space, identifying the ureters, and reflecting them off the broad ligament at the level of the cardinal ligament. Therefore, laparoscopic division of the supports of the uterus requires a deeper understanding of pelvic anatomy and retroperitoneal dissection than operations on the adnexa or in the cul-de-sac. Although we believe that a posterior dissection (division

of the uterosacral ligaments and posterior colpotomy) is to be preferred to an anterior one (bladder dissection, anterior colpotomy, division of cardinal ligaments), it would be inappropriate to restrict the term or to separate it into two categories at this stage of the operation's development. Time will tell which is the best approach, and the maturation process will not be enhanced by a plethora of technical names.

REFERENCES

1. Kadar N, Pelosi MA. Laparoscopically assisted hysterectomy in women weighing 200 pounds or more. Gynaecol Endosc 1994;3:159-162.

2. Pelosi MA, Kadar N. Laparoscopically assisted hysterectomy for uteri weighing 500 grams or more. J Am Assoc Gynecol Laparosc 1994;1:405-409.

3. Gitsch G, Berger E, Tatra G. Trends in 30 years of vaginal hysterectomy. J Gynecol Obstet 1991;172:207–210.

4. Vessey MP, Villard-Mackintosh L, McPherson K, Coulter A, Yeates D. The epidemiology of hysterectomy: findings in a large cohort study. Br J Obstet Gynaecol 1992;99:402–407.

5. Querleu D, Cosson M, Parmentier D, Derbodinance P. The impact of laparoscopic surgery on vaginal hysterectomy. Gynaecol Endosc 1993;2:89–92.

6. Summit RL, Stoval TG, Lipscomb GH, Long FW. Randomized comparison of laparoscopically assisted vaginal hysterectomy versus standard vaginal hysterectomy in an outpatient setting. Obstet Gynecol 1992;80:895–901.

7. Garry R, Reich H. Laparoscopic hysterectomy. In: Garry R, Reich H, eds. Laparoscopic Hysterectomy. Oxford: Blackwell Scientific, 1993;79–117.

8. Munro MG, Parker WH. A classification system for laparoscopic hysterectomy. Obstet Gynecol 1993;92:624-629.

9. Piver MS, Rutledge FN, Smith PJ. Five classes of extended hysterectomies of women with cervical cancer. Obstet Gynecol 1974;44:265-270.

Chapter 11
Laparoscopic Hysterectomy: The Extraperitoneal Technique

Experience is the name everyone gives to their mistakes.
—Lady Windermere's Fan, Oscar Wilde

Laparoscopic hysterectomy has become the Achilles heel of gynecological laparoscopy and the rock on which advanced laparoscopic techniques have to some extent foundered. It is arguably the most controversial major laparoscopic operation performed by gynecologists but only because it has proved to be technically much more difficult than originally imagined, and the operation is simply not as successful as, for example, laparoscopic cholecystectomy.

Surprisingly enough, more complicated operations, such as aortic lymphadenectomy, have proved to be easier to perform laparoscopically than a simple hysterectomy. This perhaps explains why gynecologic oncologists, who do not use laparoscopy regularly and who deal with much more complicated operations than simple hysterectomy, have been quick to accept, at least in principle, the possibility of managing gynecological malignancies laparoscopically. In fact, the Gynecologic Oncology Group has already initiated trials involving the laparoscopic management of endometrial and cervix cancer.

That the technical problems encountered during laparoscopic hysterectomy do not simply reflect a surgeon's lack of anatomical knowledge, surgical experience, or adequate laparoscopic training, or, indeed, even the inherent difficulty of laparoscopic surgery may be deduced from the fact that ureteric injuries, for example, have occurred during laparoscopic hysterectomy in the hands of the most experienced laparoscopic surgeons (1) as well as gynecologic oncologists proficient at performing more difficult radical opera-

tions laparoscopically and whose knowledge of pelvic anatomy is beyond dispute (2–4). What is it, then, about this operation that makes it so difficult to perform laparoscopically, more so than more complex operations that require much more extensive retroperitoneal dissection?

In our view, difficulties with laparoscopic hysterectomy stem from the fact that the operation cannot be successfully approached surgically in the same way as its open counterpart, the abdominal hysterectomy. This is the cardinal feature that distinguishes this operation from all others that are easy to perform laparoscopically once laparoscopic techniques have been mastered, such as cholecystectomy, colectomy, and pelvic and aortic lymphadenectomy. These operations are approached in exactly the same way as at laparotomy, and, in the strict sense, new operative techniques have not had to be developed. Laparoscopic hysterectomy has also been approached in the same way as at laparotomy, and this has simply not been successful.

LAPAROSCOPIC VERSUS ABDOMINAL HYSTERECTOMY: IMPORTANT DIFFERENCES

The Ureter Must Be Identified

Dissection of the retroperitoneum and identification of the ureters are seldom necessary during abdominal hysterectomy for benign pathology. A clamp can be placed safely on the infundibulopelvic ligament without visualizing the ureter if the ureter is first identified in the broad ligament by palpation. The technique for placing clamps on the uterine arteries, parametria, and the cardinal and uterosacral ligaments also ensures that only tissue directly adjacent to the cervix and, therefore, medial to the ureter will be included in the clamps, and identification of the ureter is again not required to ensure its safety. These techniques are obviously not available to the laparoscopic surgeon, and, unless the laparoscopic part of the operation is restricted to adhesiolysis, excision of endometriosis, and oophorectomy, the ureters must be identified to make the operation safe. The numerous recorded, and doubtless many more unrecorded, ureteric injuries during laparoscopic hysterectomy attest to this fact.

Open Techniques for Ureteric Identification Cannot Be Used

The ureter is easily identified during abdominal hysterectomy by blunt dissection medial to the hypogastric artery, which is, in turn, easily identified by palpation after the broad ligament is opened (see Chapter 6). The ureter cannot be identified laparoscopically by simply opening the broad ligament for it is covered by the infundibulopelvic ligament. The hypogastric arteries also cannot be seen, except in the thinnest of patients, for they are covered by fatty areolar tissue. The precise level at which to open the pararectal space is, therefore, not at first obvious, and it is all too easy to start dissecting either too proximally or too distally. Annoying bleeding then occurs, which, although rarely sufficient to be of concern in itself, stains the surrounding tissues, making it very difficult to identify the underlying ureter and hypogastric artery.

Sequence of the Operation Must be Altered

Abdominal hysterectomy begins with division of the round and then the infundibulopelvic ligaments, and many gynecologists start laparoscopic hysterectomy in the same way. If this is done, however, the parametrial tissues become increasingly floppy and difficult to place on tension, and blunt dissection of the extraperitoneal tissue planes will be extremely difficult, if not impossible. This is of no consequence so long as there are no plans to divide the uterosacral or cardinal ligaments. However, if a true laparoscopic hysterectomy is to be performed, the ureters must be identified, as we have noted, and if the hysterectomy is started in the same way as an abdominal hysterectomy, most of the time, it will not be possible to iden-

tify the ureter where it matters, in the depths of the pelvis by the cardinal ligament.

Bladder Dissection and Anterior Colpotomy Illogical

Laparoscopic dissection of the bladder off the cervix has become part of a laparoscopic hysterectomy for no apparent reason other than that this is what is done during an abdominal hysterectomy. However, it is a step that makes little sense and reveals better than any other the extent to which our approach to laparoscopic hysterectomy has been influenced by the technique of abdominal hysterectomy. During abdominal hysterectomy, the vagina is entered anteriorly simply because, when viewed through an abdominal incision, it is the anterior rather than the posterior vaginal wall that presents itself *en face* to the surgeon. There are no deeper reasons for entering the vagina by this route. Indeed, in a vaginal hysterectomy, where anterior colpotomy carries no such advantages over a posterior colpotomy, many vaginal surgeons start the operation by incising the posterior vaginal wall rather than with a circumferential incision around the cervix.

Unless total laparoscopic hysterectomy is to be performed and the vaginal cuff sutured laparoscopically, laparoscopic bladder dissection makes no sense at all. First, it is easier to make a posterior colpotomy laparoscopically than an anterior, provided a suitable vaginal manipulator is used that allows anteversion of the uterus and unless the uterus is greatly enlarged (see Chapter 13). Second, if the vaginal cuff is to be closed transvaginally, laparoscopic dissection of the bladder will only serve to bring the bladder and distal ureter down into harm's way and make closure of the cuff more difficult (2).

Steps of the Operation Undefined

Hysterectomy entails a limited number of operative steps regardless of the route by which they are carried out. For abdominal and vaginal hysterectomy, these steps are clearly defined and the sequence in which they are performed is in fact reversed. In a laparoscopic hysterectomy, it is unclear which steps must or should be carried out laparoscopically and which ones vaginally. The number of permutations is rather large and the scope for disagreement wide. There is a danger, therefore, that questions of technique will become embroiled with the rather different question of which steps to perform laparoscopically. To the extent that what is to be done affects how it can be done, the two questions are related, but it is helpful to keep them separate. The difficulties of laparoscopic hysterectomy do not stem from disagreements over what to do laparoscopically but from how to approach what is to be done laparoscopically, and this approach, as we have tried to show, cannot be the same as that used in an abdominal hysterectomy.

LAPAROSCOPIC HYSTERECTOMY: OVERALL STRATEGY

The technique of laparoscopic hysterectomy to be described evolved in stages out of the technical difficulties encountered when laparoscopic hysterectomy was approached in the same way as an abdominal hysterectomy. It incorporates two strategies that have no real parallel in abdominal hysterectomy.

First, the sequence of the steps is altered, and the uterine artery is divided before the upper blood supply and supports of the uterus to preserve the natural tension in the tissues and to facilitate dissection of the retroperitoneum.

Second, the obliterated hypogastric arteries are isolated and traced retrogradely to the origin of the uterine vessels. This seemingly circuitous step allows the uterine arteries not only to be identified, but to be completely freed, the pararectal spaces to be accurately located and opened, and the ureter to be identified.

Once this preparatory dissection has been completed, laparoscopic hysterectomy becomes a simple matter of dividing a few structures by whatever means the surgeon wishes, although, of course, we would strongly encourage traditional techniques of scissor dissection.

REVIEW OF RELEVANT ANATOMY

Relations of the Ureter

The ureters lie medial to the ovarian vessels at the pelvic brim. Here, the ovarian vessels enter the infundibulopelvic ligament, which runs medially from the pelvic brim to the ovary in the roof of the broad ligament. The infundibulopelvic ligament, therefore, crosses the ureter and lies at first above and then medial to it (Figure 11.1). These anatomic relationships have the following important practical corollaries: (1) the ureter cannot be damaged when the pelvic sidewall peritoneum is incised so long as the incision is kept lateral to the anatomic position of the infundibulopelvic ligament, which, therefore, must not be displaced medially before the incision has been extended; and (2) the infundibulopelvic ligament must be retracted medially before the ureter can be exposed at the pelvic brim.

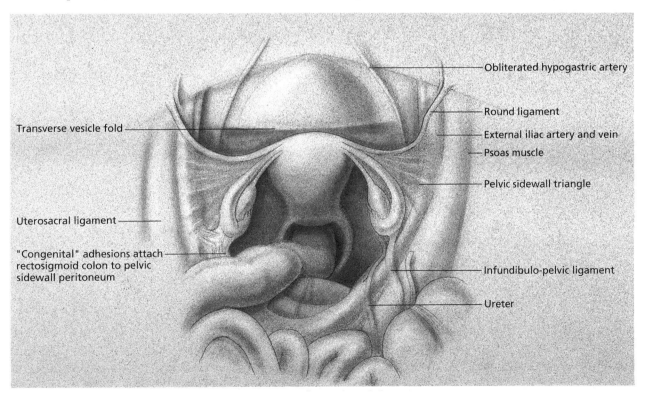

Figure 11.1 Panoramic laparoscopic view of the pelvis.

Relations of the Obliterated Hypogastric Artery

The hypogastric artery descends quite steeply into the pelvis along the pelvic sidewalls to where the uterine arteries are given off at the lateral attachments of the cardinal ligaments. They then sweep sharply upwards on either side of the bladder as the obliterated hypogastric arteries cross the superior pubic rami and run beneath the peritoneum of the anterior abdominal wall to the umbilicus.

The obliterated hypogastric arteries (lateral umbilical ligaments) are easily identified laparoscopically as prominent peritoneal folds that hang laterally on either side of the anterior abdominal wall crossed by the distal portion of the round ligaments medial to the internal inguinal ring and, more superiorly, by the transverse vesical fold (Figure 11.1). They are also relatively fixed structures and are easily dissected free of the bladder and surrounding areolar tissues in the paravesical space. The corollary is that (1) the obliterated hypogastric arteries can be traced retrogradely to identify the uterine arteries, and (2) because the uterine artery runs on top of the cardinal ligament at the caudal limit of the pararectal space, it provides an important landmark for the laparoscopic dissection of the pararectal space.

OPERATIVE TECHNIQUE

▶ STEP 1. The pelvic sidewall triangles are opened.

Right Side: The uterus is deviated to the left to delineate the triangle of the right pelvic sidewall. The base of this triangle is formed by the round ligament, the lateral border by the external iliac artery, the medial border by the infundibulopelvic ligament, and the apex by where the infundibulopelvic ligament crosses the external iliac artery. The peritoneum in the middle of the triangle is desiccated with a bipolar current, incised with dissecting scissors, and the incision extended to the round ligament, which is not divided at this time, and then to the apex of the triangle, lateral to the infundibulopelvic ligament (Figure 11.2). It is important not to displace the infundibulopelvic ligament medially before the peritoneal incision is completed, otherwise the natural anatomic relationship between the infundibulopelvic ligament and ureter, which serves to protect the ureter from injury as it lies medial to the infundibulopelvic ligament, will be lost. As the peritoneal incision is made, the broad ligament is opened by bluntly separating the extraperitoneal areolar tissues. Even tiny vessels should be coagulated because the slightest amount of bleeding can stain the extraperitoneal areolar tissues and obscure view of the

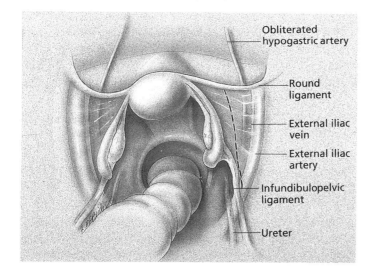
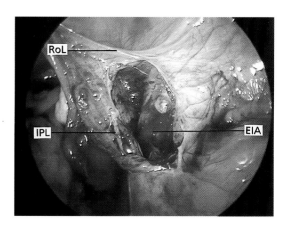

Figure 11.2 The incision in the pelvic sidewall triangle peritoneum is made along the dotted line (Step 1).

underlying structures (Figure 11.3). It is also important not to perforate the leaves of the broad ligament when the initial incision is made. If the peritoneum in the center of the triangle is difficult to pick up, the peritoneum can be incised at its apex, but the incision must be very superficial because the external iliac artery lies just below.

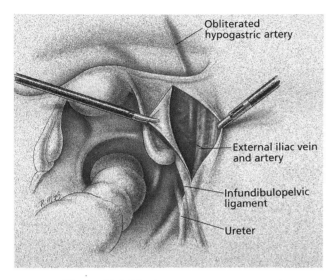

Figure 11.3 The broad ligament is opened.

Left Side: On the left side, so-called congenital adhesions, which usually cover the apex of the pelvic triangle, attach the rectosigmoid to the peritoneum laterally at or just above the pelvic brim. The dissection on the left side is begun by separating these adhesions from the underlying peritoneum, and the pelvic sidewall triangle is opened at or near its apex (Figure 11.4). (The external iliac artery will be below the plane of dissection.) The peritoneal incision is then carried distally to the round ligament, which is, again, not divided at this time.

In women who are obese or have a very deep cul-de-sac or a very redundant rectosigmoid, it is advantageous to begin the operation with an incision in the cul-de-sac peritoneum because the incision is much more awkward to make later in the operation in these patients. The incision is extended upwards on either side of the broad ligament to the point where the peritoneum is adherent to the uterosacral ligaments, and the operation is then continued in sequence from Step 1. The ureters are always superior to the uterosacral ligaments at this point and do not have to be identified, although they may be seen on the medial leaf of the broad ligament.

Figure 11.4 The attachments of the sigmoid colon are divided, and the incision on the left is started at the apex of the pelvic sidewall triangle.

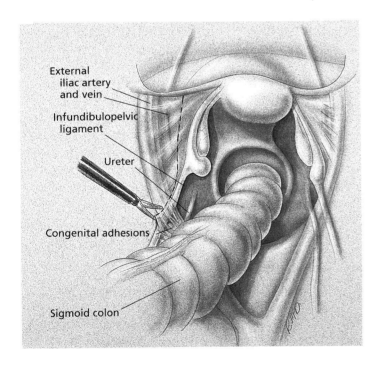

▶STEP 2. The ureter is identified at the apex of the pelvic triangle.

Right Side: The infundibulopelvic ligament is pulled medially with grasping forceps to expose the ureter at the pelvic brim, where it crosses the common or external iliac artery (Figure 11.5). This is a crucial step, and a good, atraumatic instrument is invaluable here. Rarely, it may be necessary to reflect the ureter off the medial leaf of the broad ligament for a short distance to aid in its identification.

It is important to mobilize the infundibulopelvic ligament adequately; otherwise, it will not be possible to retract its proximal end sufficiently medially to expose the ureter at the pelvic brim. To achieve this, the peritoneal incision has to be extended much further proximally than is necessary in an open case, frequently to the mesentery of the cecum (on the right) or the descending colon (on the left). Failure to achieve adequate mobilization of the infundibulopelvic ligament is the most common error in carrying out the dissection. The operator then searches for the ureter distal to the pelvic brim and lateral to the infundibulopelvic ligament but frequently fails to find it for the ureter is at that point covered by fatty areolar tissue, or, more distally, by the infundibulopelvic ligament itself and cannot be seen except in the thinnest of patients.

Left Side: The dissection of the apex is more difficult on the left side, partly because the ureter is covered by the mesentery of the sigmoid colon, but mainly because it crosses the iliac vessels higher (more proximally) and, consequently, lies more medial than the right ureter. As a result, it is more difficult to expose the left ureter by retracting the infundibulopelvic lig-ament medially. The peritoneal incision usually has to be extended to the white line of Toldt in the paracolic gutter to mobilize the sigmoid colon, and, with it, the infundibulopelvic ligament, which at this point lies extraperitoneally, under the mesentery (Figure 11.6). Occasionally, it is necessary to mobilize the medial leaf of the broad ligament from the pelvic brim and sacrum. To do this, the operator has to dissect bluntly in a medial direction under the infundibulopelvic ligament, taking care not to perforate the medial leaf of the broad ligament, or the right plane of dissection will be lost. Finally, the operator needs to be aware that the external iliac artery will be below the plane of dissection much of the time.

▶STEP 3. The obliterated hypogastric arteries are identified extraperitoneally.

The dissection is continued bluntly underneath and caudad to the round ligament, until the obliterated hypogastric artery is identified extraperitoneally (Figure 11.5). Although the anatomy will be unfamiliar to most general gynecologists, this step is, in fact, the most straightforward part of the dissection. If any difficulty is encountered, the artery should first be identified intraperitoneally, where it hangs from the anterior abdominal wall, traced proximally to where it passes behind the round ligament, and then, with both its intraperitoneal portion and the dissected space under the round ligament in view, the intraperitoneal part of the ligament should be moved back and forth. It will always be possible to detect corresponding movements in the extraperitoneal portion of the ligament.

In approximately 10% of individuals, the obliterated hypogastric artery will not be prominent, but it

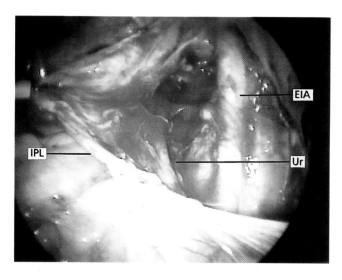

Figure 11.5 The infundibulopelvic ligament has been pulled medially to expose the ureter at the pelvic brim.

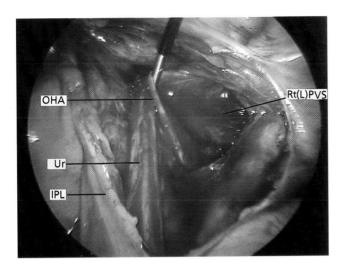

Figure 11.6 Mobilization of the left infundibulopelvic ligament.

can still be located from its relationship to the round ligament and transverse vesical fold (Figure 11.1). If a probe is pressed lightly against the peritoneum and moved back and forth over a spot just above the transverse vesical fold and about 1 inch medial to and vertically above where the round ligament crosses the psoas muscle, corresponding movements in the extraperitoneal part of the ligament will still be visible through the peritoneum of the pelvic triangle.

▶STEP 4. The paravesical spaces are developed.

Once the obliterated hypogastric arteries have been identified extraperitoneally, it is a simple matter to develop the paravesical space by bluntly separating the areolar tissue on either side of the artery. The dissection is started lateral to the artery, mindful that the external iliac vein is just lateral to it. The tips of the closed dissecting scissors are placed against the lateral edge of the artery and the artery is simply pulled medially, whereupon a bloodless plane will open lateral to it (Figure 11.7). The medial border of the artery is then freed in an identical manner but working in the opposite direction. During this maneuver, the operator must take care not to press on the external iliac vein as the artery is displaced laterally (Figure 11–8). It is, in fact, best to dissect in a medial direction against the bladder while holding the umbilical ligament fixed and deviated slightly laterally rather than against the ligament itself.

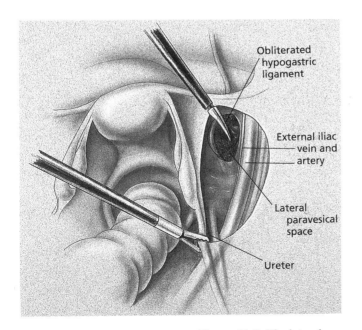

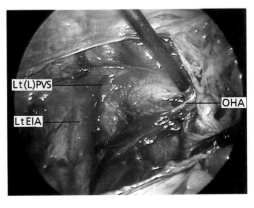

Figure 11.7 The lateral paravesical space is opened.

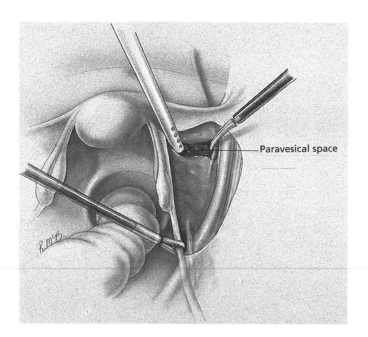

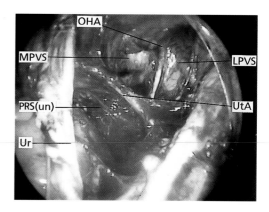

Figure 11.8 *The medial paravesical space is opened.*

The purpose of the dissection is to free the obliterated hypogastric artery completely from the surrounding areolar tissues so that it can be clearly traced proximally. However, it is advantageous to develop the paravesical spaces widely even for a simple hysterectomy; it literally takes only a minute or so, and the uterine arteries and cardinal ligaments will be much better exposed. This is especially helpful if the artery bleeds when it is divided, which can occur despite what appears to be adequate bipolar desiccation, because the bleeding points will be easy to visualize and coagulate.

Steps 3 and 4 can be executed before Step 2, i.e., the umbilical ligament identified before the ureter, and this may be a more natural sequence in thin patients in whom the obliterated hypogastric artery is only sparsely covered with areolar tissue. Once the incision in the pelvic sidewall triangle peritoneum has been extended to the round ligament, the dissection is continued under the round ligament to free the obliterated hypogastric artery in the paravesical space before proceeding proximally to identify the ureter (Step 2).

▶STEP 5. The pararectal spaces are developed.

The obliterated hypogastric arteries are next traced proximally to where they are joined by the uterines, and the pararectal spaces are opened by blunt dissection proximal and medial to the uterine arteries, which lie on top of the cardinal ligaments. Once the pararectal spaces have been opened, the ureter on the ipsilateral side is easily identified on the medial leaf of the broad ligament, which forms the medial border of the pararectal space. This step also clearly identifies the uterine artery and cardinal ligament at the distal (caudal) border of the space and the internal iliac artery on its lateral border (Figure 11.9). Starting proximal to the cardinal ligaments, the ureters are then dissected off the medial leaf of the broad ligament for a short distance in preparation for division of the uterosacral ligaments.

The pararectal space can be opened before the uterine arteries have been identified, especially in thin patients, after the ureters have been identified at the pelvic brim. The ureter is simply pushed gently medially with the tip of the suction irrigator and the pararectal space lateral to it opened by blunt dissection (see Chapter 7). The uterine artery will not, however, be cleanly dissected unless the paravesical space is also opened to expose the caudal surface of the artery.

▶STEP 6. The uterine arteries, round ligaments, and infundibulopelvic ligaments are divided.

Areolar tissue still covers the anterior aspect of the uterine artery and cardinal ligament, and this is bluntly dissected off at this time by pushing the uterine artery backwards and medially and the areolar covering forwards and laterally. A wall of tissue will separate off the anterior surface of the uterine artery and cardinal ligament, and it is at this point that the superior vesical artery will be seen lying in this

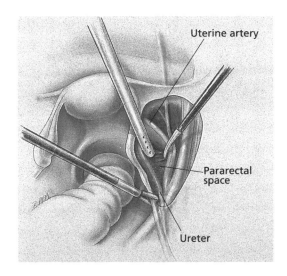
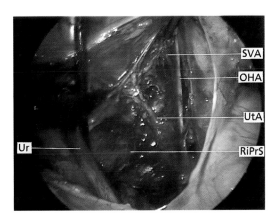

Figure 11.9 The pararectal space is developed.

areolar tissue as the tissue is placed on tension by pushing the umbilical ligament laterally (Figure 11.9). The uterine arteries are next desiccated with bipolar forceps or clipped with Laproclips and divided (Figure 11.10). Our preferred method is now to clip the uterine arteries (and infundibulopelvic ligaments) with Laproclips because this is quicker, and more reliable hemostasis is obtained. The round ligament is next divided and the incision continued along the anterior leaf of the broad ligament and the bladder peritoneum to the contralateral side, but the bladder is not dissected off the vagina. Finally, the infundibulopelvic ligaments are desiccated, ligated with silk, or doubly clipped with Laproclips and divided, and the incision is continued along the medial leaf of the broad ligament toward the uterus to where the ureters have been reflected laterally (Figure 11.11). If bipolar coagulation is used, it is important to use the forceps efficiently, and rather than repeatedly taking it in and out of the peritoneal cavity, we generally coagulate the uterine artery and round and infundibulopelvic ligaments in sequence before dividing them. The smoke generated must be continuously suctioned during desiccation.

▶STEP 7. The posterior dissection: the uterosacral ligaments are divided and posterior vaginal wall incised.

A plane is developed between the peritoneum and the uterosacral ligaments. The peritoneum is incised, and the incision extended to the pouch of Douglas, which is opened. The incision is continued across the midline to meet a similar incision in the peritoneum of the opposite broad ligament. The ureters are retracted laterally, and the uterosacral ligaments are divided with the closed tips of the dissecting scissors using a monopolar current (Figure 11.12).

The uterus is sharply anteflexed with the uterine mobilizer to an almost vertical position, whereupon a bulge resembling the cervix, which is, in fact, the hub of the instrument against the posterior vaginal wall, will appear at its lower end. The posterior vaginal wall is incised against this bulge with the points of the dissecting scissors closed using a monopolar current (Figure 11.13). The incision should not be too close to the cervical attachment of the posterior vaginal wall; otherwise, the incision will be too proximal to facilitate the vaginal part of the procedure. Contact between the dissecting scissors and the hub of the mobilizer is of no consequence because the surface area is large and any current that flows down the instrument will be dissipated along low current density pathways (see Chapter 3).

▶STEP 8. The hysterectomy is completed vaginally.

The cervix is grasped with two single-toothed tenacula and elevated to expose the incision in the posterior vaginal wall, and a long, self-weighted speculum is placed in the peritoneal cavity. The incision is then continued across the front of the cervix with a scalpel, the bladder dissected sharply off the cervix, the anterior cul-de-sac entered, and the bladder retracted with a deaver. A Zeppelin clamp is placed on each cardinal ligament, then the ligaments are divided, and sutured. The vagina is closed horizontally with a running, non-locking stitch. The pneumoperitoneum is reestab-

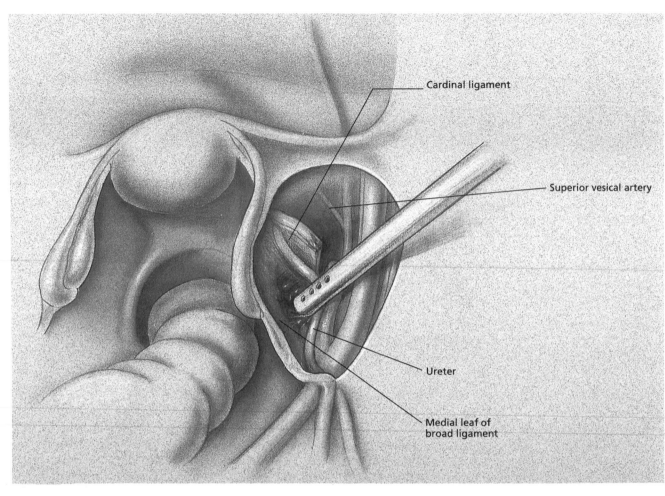

Cardinal ligament

Superior vesical artery

Ureter

Medial leaf of
broad ligament

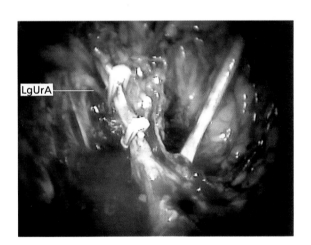

LgUrA

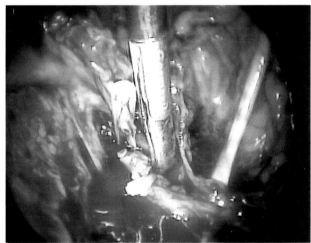

Figure 11.10 The uterine arteries are divided.

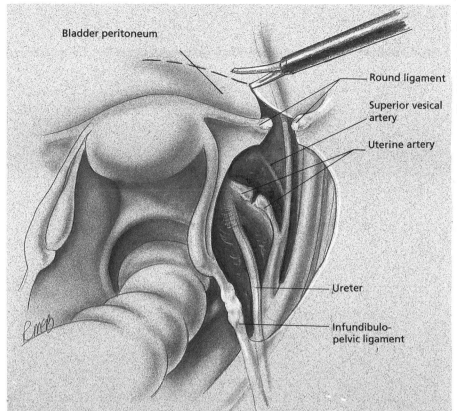

Bladder peritoneum

Round ligament

Superior vesical artery

Uterine artery

Ureter

Infundibulo-pelvic ligament

Figure 11.11 The infundibulopelvic ligament has been dessicated and the round ligament divided, and the incision is being extended along the anterior broad ligament and bladder peritoneum (Step 6).

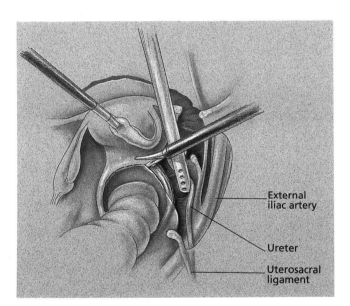

External iliac artery

Ureter

Uterosacral ligament

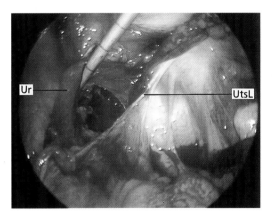

Ur

UtsL

Figure 11.12 The infundibulopelvic ligament has been divided and the incision extended along the broad ligament to the uterosacral ligament. The ureter is retracted laterally as the uterosacral ligament is divided.

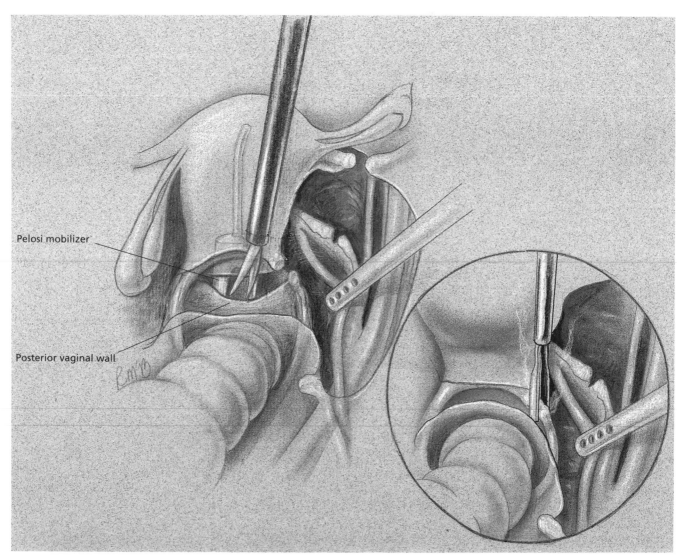

Pelosi mobilizer

Posterior vaginal wall

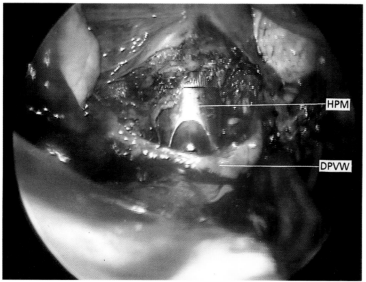

HPM

DPVW

Figure 11.13 The posterior vaginal wall is opened against the hub of the Pelosi uterine mobilizer.

lished, the pelvis is irrigated copiously and checked for hemostasis.

Discussion

Robbed of the ability to palpate tissues, the laparoscopic surgeon must rely entirely on visual recognition to identify normal structures in the pelvis. Anyone who approaches laparoscopic hysterectomy in the same way as an abdominal hysterectomy, however, will quickly discover that it is very difficult to visualize important retroperitoneal structures by simply opening and spreading apart the leaves of the broad ligament. The reasons are to be found in the subtle anatomic relationship between these structures. The infundibulopelvic ligament, for example, hides the ureter that lies beneath it and will continue to do so throughout the operation unless the ligament is mobilized at least up to the pelvic brim, and often beyond, and pulled medially. With each step of the operation, it will also be increasingly more difficult to place tissues on sufficient tension to open critical tissues planes, such as the pararectal space. The technique for laparoscopic hysterectomy described here was developed specifically to overcome these difficulties, and the logic of the operation can only be followed if these difficulties are appreciated.

The goal in Step 1 is to enter the retroperitoneum without dividing the round or infundibulopelvic ligaments because these will then provide countertraction on the broad ligament when the uterus is deviated to the contralateral side. Step 2 ensures that once the pararectal space has been developed, the ureter will be fully exposed throughout the operation and will not be obscured by the infundibulopelvic ligament. Steps 3 and 4 prepare the way to identify the uterine arteries and pararectal spaces and allow the latter to be opened accurately without bleeding (Step 5), which, in turn, permits the ureters to be identified where it matters, in the depths of the pelvis in the vicinity of the cardinal ligaments.

Once the retroperitoneal dissection has been completed, one must decide which structures, besides the uterine arteries, round ligaments, and infundibulopelvic ligaments (Step 6), to divide laparoscopically. Before settling on the uterosacral ligaments and the posterior vaginal wall (Step 7), the author tried completing the entire hysterectomy laparoscopically as well as opening the anterior vaginal wall after dissecting the bladder off the cervix and vagina. Several conclusions were reached.

Total Laparoscopic Hysterectomy

It is both time-consuming and unnecessary to divide the cardinal ligaments laparoscopically. After the uterosacral ligaments have been divided (Step 7), the hysterectomy can always be completed vaginally, even in morbidly obese nulligravidas, and completed more easily than laparoscopically. It is unclear to this author at this time that absolute indications for total laparoscopic hysterectomy (TLH) in fact exist, or that it is ever advantageous to perform a TLH instead of a laparoscopic hysterectomy.

Bladder Dissection and Anterior Colpotomy

The vaginal part of the operation is not facilitated very much by opening the anterior vaginal wall laparoscopically. Moreover, if the vagina is to be closed from below, laparoscopic dissection of the bladder off the cervix is not advisable. The reason is that the bladder will be dissected distally (caudad), and this will not make it easier to suture the vaginal cuff from below. Indeed, by bringing the bladder and distal ureter closer to where the sutures are being placed, the dissection places the bladder and ureter at risk of suture entrapment, and this has happened to the author and others (2,5).

Laparoscopically Assisted Versus Laparoscopic Hysterectomy

We defined total laparoscopic, laparoscopically assisted, and laparoscopic hysterectomies in Chapter 10. We find very few indications for laparoscopically assisted vaginal hysterectomy, but when they arise, the operation does not really call for the laparoscopic techniques described in this chapter so much as the techniques for adhesiolysis, excision of endometriosis, and adnexectomy to be described in subsequent chapters. The single-puncture approach described by Dr. Pelosi, in my view, has its greatest potential application in these cases.

REFERENCES

1. Hourcabie JA, Bruhat M-A. One hundred and three cases of laparoscopic hysterectomy using endo-GIA staples and a device for presenting the vaginal fornices. Gynaecol Endosc 1993;2:65–72.

2. Kadar N, Lemmerling L. Urinary tract injuries during laparoscopically assisted hysterectomy: causes and prevention. Am J Obstet Gynecol 1994;170:47–48.

3. Hunter RW, McCartney AJ. Can laparoscopic assisted hysterectomy safely replace abdominal hysterectomy? Br J Obstet Gynaecol 1993;100:932–934.

4. Childers JA, Brzechffa PR, Hatch KD, Surwit EA. Laparoscopically assisted surgical staging (LASS) of endometrial cancer. Gynecol Oncol 1993;51:33–38.

5. Blecharz A, Rzempoluch J, Zamlynski J. Laparoscopic hysterectomy; review of 33 cases (Abstract). Presented at the 2nd European Congress in Gynaecologic Endoscopy and New Surgical Techniques, Heidelberg, October 21–23, 1993. Gynaecol Endosc 1994;3:21.

▼ ▼ ▼ ▼ ▼ ▼ ▼ ▼ ▼

Chapter 12
Supracervical Hysterectomy

Marco Pelosi

The handwriting on the wall may be a forgery.
—Hodgson

Total abdominal hysterectomy has been the preferred method of removing the uterus for benign disease since the 1940s. At that time, the operation replaced supracervical hysterectomy because it was felt that the cervix should be removed prophylactically to prevent cancer from developing in the cervical stump. However, there is evidence to show that cervix cancer is no more likely to develop in a cervical stump than it is in the cervix of an intact uterus, and the incidence of stump carcinoma can be reduced by coagulating the endocervix at the time of a supracervical hysterectomy (1). This fact, coupled with increasing awareness that subtotal hysterectomy has many advantages over a total hysterectomy, has increased the popularity of laparoscopic supracervical hysterectomy, which is beginning to replace total hysterectomy as a means of removing the uterus in some patients.

The author had the opportunity to perform the first laparoscopic supracervical hysterectomy and to publish the first preliminary report of the technique in the English literature (2). Other investigators have also rediscovered this operation and have found it to be technically easier and less morbid than laparoscopic total hysterectomy. The procedure has been advocated by Semm in Germany (3), Lyons in Atlanta (4), and Hasson in Chicago (5). Hasson (1), in an excellent and exhaustive review of the literature, concluded that in the presence of benign disease, supracervical hysterectomy is a valid alternative to total hysterectomy.

Subtotal hysterectomy is technically easier to perform. It has been associated with decreased blood loss, operating time, and surgical complications compared

with laparoscopic total hysterectomy. Additional advantages claimed for the supracervical operation include: (1) preservation of the anatomy and integrity of the pelvic floor, which minimizes the risk of subsequent vault prolapse and enterocele formation; (2) avoidance of granulation tissue formation at the vaginal cuff and prolapse of the fallopian tubes; (3) less shortening of the vagina; (4) preservation of the paracervical ganglia, which minimizes postoperative bladder and bowel dysfunction and loss of vaginal orgasm and lubrication; and (5) less dyspareunia and less long-term psychiatric complications.

OPERATIVE TECHNIQUES

Common to all current techniques of laparoscopic subtotal hysterectomy are supracervical amputation of the uterus and thermal destruction of the endocervix and ectocervix.

Multiple-Puncture Techniques

After careful exploration of the upper abdomen and pelvis, adhesiolysis is carried out as indicated. In the presence of large myomas, access to the upper uterine attachments and vascular pedicles may be compromised. Under these circumstances, myomectomy sometimes needs to be carried out as the first step. We now start the operation with Kadar's superior approach to ureteric identification described in Chapter 7. The pelvic peritoneum is opened lateral to the infundibulopelvic ligament, and the infundibulopelvic ligament is mobilized to expose the ureter

(Figures 12.1A,B). The infundibulopelvic or utero-ovarian ligaments, and then the round ligaments are successively coagulated with bipolar forceps and divided. The peritoneal incision in the anterior leaf of the broad ligament is continued along the vesicouterine fold to the contralateral side and the bladder dissected off the cervix to the level of the internal os sharply with scissors. The posterior leaf of the broad ligament is then incised down to the uterosacral ligament. Meticulous hemostasis should be maintained throughout the dissection as this simplifies identification of the uterine vessels. The ureter is pushed downwards with the suction irrigator and the uterine arteries (or, more properly, their anterior branch) coagulated at the level of the internal os on the side of the uterus (Figure 12.1C).

The cervix is incised anteriorly with a knife electrode, and the incision is continued in the same plane until the metal tip of the uterine manipulator is encountered (Figure 12.1D). The incision is then continued circumferentially around the cervix somewhat in a cone-shaped fashion to ensure removal of both the endocervix and any endometrial remnants (Figure 12.1E). After the fundus has been amputated, the manipulator is removed and the endocervix is ablated transvaginally, laparoscopically, or by a combined approach using unipolar electrocoagulation or lasers. We find no need to reperitonealize this area.

The amputated uterus is then removed either abdominally or vaginally. Vaginal extraction through a colpotomy incision is preferred if there is enough room; otherwise, the amputated fundus is removed abdominally through an extended umbilical or suprapubic incision. If the uterus is large, the fundus may need to be morcellated laparoscopically before it can be removed.

Classic Abdominal Serrated Morcellator Hysterectomy (CASH)

The CASH procedure described by Semm (3) is a laparoscopic supracervical hysterectomy with transvaginal coring out of the cervix. Under laparoscopic visualization, the uterus is perforated centrally with a large probe. The infundibulopelvic and round ligaments are ligated and transected. Endoloops are applied to the transected pedicles to achieve additional hemostasis. The utero-ovarian ligament and fallopian tube are ligated and transected if the ovaries are to be preserved. The leaves of the broad ligament are separated. Dilute Pitressin is injected prior to separating the bladder from the upper cervix. The vesicouterine

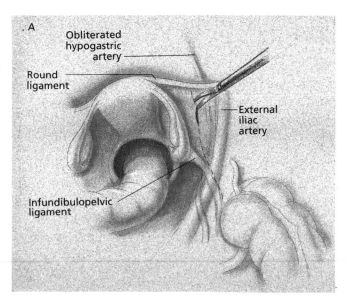

Figure 12.1A The peritoneum of the pelvic sidewall triangle is opened to gain access to the retroperitoneum.

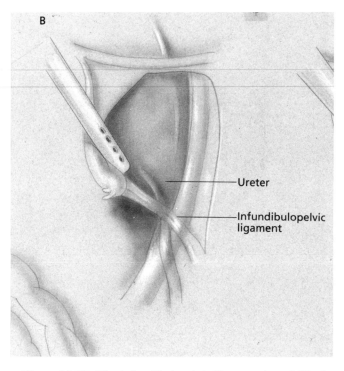

Figure 12.1B The infundibulopelvic ligament is mobilized and pulled medially to expose the ureter at the pelvic brim.

fold is then separated with sharp dissection and the bladder flap is suspended using a long needle pushed through the abdominal wall. Both ends of the suture are clamped with forceps.

After adequate paracervical dissection, a large Roeder loop is placed over the uterine fundus and is pushed down toward the cervix, and the ligature is tied. The purpose of the suture is to avoid loss of pneu-

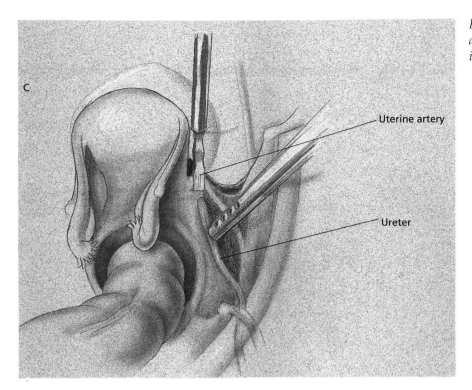

Figure 12.1C The uterine arteries are coagulated at the level of the internal os.

Uterine artery

Ureter

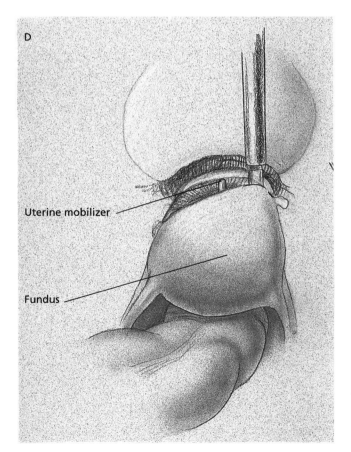

Uterine mobilizer

Fundus

Figure 12.1D The fundus is transected at the level of the internal os.

moperitoneum, to ligate the paracervical vessels, and to prevent CO_2 embolism.

A transvaginal central coring out of the cervix and uterus is then performed using the serrated macromorcellator, which is placed over the perforation probe. A large tissue cylinder is removed, the fundus is grasped with large claw forceps, and three more endoloops are placed around the cervix. Transvaginal thermocoagulation is used to achieve hemostasis of the cored-out cervix. The uterus is then transected laparoscopically using scissors or a knife. To avoid the possibility of losing the amputated uterus in the abdominal cavity, the uterus is temporarily sutured to the anterior abdominal wall using a suture placed transabdominally.

The round ligaments are sutured to the cervical stump, and the pelvis is reperitonealized, the uterus morcellated with a morcellator, and a Robinson's drain placed through one of the puncture sites. Semm recommends the CASH procedure only for a uterus that is no bigger than 12 weeks in size. One drawback of the technique is that it is associated with significant blood loss.

Vaginal Techniques of Subtotal Hysterectomy

Supracervical hysterectomy was first performed vaginally by Döderlein of Munich in the 19th century. The operation has been rediscovered by Semm who has

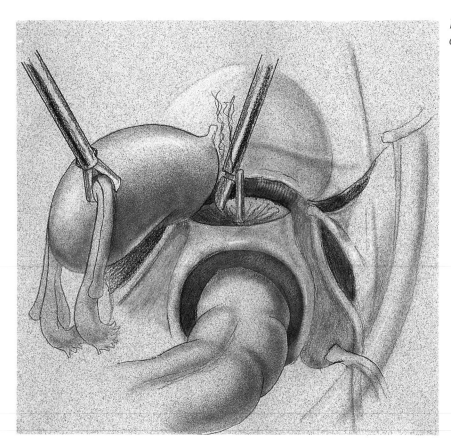

Figure 12.1E The cervix is cored out as the fundus is transected.

reported an isolated case of this operation (6). This author has performed six vaginal subtotal hysterectomies for recurrent dysfunctional uterine bleeding refractory to hormone therapy in women with normal sized or minimally enlarged uteri (mean weight 135 grams). The operation is very straightforward and provides a more effective and less costly alternative to endometrial ablation in these women. The technique is as follows.

An anterior cervical incision is made in the vaginal mucosa using diathermy (Figure 12.2A), the bladder is dissected free, and the anterior cul-de-sac is entered. The fundus is delivered through the anterior cul-de-sac (Figure 12.2B) and the upper attachments and blood supply of the uterus are clamped, divided, and suture ligated (Figure 12.2C). The uterine vessels are then divided and ligated (Figure 12.2D), and the uterus is transected at the cervical-uterine junction using diathermy (Figure 12.2E). The anterior and posterior edges of the proximal cervical stump are then approximated with a running suture (Figure 12.2F). The anterior cul-de-sac and vaginal wall are closed, and the endocervix coagulated with diathermy. If the patient has occult prolapse, as many do, the uterosacral ligaments are plicated before the vagina is closed.

The indications for subtotal vaginal hysterectomy are limited to women who have abnormal uterine

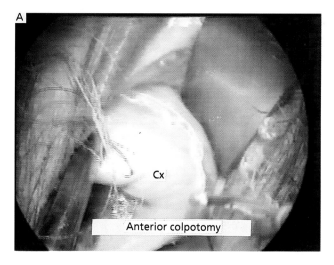

Figure 12.2A The anterior vaginal wall is incised.

bleeding of benign etiology, minimal uterine enlargement, and no present or prior cervical abnormalities. Uteri larger than 10–12 weeks are technically difficult to deliver through the anterior cul-de-sac, especially when the adnexa and round ligaments have not been previously divided laparoscopically and a large uterus requires a cumbersome and time-consuming laparoscopic morcellation or myomectomy prior to its delivery through the anterior cul-de-sac.

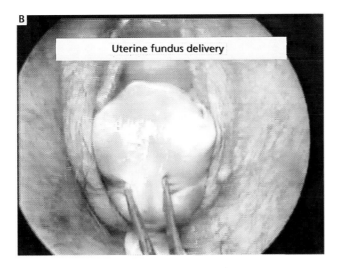

Figure 12.2B *The uterine fundus is delivered through the anterior fornix after the anterior cul-de-sac is opened.*

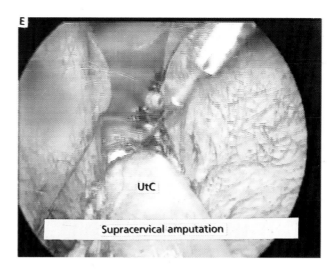

Figure 12.2E *The uterus is transected at the cervico-isthmic junction.*

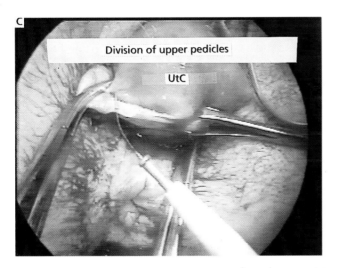

Figure 12.2C *The adnexal pedicle is divided.*

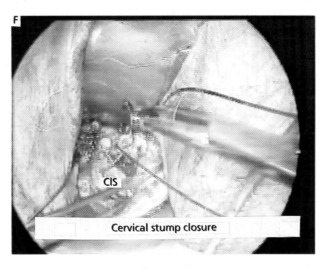

Figure 12.2F *The proximal end of the cervical stump is sutured.*

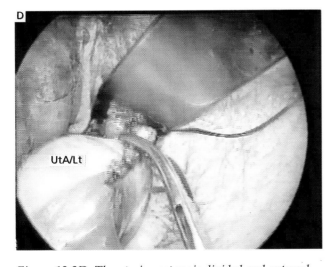

Figure 12.2D *The uterine artery is divided and sutured.*

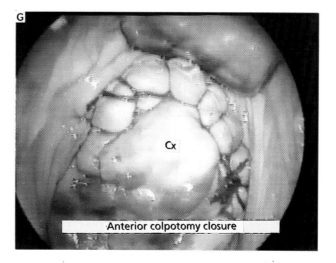

Figure 12.2G *The anterior colpotomy incision is closed.*

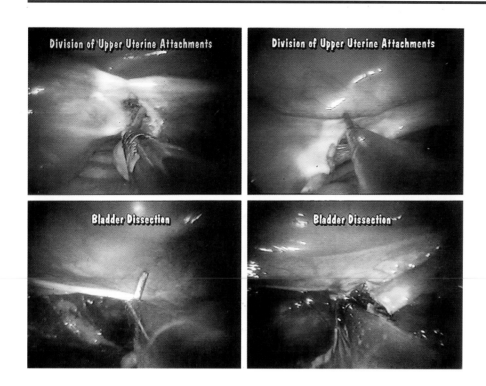

Division of Upper Uterine Attachments

Division of Upper Uterine Attachments

Bladder Dissection

Bladder Dissection

Figure 12.3 The round ligament is transected and the bladder peritoneum divided.

Single-Puncture Laparoscopic Supracervical Hysterectomy

In January 1990, the author performed the first laparoscopic subtotal hysterectomy in a patient who specifically requested preservation of the cervix. The procedure was accomplished successfully using solely the operative laparoscope (2). Since then, over 40 supracervical hysterectomies have been performed using the same approach, and many uteri have weighed over 1 kg.

As is true for almost all laparoscopic operations, single-puncture supracervical hysterectomy follows the same surgical steps as are used in the multiple-puncture techniques. The mid portion of the round ligaments are coagulated with bipolar forceps and divided with hook scissors, and, then, either the infundibulopelvic or the utero-ovarian ligaments are coagulated and divided in exactly the same way, depending on whether the ovary is to be preserved or removed. With the bladder partly distended with methylene blue solution, the vesicouterine fold of peritoneum is opened with scissors and, using sharp and blunt dissection, the bladder is dissected off the uterus and carried to the level of the internal os (Figure 12.3). This anterior dissection simplifies the identification of the uterine vessels.

The posterior leaf of the broad ligament is then dissected free and incised down to the level of the uterosacral ligaments (Figure 12.4A). If carried out properly, this maneuver releases the ureter from the operative field. Laparoscopic supracervical hysterectomy does not require routine dissection of the ureter, but if the anatomy is distorted by fibroids, adhesions, endometriosis, or previous surgery, the ureters must be identified.

The uterine arteries are now skeletonized, desiccated, and transected (Figure 12.4B), and the uterus amputated at the level of the internal os. Using unipolar scissors or a knife or needle electrode passed down the operating channel of the laparoscope, the cervix is incised anteriorly, and the incision is continued in

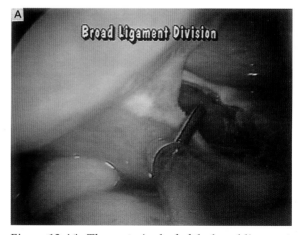

A

Broad Ligament Division

Figure 12.4A The posterior leaf of the broad ligament is incised.

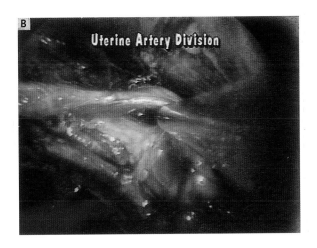

Figure 12.4B *The uterine artery is coagulated.*

the same plane until the tip of the Pelosi mobilizer is encountered. A circumferential incision is then made around the tip of the instrument. This circumferential incision is made at an angle to the cervix, with the plane of dissection coned inwards to remove any endometrial remnants and the upper portion of the endocervix. The cervical cuff is carefully inspected and bleeding points are coagulated with bipolar forceps. The amputated uterus is then bisected or morcellated to facilitate its later abdominal or vaginal removal.

The author's surgical technique has been recently modified. We have found that bisection or morcellation of the uterus is greatly simplified if these are carried out *before* the cervix is amputated (Figure 12.5A,B). It is technically easier to bisect the fundus when it is fixed by its attachment to the cervix rather than free, and, with the help of the manipulator, the uterus can be easily fixed in a position that is optimal

for the fundus to be split along the vertical axis of the metal tip of the mobilizer. After the fundus is divided, each half is amputated at the level of the internal os. This modification has reduced operating time considerably. The uterine manipulator is then removed and the remainder of the endocervix desiccated partly laparoscopically and partly transvaginally. We have not found it necessary to close the peritoneum over the cervical stump, and to judge from the second-look laparoscopies that have been performed in a few patients, healing is excellent and accompanied by little adhesion formation.

If the vagina is pliable and the uterus only moderately enlarged, the fundus is most easily removed through a colpotomy incision. If vaginal access is compromised, however, or the fundus is very large, it is better to remove it abdominally either through an enlarged umbilical incision or through a separate suprapubic minilaparotomy incision. The fundus is then morcellated through the abdominal incision (see Chapter 17). The author's preference is to remove the fundus through the extended umbilical puncture site (Figures 12.6A–C), and he has encountered no significant technical difficulties in removing myomatous uteri weighing even as much as 2,375 grams, although such extractions are, to be sure, tedious.

The surgeon must be aware that misplacement of the amputated fundus is a real possibility, and, occasionally, the misplaced fundus can be very difficult to find, necessitating a frustrating and prolonged search, and even ultimately a laparotomy (3). This has happened to the author on one occasion, when he lost one half of an 800-gram fibroid uterus. The specimen was finally located in the cul-de-sac but only after a

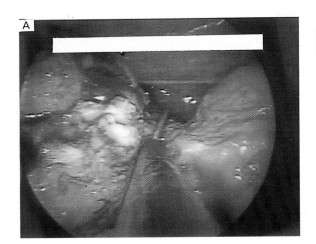

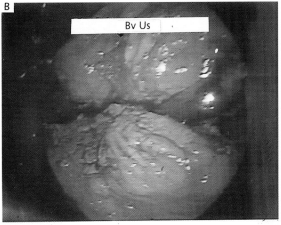

Figure 12.5A,B *The uterine fundus is bivalved while it is still attached to the uterus.*

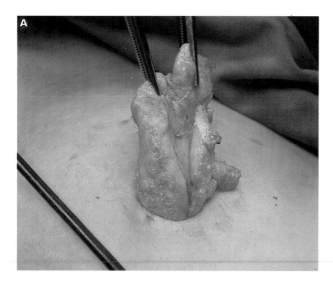

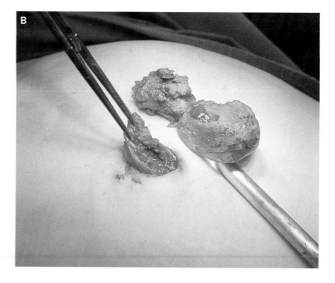

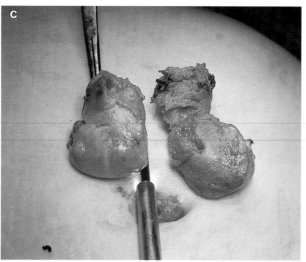

Figure 12.6A–C Each half of the uterine fundus is removed through an extended umbilical incision.

90-minute search, during which the abdomen was irrigated copiously, the patient placed in a steep reverse Trendelenburg position, and the bowel "stirred" with the operative laparoscope.

DISCUSSION

Current interest in supracervical hysterectomy by laparoscopists can be attributed to two factors: (1) supracervical hysterectomy is technically easier and safer to perform laparoscopically than total laparoscopic hysterectomy, and (2) supracervical hysterectomy is believed to have certain advantages over total hysterectomy.

It is well known that *abdominal* supracervical hysterectomy is associated with less morbidity and

shorter hospital stay than total abdominal hysterectomy (1), and recent data appear to indicate that the same is true of the laparoscopic route. Laparoscopic supracervical hysterectomy is not only associated with shorter operating time, less blood loss, and less morbidity than laparoscopic total hysterectomy, but it may also be more cost-effective (2,4,5).

Laparoscopic supracervical hysterectomy is not an innocuous procedure, however, and several immediate and late major and minor complications have been reported (5,8,9). Complications associated specifically with the retained cervical stump include the continuation of light menses and the need for later removal because of endometriosis or an abnormal Papanicolaou smear (5,9).

To justify laparoscopic supracervical hysterectomy solely on the grounds that it is easier to perform than total hysterectomy is inappropriate. However, some data show that retention of the cervix may be beneficial to some patients. At the present time, specific indications for laparoscopic supracervical hysterectomy have not been defined, but we consider the subtotal operation an attractive and effective alternative for a select group of women who have a healthy cervix and no genital prolapse and who are reliable, highly motivated, and well-informed about the need for subsequent cytologic follow-up.

Although in our preliminary report, we surmised that uteri larger than 12 weeks in size were probably not suitable for laparoscopic supracervical hysterectomy (2), further experience has shown this prediction to be not only very conservative but, frankly, incorrect. Indeed, we have found that in women who have large myomatous uteri and narrow, long vagina, narrow

COMMENT
Nicholas Kadar

I asked Dr. Pelosi to describe the subtotal operations that are used to remove a uterus because there is clearly interest in these techniques, but these are operations I am rarely called upon to perform. My concern about laparoscopic supracervical hysterectomy is that it is being undertaken for the wrong reasons, as a means of avoiding proper dissection of the retroperitoneum and identification of the ureters. This concern may appear somewhat theoretical and even contrived, but, in my view, laparoscopic supracervical hysterectomy is not so different from its total counterpart that it can be safely undertaken in all cases by a surgeon handicapped by the inability to identify the ureter laparoscopically. Supracervical hysterectomy is undoubtedly an easier operation when it is performed via a laparotomy, but when it is performed laparoscopically, any advantages of the operation are offset by the difficulties of removing the fundus from the peritoneal cavity and by the need to coagulate the endocervical canal. Thus, I am very doubtful that in indicated cases, supracervical hysterectomy is likely to be either quicker or easier than a total hysterectomy if the operation is performed laparoscopically. I can accept that, occasionally, the supracervical removal of a large uterus can be slightly less tedious than total hysterectomy if the vagina is narrow, etc., as Dr. Pelosi has described, but I regard these as exceptions that prove the rule.

I am equally puzzled by the finding that operative blood loss is reduced by this operation, for everyone who has performed a subtotal hysterectomy abdominally will know that bleeding from the transected cervix is the rule, and it can often be difficult to control. It seems to me that if supracervical hysterectomy is being undertaken to avoid the need to identify the ureter, the cervix is likely to be transected higher than in the open operation, and this will simply make the problem worse.

I cannot allow my great admiration and respect for Professor Semm's genius to silence my objections to his CASH procedure, which seems to me to be just a complicated way of destroying the lining of the endocervical canal and performing a supracervical hysterectomy. Moreover, fixation of the vaginal vault to the round ligament is a long discredited tactic that anteverts the vaginal axis and predisposes to enterocele formation.

If one accepts that leaving the cervix behind is advantageous so far as sexual function is concerned (and which I am hesitant to do at this time) then it must surely be advantageous to leave it behind regardless of the route by which the uterus is removed. This provides a rationale for supracervical vaginal hysterectomy. However, the operation is likely to be feasible only if there is some degree of prolapse, and limited uterine enlargement. Therefore, it is essential to obtain good support of the vaginal vault to avert subsequent vault prolapse. It is not the presence of the cervix per se that predisposes to vault prolapse, but the pre-existing weakness in the supports of the upper vagina. It should, however, be possible to support the vaginal vault equally well regardless of whether the cervix is in situ or not.

There is no question that during vaginal supracervical hysterectomy one obtains much better access to the adnexa if the uterus is delivered anteriorly rather than posteriorly, but I must confess to never having understood the mechanism whereby delivery of the fundus through the anterior vagina during a vaginal hysterectomy (the Döderlein hysterectomy) is supposed to prevent subsequent vault prolapse compared with posterior delivery of the fundus. It seems to me that we all sometimes deliver the uterus in this way when that seems to be the more natural thing to do, and I always do this in a Schauta operation. In as much as the same structures must be divided to remove the uterus whichever way the fundus is delivered from the peritoneal cavity, it is difficult for me to see how this could possibly affect the risk of subsequent vault prolapse. Of all the technical modifications to the subtotal operation that Dr. Pelosi has described, the one that strikes me as the most advantageous is his own. Although I have never had occasion to do this, it seems to me that dividing the fundus while it is still attached to the cervix is a clever way to fix the uterus, and this must make it easier to cut it in half.

Of the potential advantages listed for laparoscopic supracervical hysterectomy, the only ones that can be accepted unreservedly are granulation tissue at the vaginal cuff, prolapse of the fallopian tubes, and, probably, reduced risk of

COMMENT

ureteric injury. Total simple hysterectomy does not cause any significant postoperative disturbances of bowel and bladder function or shortening of the vagina, and the claim that it predisposes to subsequent vault prolapse or sexual dysfunction has yet to be convincingly demonstrated. With that said, we should embrace this operation if the advantages claimed for it are demonstrated to be valid, but, in that case, I would recommend identification of the ureter by one of the techniques discussed in Chapter 7 before the uterine arteries are divided and the cervix transected.

subpubic arch, or massive thighs or protuberant buttocks, the technique is not only a practical alternative to total hysterectomy but, in our opinion, a preferable approach that avoids an otherwise very difficult, time-consuming and potentially bloody transvaginal completion of a laparoscopic total hysterectomy.

REFERENCES

1. Hasson HM. Cervical removal at hysterectomy for benign disease: risks and benefits. J Reprod Med 1993; 38:780–790.

2. Pelosi MA, Pelosi MA III. Laparoscopic supracervical hysterectomy using a single umbilical puncture (minilaparoscopy). J Reprod Med 1992;37:774–784.

3. Semm K. Hysterectomy by pelviscopy: an alternative approach without colpotomy (CASH). In: Garry R, Reich H, eds. Laparoscopic Hysterectomy. Oxford: Blackwell Scientific, 1993;118–132.

4. Lyons T. Supracervical laparoscopic hysterectomy: a comparison: Morbidity and mortality results with LAVH. J Reprod Med 1993;38:763–767.

5. Hasson HM, Rotman C, Rana N, Asakura H. Experience with laparoscopic hysterectomy. J Am Assoc Gynecol Laparosc 1993;1:1–11.

6. Semm K. Subtotal vaginal hysterectomy. Presented at the World Congress of Gynecologic Endoscopy AAGL 22nd Annual Meeting, San Francisco, CA, November 10–14, 1993.

7. Mettler L, Semm K. Intrafascial supracervical hysterectomy without colpotomy and transuterine mucosal resection by pelviscopy and laparotomy, our first 100 cases. Presented at the Third Biennial Meeting of the International Society of Gynecologic Endoscopy, Washington, DC, June 23–26, 1993

8. Schwartz RO. Complications of laparoscopic hysterectomy. Obstet Gynecol 1993;81:1022–1024.

Chapter 13
Laparoscopic Hysterectomy Techniques for the Large Uterus

Young people are always more given to admiring what is gigantic than what is reasonable.
—Delacroix

The laparoscopic removal of uteri at least the size of an 18-week gestation and reaching the lower border of the umbilicus is considered separately because it presents a number of technical difficulties unique to this setting. First, because the uterine fundus is close to the umbilicus, it can easily be injured during trocar insertion, and the technique for inserting trocars must, therefore, be modified. Second, because exposure is often problematic, the sequence of operative steps often needs to be changed and, to some extent, improvised to meet individual circumstances. It is particularly difficult to expose the pouch of Douglas properly and, hence, the uterosacral ligaments and posterior vaginal wall. Third, removal of the uterus requires morcellation, which has to be approached in an organized manner if it is to be successful and excess blood loss avoided.

FEASIBILITY OF THE OPERATION

With the patient under anesthesia, the feasibility of laparoscopic hysterectomy should be reassessed. A careful vaginal examination is carried out before the uterine manipulator is inserted into the uterus, and particular attention is paid to the capacity of the vagina and the angle subtended by the subpubic arch. The size and mobility of the uterus are next determined, and special attention is paid to the amount of room lateral to the cervix. The cervix itself is also palpated to ensure that it has not been effaced by a submucous fibroid. Finally, the size of the patient and particularly the size of her buttocks is also taken into

consideration. Adverse features on this examination may sway one towards abandoning the laparoscopic approach as, for example, when the cervix is completely effaced, the vagina and subpubic arch are extremely narrow, or there is little if any room lateral to the cervix.

Once the pneumoperitoneum has been established, feasibility of a laparoscopic hysterectomy is assessed once more, this time from an abdominal viewpoint. Laparoscopic hysterectomy should be reconsidered if there are any other adverse technical features present besides the large uterus. These would include significant adhesions, obliteration of the cul-de-sac, endometriosis, and massive obesity, which would all render laparoscopic hysterectomy inefficient and impractical.

STEPS OF THE OPERATION

The overall strategy used to remove greatly enlarged uteri laparoscopically is to detach the upper attachments of the uterus, control its proximal blood supply, coagulate the uterine arteries, and incise the bladder peritoneum. It will generally not be possible to divide the cervical ligaments, although the uterosacral ligaments can sometimes be accessed by rotating the uterus on its long axis to the contralateral side while anteverting as much as possible at the same time.

Trocar Insertions

A blunt-ended trocar is introduced at the umbilicus using Hasson's open technique (Chapter 12), which is particularly easy in these cases because the uterine fundus gives one a firm base to work against. The uterus must be manipulated with a hinged uterine mobilizer, and an extra long uterine attachment specifically designed for the large uterus is presently being developed for the Pelosi uterine mobilizer.

An alternative way to insert the first trocar is to make an intraumbilical incision, open the peritoneum bluntly with a clamp or finger, and then introduce the cannula of the trocar, without the sharp obturator (Figures 13.1A–E). Quite frequently, the trocar has to be directed toward the patient's head rather than her feet (Figure 13.2).

It is essential to use sharp trocars, which require minimal force to insert, for the auxiliary ports so that the anterior abdominal wall is not compressed toward

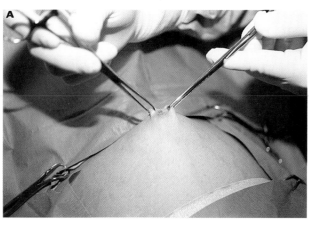

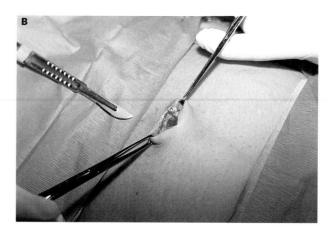

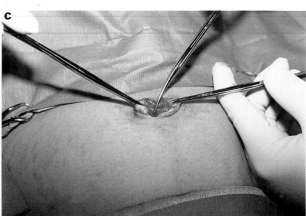

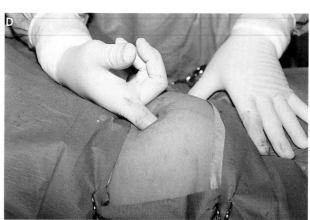

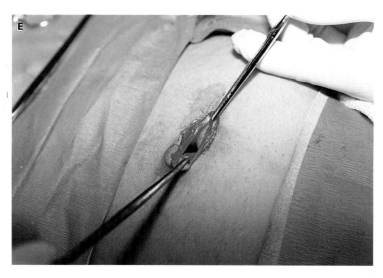

Figure 13.1 A–E Modified technique for making an intraumbilical incision for open laparoscopy.

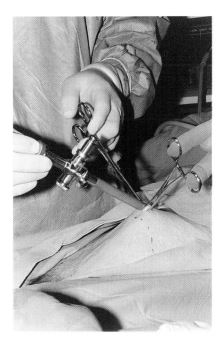

Figure 13.2 The cannula of a 10-mm trocar is inserted into the peritoneal cavity in the direction of the patient's head.

the enlarged uterus. The Hunt-Reich trocars are particularly suitable for this purpose. These trocars are so sharp that they can be "screwed" through the anterior abdominal wall with almost no pressure. Unfortunately, despite having a screw-fixing device threaded onto their shaft, they frequently pull out during prolonged procedures that require extensive dissection and trocar manipulation, but this is rarely required during the removal of large fibroid uteri. The Ethicon Tristar trocar, by contrast, is quite unsuitable for this purpose because it requires an inordinate amount of force to insert. The uterus must be deviated away from the trocar insertion site as much as possible and the trocar introduced with minimum force. The preset intra-abdominal pressure on the automatic insufflator can also be increased temporarily to 20–25 mm of mercury.

Laparoscopic Part of the Operation

After a pneumoperitoneum has been obtained, the feasibility of the operation established, and all auxiliary ports placed, the steps of the operation are executed as much as possible in the sequence outlined in Chapter 11, although this is often not possible. The pelvic sidewall triangle is delineated, but to view the apex, the laparoscope must be directed upwards, toward the patient's head rather than her feet. The peritoneum is incised parallel and lateral to the in-

fundibulopelvic ligament. In making this incision, the surgeon will be working vertically downward from the cornua of the enlarged uterus toward the pelvic brim. The infundibulopelvic ligament is mobilized medially as much as possible, but sufficient mobilization may not be achieved to identify the ureter at the pelvic brim. Nonetheless, if the medial leaf of the broad ligament is incised well away from the pelvic brim, toward the ovary, the infundibulopelvic ligament can be safely isolated and divided because the ureter will be much deeper in the pelvis and far away from the point of dissection. The same is true of the relationship between the ureter and the ovarian ligament. Therefore, if the ovary is to be preserved, the adnexal pedicle can be safely divided without fear of ureteric injury because, at this point, the ureter will be far below the point of dissection.

The larger the uterus and the less side-to-side mobility, the less likely is it that the steps of an extraperitoneal hysterectomy (see Chapter 11) can be followed closely. In these cases, the operation proceeds very much in the same way as an abdominal hysterectomy. The round ligaments are divided and the peritoneal incision continued across the front of the uterus to the contralateral side, the peritoneum is incised parallel and lateral to the infundibulopelvic ligament, and either the infundibulopelvic ligament or the uteroovarian ligament is coagulated with bipolar forceps and divided. The medial leaf of the broad ligament is then incised until the side of the uterus is reached and the uterine vessels skeletonized as in an open operation. The uterine vessels are then coagulated with bipolar forceps at several points high up on the fundus of the uterus, but they are only divided if there is complete control of the operative field so that, should there be any bleeding, this can be arrested with further coagulation without difficulty.

A decision must be made about a colpotomy. A posterior colpotomy will rarely, if ever, be possible even if the uterosacral ligaments can be partly divided by rotating the uterus to the contralateral side along its long axis. An anterior colpotomy may, however, be feasible, in which case the bladder needs to be dissected off the cervix and vagina caudally. However, if an anterior colpotomy is made, great care must be exercised when the vagina is closed, and the bladder may need to be dissected off the cut edge of the vagina toward the surgeon to ensure that it will not be injured during cuff closure (1). Sometimes, it is difficult to make a colpotomy even vaginally. In these cases, grasping forceps can be passed laparoscopically behind the uterus into the cul-de-sac, pressed against the posterior vaginal wall, and its tip palpated vaginally by the assistant. The jaws of the forceps are opened, and the assistant incises the vagina between the open jaws of the forceps. The forceps are then inserted through the incision into the vagina and a colpotomy fashioned around this site when the operation is continued vaginally.

Vaginal Component of the Operation

A circumferential incision is made around the cervix and the vesicocervical and rectovaginal spaces developed by sharp-scissor dissection (Figures 13.3A,B). The peritoneum of the posterior cul-de-sac is incised with scissors and a long weighted speculum is placed into the pouch of Douglas. It is important to stop all bleeding, however minor, from the cut edge of the vagina because the procedure is likely to be prolonged and the cumulative blood loss from the vagi-

nal cuff can be considerable. The anterior cul-de-sac can then be entered by blunt finger dissection because the anterior peritoneum has already been incised laparoscopically and deaver retractors placed into the peritoneal cavity. Obviously, the incision must be tailored to the circumstances present. If, for example, there is a large anterior fibroid, the operation will start with a posterior colpotomy, and if there is a low cervical fibroid, this may first need to be enucleated before the peritoneal cavity can be entered. It is sometimes useful to infiltrate the serosa with a vasopressin solution (20 ml/100 ml saline) before enucleating a fibroid to reduce blood loss.

Next, the cardinal and uterosacral ligaments are clamped, divided, and suture ligated (Figures 13.4A,B). If access to the peritoneum is difficult, however, the uterosacral and cardinal ligaments are first divided extraperitoneally, and the peritoneal cavity entered afterwards. Because the region of the isthmus is gener-

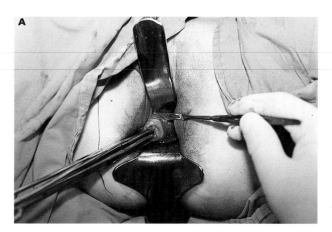
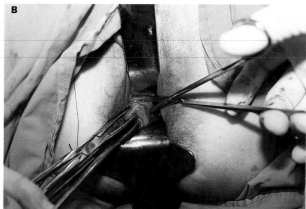

Figures 13.3A,B A circumferential incision is made around the cervix and the vesicovaginal and rectovaginal spaces developed by sharp-scissor dissection.

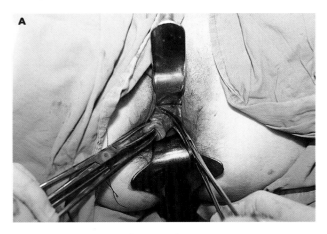
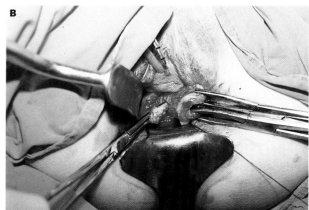

Figures 13.4A,B The cardinal ligament is clamped and divided.

ally enlarged, it is usually necessary to clamp these ligaments separately, and often, several bites may need to be taken of each ligament. Once the tissues adjacent to the cervix and just above the cardinal ligament have been clamped, divided, and suture ligated, the blood supply to the uterus will have been sufficiently controlled for morcellation to begin. The uterine vessels are often not seen clearly and taken as a separate pedicle, but because the upper uterine blood supply to the uterus and most of that coming from the uterine arteries can be controlled laparoscopically, significant hemorrhage is much less likely than would be the case if a purely vaginal approach was used. Depending on the circumstances, the cervix can be excised or bivalved to gain access to the isthmus and lower portion of the uterus. Morcellation of the uterus then begins using three basic strategies usually in combination and at different stages of the operation.

MORCELLATION OF THE UTERUS

Bivalving, as the name implies, consists of cutting the uterus into two halves by incising its anterior and posterior walls in the midline, first with a scalpel (Figure 13.5A) and then with scissors. The incision is made anteriorly first and then posteriorly, after the posterior wall of the uterus has been elevated or a finger placed behind it to ensure that there is nothing in between the long weighted speculum in the pouch of Douglas and the back of the uterus. For relatively small uteri, i.e., those the size of a 12- to 14-week pregnancy (many of which can usually be treated by vaginal hysterectomy alone), bivalving is usually all that is necessary to excise the uterus after the cervical ligaments and uter-

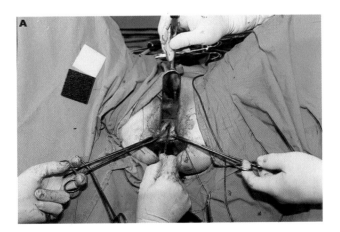

Figure 13.5A Bivalving of the uterus begins with an incision in the anterior wall of the cervix and uterus.

ine arteries have been ligated (Figures 13.5B–D). Stepwise bivalving is also part of the morcellation technique used to reduce the size of larger uteri, the purpose of the midline incisions in the anterior and posterior uterine walls being to gain access to the wall of the uterine cavity at successively higher points.

Enucleation of individual fibroids is the easiest part of morcellation and simply consists of grasping a fibroid with a strong toothed clamp to put it on tension, developing the usual plane of dissection between the fibroid and the surrounding myometrium (Figure 13.6), and extracting the fibroid as in a myomectomy (see Chapter 17). Large multiple fibroid uteri are, therefore, the easiest to remove by morcellation because the size of the uterus is readily reduced by the extraction of a few large fibroids.

Wedge resection, as the name implies, consists of excising large V-shaped segments of the uterine wall. The apex of the V-shaped segments should always lie in the midline, and the excision should be done under direct vision rather than by feel to ensure that vital structures, particularly the bladder and the rectum, are not injured in the process (Figure 13.7). This is the least satisfying, usually the bloodiest, and the most difficult strategy by which to reduce the size of a uterus. Thus, smoothly enlarged uteri are, in general, much more difficult to remove than those containing multiple fibroids.

Lash has described a *coring* technique whereby a globular uterus is converted into a tubular structure, which is easily excised. The technique consists of placing the cervix on tension and then incising the uterus subserosally more or less parallel to the serosa but with the knife inclined slightly inward. It is important to stay in the same plane and not to start multiple planes as one works one's way around the uterus with the scalpel (Figures 13.8A,B). I have personally not found this technique to be very helpful. Either the uterus is too large for it to work or, in smaller uteri, simple bivalving provides a much more expeditious method of removal. The technique does, however, come in use when bivalving is impeded by a narrow subpubic arch, and a smoothly enlarged uterus, about 12–16 weeks in size, is present.

Morcellation through Microceliotomy

Suprapubic incisions 3–5 cm in length have been used to extract fibroids from the peritoneal cavity following myomectomy (see Chapter 17). Recently, I have had occasion to use the same idea to morcellate an extremely large uterus that otherwise could not be

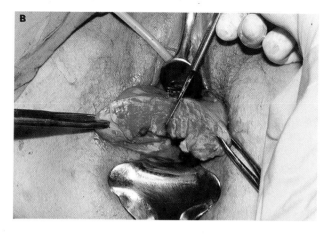

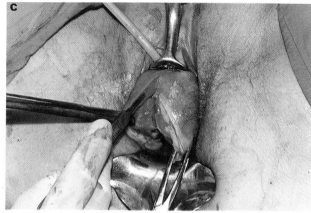

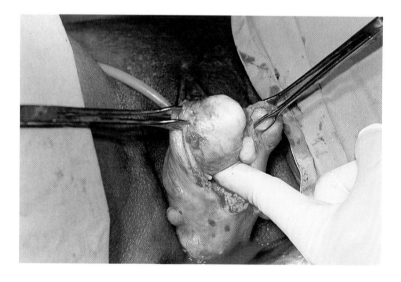

Figures 13.5B–D The uterus is completely bivalved before it is removed.

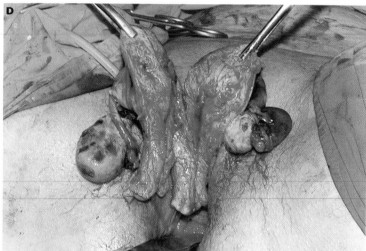

Figure 13.6 Enucleation of a fibroid during morcellation.

removed by laparoscopically assisted vaginal techniques. The patient had a 26- to 28-week size fibroid uterus, weighing 2.4 kg and containing a large submucous fibroid that effaced and dilated the cervix, making it difficult to place clamps on the cardinal lig-

ament (Figure 13.9). After it became apparent that vaginal morcellation was not going to succeed, a small suprapubic incision was made about 4 cm in length through which the uterus was morcellated by a combination of wedge resection and enucleation, with

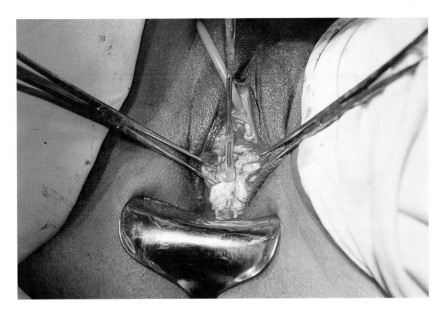

Figure 13.7 Wedge resection of the uterus during morcellation. Note that the incision is in the midline and made under direct vision.

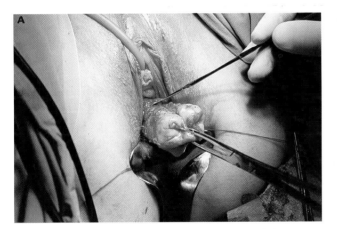

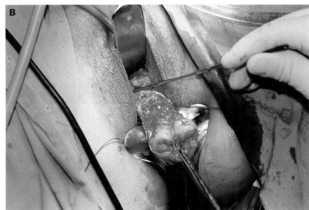

Figures 13.8A,B Coring of the uterus.

gratifying results. Marco Pelosi has also recently used this technique to remove a supracervical hysterectomy specimen (Figure 13.10).

Other Strategies

There are occasions when two other strategies, laparoscopic myomectomy and laparoscopic morcellation, are useful. Laparoscopic myomectomy (see Chapter 17) is helpful whenever one or more fibroids impede the laparoscopic part of the procedure, and prevent access to, for example, the uterine arteries. Laparoscopic morcellation, which usually consists of simply bivalving the uterus laparoscopically, is used in conjunction with vaginal morcellation when vaginal access to the fundus is seriously restricted. A combination of both techniques may be necessary. Thus, a uterus that may at first seem impossible to remove may, for example, be easily (even if laboriously) removed by laparoscopic enucleation of one or two myomata and enucleation of a cervical fibroid, prior to conventional vaginal morcellation of the uterus.

DISCUSSION

Large fibroid uteri can be very easily removed by abdominal hysterectomy because the vascular pedicles are elevated out of the pelvis as the uterus enlarges. However, a midline incision frequently has to be made and the recovery time from the operation can be substantial, ranging between six weeks to three or more months. Although it is a difficult area to study and there are not much good data available, everyone involved in the care of patients who have undergone laparoscopic hysterectomy for myomatous uteri, including the patients themselves, perceive this to be of

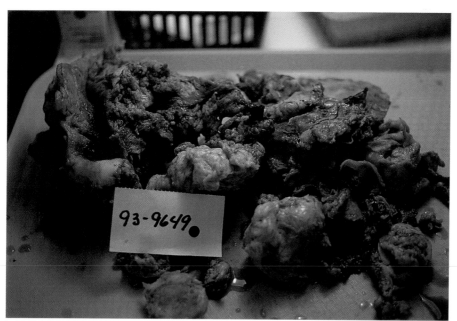

Figure 13.9 Large fibroid uterus weighing 2.4 kg was removed from a nulliparous woman by morcellation that required suprapubic microceliotomy.

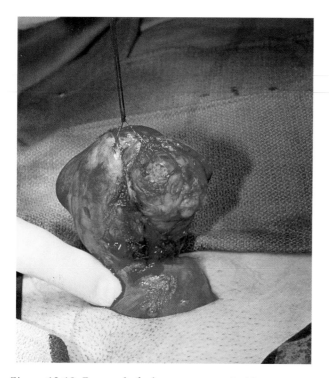

Figure 13.10 Removal of a large supracervical hysterectomy specimen with the aid of a suprapubic microceliotomy.

great advantage to them. Those who are not involved with the patient postoperatively all too frequently contrast the surgeon's seeming struggle to remove a large uterus vaginally with the effortless way in which they can be removed through a large midline incision and erroneously assume that what is easier for the surgeon (and for them) is also easier for the patient. This, how-

ever, is simply not the case, and, as Krige (2) observed many years ago, "it is a peculiar fact that the struggle in a really difficult vaginal hysterectomy is often not reflected in the patient's postoperative course." This is equally true for laparoscopic hysterectomies.

Evidence has been presented by Stovall et al. (3) purporting to show that preoperative treatment of patients with 14- to 18- week size fibroid uteri with leuprolide acetate (Lupron) induces sufficient shrinkage of the fibroids and uterus to enable a vaginal instead of an abdominal hysterectomy to be performed. This study has convinced some to use this very expensive drug for a questionable (and not FDA-approved) indication, which has become one of the biggest markets for the compound. Furthermore, the findings of this study have been used as presumptive evidence against the need for laparoscopic hysterectomy to treat fibroid uteri. Clearly, this is a study that merits careful scrutiny.

Fifty patients with fibroid uteri 14–18 weeks in size (mean ~15.5 weeks) were randomly assigned to receive Lupron or no preoperative therapy. In the control group, 21/25 (84%) women underwent an abdominal hysterectomy "as a result of uterine size more than 14 weeks gestation." In the treatment group, all women had uteri >14 weeks in size prior to treatment with Lupron, and all had uteri <14 weeks in size after treatment, although four were still considered not to be candidates for hysterectomy. Two of the 21 women in whom vaginal hysterectomy was attempted failed the attempt and sustained lacerations to the bladder or rectum. The first point to note, then, is that these authors regarded a uterine size >14 weeks as an automatic contraindication to vaginal hysterectomy, a premise that neither we nor any other experienced vaginal surgeon would accept. Moreover, 10% of the patients with uteri <14 weeks failed the attempt and sustained injuries to the bladder or rectum. Thus, Lupron allowed the vaginal hysterectomy rate to be increased from 16% to 76% but only at the risk of lacerating the bladder or rectum in 10% of cases.

Examination of the authors' Table II is revealing. Ultrasonographically determined uterine volume was reduced from a mean of 1087 ml to 723 ml by treatment, but this was not significantly different from the uterine volume in the control group (888 ml). The weight and volume (measured by water displacement) of the uteri were also measured postoperatively in the treatment and control groups, and the differences between them (65 grams and 90 ml, respectively) were again not statistically significant. In other words, the only significant difference between the treatment and control groups was in the size of the uterus as measured by palpation, i.e., subjectively. There was no significant difference in any objective measure of uterine size between the two groups.

With what then are we left? First, we have a nonblinded study sponsored by a pharmaceutical company in which large differences are claimed for therapy (a 60% difference in the vaginal hysterectomy rate), yet no objective measure of uterine size reached statistical significance between the two groups, and, *much more important*, the differences in weight and volume that were observed between the two groups were quantitatively minor (65 grams and 90 ml, respectively).

That Lupron induces a hypoestrogenic state and reduces uterine volume by 30–40% is incontestible. Whether this helps to "convert" abdominal hysterectomies into vaginal ones is, however, highly questionable and the study by Stovall et al. (3) certainly provides no support for the proposition. What this study has shown is that Lupron reduces the size of the uterus beyond an arbitrary value (14 weeks), and the authors already decided that above that arbitrary value, vaginal hysterectomy will not be performed. Thus, all the study demonstrated was that Lupron reduces the size of the uterus, which we knew already; the rest of the argument is tautologous and its premise untested.

From the volume of a sphere, it follows that to reduce volume by 30–40% requires a reduction in the radius (or diameter) of only 12–15%. For a sphere, *Volume (V)* $= 4/3\pi r^3$. Therefore, if $V_2 = 0.6 \times V_1$ (i.e., a 40% reduction), then $4/3\pi r^3 = 0.6 \times 4/3\pi r^3$ or, $r_2/r_1 = \sqrt[3]{0.6} = 0.85$, i.e., $r_2 = 0.85\,r_1$. We do not accept that a 15% difference in the radius (or diameter) of a uterus or fibroid is what separates those that can be removed vaginally from those that cannot. Moreover, there is some evidence that shrinkage of the myometrium contributes more to the reduction in volume of a fibroid uterus than shrinkage of the fibroid(s) (3).

Finally, the above study provides a perfect example of one that has a subjective end point (in this case the feasibility of vaginal hysterectomy) in which blinding was impossible (because Lupron causes amenorrhea and placebo does not), and, therefore, bias could not be eliminated, despite the fact that treatment was assigned randomly (see Chapter 25). Clearly, postrandomization decisions by the investigators can influence treatment outcome, and if the authors know which treatment the patient received, decisions that affect outcome can be influenced by that knowledge. It is impossible to be convinced by an unblinded study in which both the sponsors and the investigators have a vested interest in a positive result, especially when large differences in treatment are attributed to nonsignificant differences in objective measures of variables (in this case, uterine size) that affect outcome.

REFERENCES

1. Kadar N, Lemmerling L. Urinary tract injuries during laparoscopically assisted hysterectomy: causes and prevention. Am J Obstet Gynecol 1994;170:47–48.

2. Krige CF. The repair of genital prolapse combined with vaginal hysterectomy. J Obstet Gynaecol Br Commonw 1962;69:570–579.

3. Stovall TG, Ling FW, Henry LC, Woodruff MR. A randomized trial evaluating leuprolide acetate before hysterectomy as treatment for leiomyomas. Am J Obstet Gynecol 1991;164:1420–1425.

Part C
Operations for Benign Gynecologic Disease

Chapter 14
Laparoscopic Management
of Adnexal Masses

Nothing is so firmly believed as what we least know. —de Montaigne

The laparoscopic management of ovarian cysts and masses raises more questions than technical problems, for laparoscopic ovarian cystectomy, oophorectomy, and salpingo-oophorectomy are all very straightforward procedures, even if, as we shall see, laparoscopic ovarian cystectomy usually entails cyst rupture. If the adnexal mass is a chronic tubo-ovarian abscess or an extraperitoneal residual ovary buried in adhesions, removal of the mass may require an extensive, difficult dissection, but this would also be the case if a laparotomy was performed instead, and the dissection is no more difficult laparoscopically than at a laparotomy.

OOPHORECTOMY, SALPINGO-OOPHORECTOMY

Originally described by Semm using a Roeder (tonsillectomy) loop, removal of an ovary can easily be accomplished by placing three preknotted loops around the utero-ovarian and infundibulopelvic ligaments and dividing the ligaments with scissors (Figure 14.1). Our mistrust of the Roeder knot has swayed us away from this technique, and we use bipolar coagulation—or, more recently, Laproclips (Davis & Geck)— to desiccate (or clip) the ovarian and infundibulopelvic ligaments before dividing them. Semm's technique may, however, be somewhat quicker and worth considering if the ovaries are essentially normal, as when they are removed prophylactically, for example, in cases of familial ovarian cancer.

Salpingo-oophorectomy is no more difficult. The proximal part of the fallopian tube is desiccated with bipolar forceps and divided. The broad ligament is successively coagulated and divided until the infundibulopelvic ligament is reached and isolated. The ligament can again be either desiccated or clipped with Laproclips and divided (Figures 14.2A–C).

The ureter can be injured at two points during oophorectomy, by the infundibulopelvic ligament and below the ovarian fossa. This is most likely to occur if the ovary or pelvic sidewall is distorted and/or covered in dense adhesions, and the ureter should be

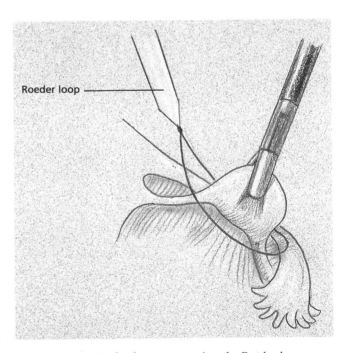

Figure 14.1 Oophorectomy using the Roeder loop.

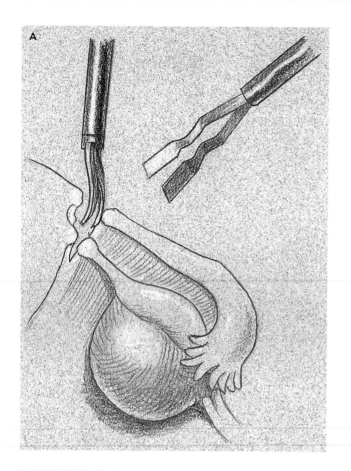

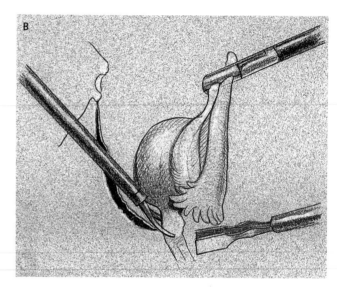

Figures 14.2A–C Salpingo-oophorectomy.

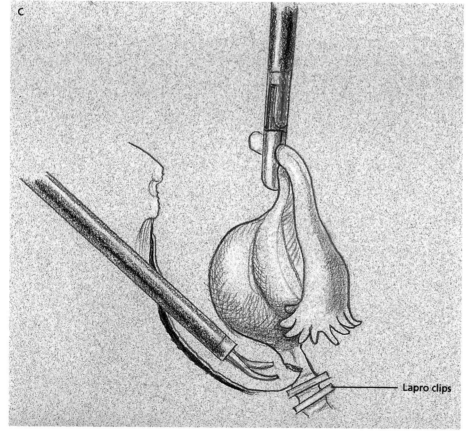

Lapro clips

identified under these circumstances. It is unlikely that the ureter will be visible through the broad ligament when the pelvic sidewall is distorted by adhesive disease, and the most expeditious way to identify it is to use the superior approach described in Chapter 7.

The pelvic sidewall peritoneum is incised lateral to the infundibulopelvic ligament, and the incision extended along the middle of the pelvic sidewall triangle in the usual way, and proximally above the pelvic brim toward the cecum (Figure 14.3A). The infundibulopelvic ligament is retracted medially and the ureter identified at the pelvic brim (Figure 14.3B). The peritoneum between the infundibulopelvic ligament and the ureter is incised and the infundibulopelvic liga-

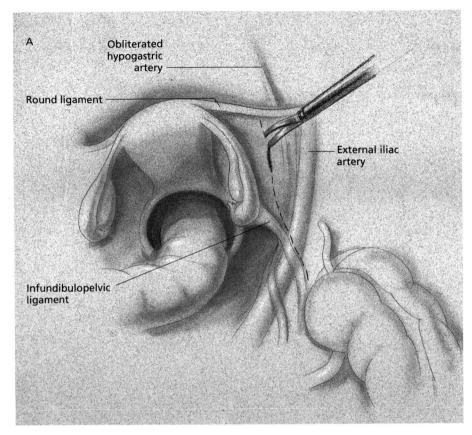

Figures 14.3A,B The pelvic sidewall triangle is opened and the ureter is identified at the pelvic brim.

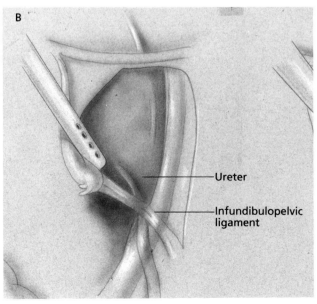

ment clipped or desiccated and divided (Figure 14.3C). The ligament is then elevated and the broad ligament incised distally to a point just beyond the ovary. The ovarian ligament ± tube are then clipped, ligated or desiccated, and the ovary ± tube are excised (Figure 14.3D).

The specimen is placed in an appropriately sized LapSac (Cook OB/GYN, Spencer, IN, USA), an impervious, polyurethane-lined nylon pouch with a drawstring (Figure 14.4). A colpotomy incision is made as described in Chapter 8, and the neck of the pouch delivered by pulling on its drawstring. If the mass is too large to extract through the colpotomy incision intact,

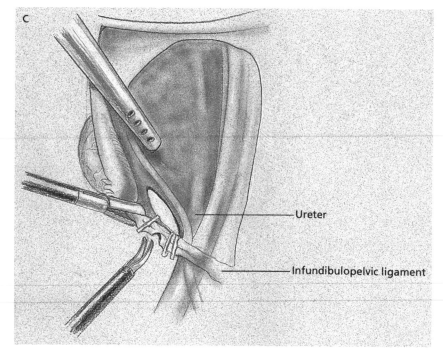

Figure 14.3C The infundibulopelvic ligament is isolated, coagulated, or clipped with Laproclips, and divided.

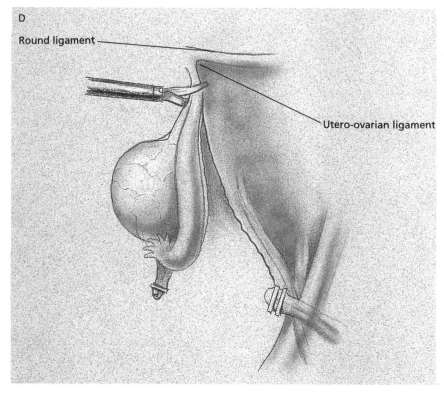

Figure 14.3D The broad ligament is incised, the tube and ovarian ligament coagulated and divided.

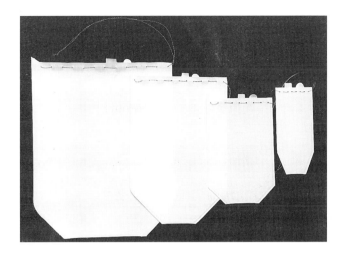

Figure 14.4 Impermeable endoscopic bags are available in varying sizes (Cook Urological).

the neck of the pouch is opened and the cyst aspirated within the pouch and, if need be, morcellated just sufficiently to deliver the pouch with its contents. The colpotomy incision is then closed with a running, nonlocking chromic stitch. The pneumoperitoneum is reestablished and the pelvis irrigated copiously.

OVARIAN CYSTECTOMY

Ovarian cysts cannot be shelled out laparoscopically as easily or as successfully as at laparotomy, and although one can attempt to remove them intact, this is usually not successful. Even if the cyst is shelled out intact, it usually ruptures on excision, although it can be placed in a LapSac and ruptured inside it to prevent spillage of its contents into the peritoneal cavity.

Before proceeding with the cystectomy, the abdomen and pelvis must be inspected and evidence of malignancy looked for, particularly on the peritoneal surfaces of the paracolic gutters, right hemidiaphragm, bowel, and greater omentum, as well as on the surface of the ovary. Washings should be taken, but they can be discarded if an obvious benign process is encountered. Adhesions should be lysed and the ovary freed.

There are two quite different ways to start the cystectomy. The cyst fluid can be aspirated or, as at laparotomy, the cortex of the ovary can be incised with a needle electrode using a low wattage, nonmodulated current. The advantages of aspiration are that release of the cyst fluid is controlled, and although spillage of the cyst contents cannot be prevented entirely, it is likely to be much less than if uncontrolled rupture of the cyst takes place. We prefer the second approach be-

cause it provides a better plane of dissection, but as soon as enough of the cyst wall has been exposed to get a good grasp, it is incised with the scissors with the suction irrigator poised to aspirate the fluid and then to be inserted into the cavity of the cyst as soon as egress of fluid stops after its wall is opened.

The ovary is stabilized by grasping the ovarian ligament, and an incision is made in the ovarian cortex with a needle electrode (Figure 14.5A). The incision should be long enough to allow the specimen to be extracted, and it usually needs to be at least half as long as the diameter of the cyst. A cleavage plane between the cyst wall and the ovarian cortex is started at the most natural point, avoiding very thinned out areas, and the plane developed bluntly as much as possible before the cyst is opened. The ovarian cortex is grasped on either side of the incision with grasping forceps and traction applied (Figure 14.5B). As the cyst wall separates from the ovary, the graspers have to be reapplied at successive points along the incision. Blunt dissection is used deeper within the ovary (Figure 14.5C). If a plane cannot be found, saline can be infiltrated under the ovarian cortex with a size 18 spinal needle (aquadissection), but we have not found this necessary, and the technique is probably more useful when the cyst is drained or ruptures prior to finding the cleavage plane.

Once a good plane has been developed, the capsule is grasped with forceps, incised with scissors, and its contents suctioned. Using two grasping forceps, the cyst wall is separated from the ovarian bed by a constant gradual pulling motion, alternating between the forceps (Figure 14.6A). If the cyst wall does not separate easily, this may be facilitated by rotating the grasping forceps and twisting the cyst wall in the same way as a hernia sac is twisted to bunch it up before its neck is ligated and divided (Figure 14.6B). Once it is excised, the cyst wall is examined for excrescences and solid areas and sent for frozen section examination. Bleeding areas within the ovary are coagulated with bipolar forceps. The edges of the ovary are trimmed back and then "inverted" by desiccating the capsule just below the cut edge (Figure 14.6C). This shrinks the tissues and causes the cut edge to curl inwards.

DISCUSSION

A great deal of controversy has surrounded the laparoscopic management of adnexal masses (1–3). That the laparoscopic management of these masses is less morbid, less costly, and causes fewer adhesions

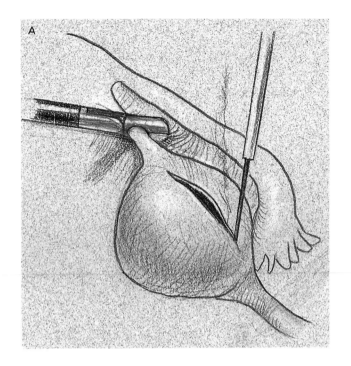

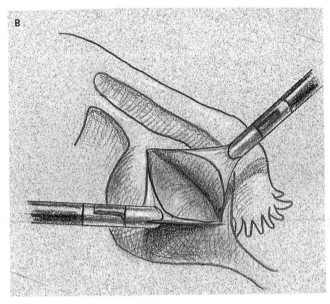

Figures 14.5A–C Ovarian cystectomy. (A) an incision is made in the cyst wall; (B) the ovarian cortex on either side of the incision is grasped and a cleavage plane developed with gentle traction; and (C) deeper layers are separated bluntly with the suction irrigator.

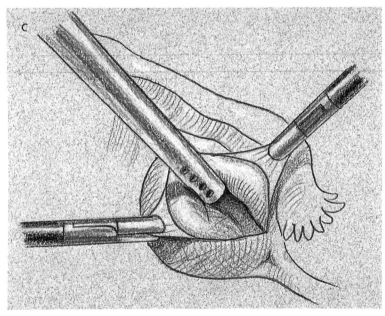

than management by laparotomy cannot be seriously questioned, nor can the potentially detrimental consequences of cyst rupture be ignored. Cysts are, of course, ruptured at laparotomy as well, but this is much more likely, indeed almost guaranteed, to occur with a laparoscopic approach, unless an oophorectomy is carried out.

The concern that rupture of a dermoid cyst would cause chemical peritonitis has been shown to be groundless, provided the pelvis is irrigated copiously after cystectomy (4,5). Indeed, to judge by the findings at second look laparoscopy, rupture of a dermoid even leaves few adhesions in its wake. The main concern, therefore, is that laparoscopic management may adversely affect the survival of the women who prove to have ovarian cancer. Presumably, this concern is based on the higher frequency of cyst rupture following laparoscopic cystectomy (and this would certainly be this author's concern), but the precise reasons have not been clearly articulated.

For example, Parker (6) has written, "Laparoscopy should not be performed in any patient with clinical or

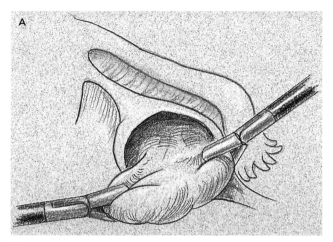

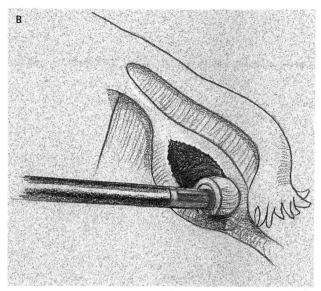

Figures 14.6A,B *The cyst wall is peeled away from the ovarian bed by (A) simple traction with grasping forceps and (B) twisting the cyst wall on itself (sardine can method).*

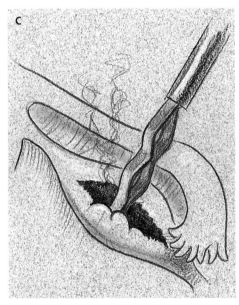

Figure 14.6C *The edges of the ovary are inverted using bipolar coagulation.*

ultrasonographic characteristics suspected of being malignant, or in any postmenopausal woman with an elevated CA-125 level," but he gave no reasons for this opinion other than to aver that "Operative laparoscopy is not appropriate when cancer is suspected," a proposition that merely begs the question, "Why?" His position is particularly difficult to understand because, by citing Dembo's (7) study, which showed no significant impairment of survival by cyst rupture in women with Stage I ovarian cancer, he pre-

sumably would not base his proscription on the possibly adverse effects of cyst rupture in the presence of a malignancy. Bruhat's group believes that cyst rupture is detrimental only if definitive therapy is delayed (8).

Whatever the precise reason, the belief that laparoscopy is inappropriate in the presence of ovarian cancer has resulted in a preoccupation with the preoperative differentiation of malignant cysts from benign ones. It is well known that this cannot be done with great precision (9–12), but what seems to be less well recognized is that the use of criteria that have a high negative predictive value necessarily entails denying women who could be managed perfectly safely without a laparotomy the benefits of laparoscopic therapy. It seems, therefore, worth reflecting on whether the laparoscopic treatment of known ovarian cancer should be considered such an anathema.

CAN OVARIAN CANCER BE MANAGED LAPAROSCOPICALLY?

Most oncologists would not countenance even the idea of treating ovarian cancers laparoscopically on the grounds that (A) one could not "debulk" the cancer through the laparoscope, and (B) one would end up rupturing localized malignancies and disseminating the cancer. These concerns are, of course, mutually exclusive, so let us explore them separately.

Tumors Cannot Be "Debulked" Laparoscopically

There is no question that huge, fixed pelvic masses that require extensive retroperitoneal dissection and often proctocolectomy and retrograde hysterectomy to remove them cannot be removed laparoscopically. But, one can usually identify women who have this type of lesion before surgery, or if not, certainly after assessing the pelvis laparoscopically. Moreover, the value of neoadjuvant chemotherapy in this setting is currently being investigated (13). Final answers are not available as yet, but we may find that neoadjuvant therapy, by shrinking the malignancy, allows us to circumvent this type of surgery altogether in many patients. Even if the disease cannot be treated laparoscopically after neoadjuvant chemotherapy has done its work, the laparoscope will still have spared the patient one laparotomy, which, given what these patients usually have to go through, is not a respite that should be dismissed lightly.

At the other extreme are cases of advanced ovarian cancer with normal-sized ovaries, a situation also referred to as primary peritoneal carcinomatosis. "Debulking" plays no part in the management of these tumors, and, although these women do usually undergo laparotomy, hysterectomy, oophorectomy, and omentectomy, it is legitimate to question what is actually being achieved by this. We would argue that surgery achieves nothing besides a diagnosis, and that these women are ideal candidates for laparoscopic management.

The majority of women with advanced ovarian cancer, probably 60–80%, have lesions in between these extremes. A proportion of these patients will have a large omental cake or large plaques of tumor involving small bowel, which will also not be suitable for laparoscopic resection. In many other cases, however, the term "debulking" is simply a way of saying total abdominal hysterectomy, bilateral salpingo-oophorectomy, and omentectomy. Although these women are often also subjected to pelvic and aortic lymphadenectomy (which, parenthetically, can be done just as well laparoscopically as we shall see), there is no evidence that this will actually benefit the patient or alter her treatment, even if it changes her stage. One report has suggested that "radical lymphadenectomy" may enhance survival in women with ovarian cancer, the implied reason being that chemotherapy cannot sterilize metastatic disease in the pelvic nodes (14). However, in as much as the survival comparison between women who had and who did not have lymphadenectomy was not adjusted for other known risk factors (besides stage), and the authors' thesis is at loggerheads with current knowledge about the pathophysiology of ovarian cancer,

these findings cannot be accepted at face value without confirmation.

Experience with laparoscopic hysterectomy in women with benign pelvic masses suggests that many of these patients could almost certainly be "debulked" laparoscopically, i.e., undergo hysterectomy, oophorectomy, and omentectomy. Although this would clearly need to be demonstrated by actual experience, it is clearly far from self-evident a priori that the laparoscopic management of advanced ovarian cancer is either misplaced or doomed to failure in most cases, as has been suggested. Tumor seeding of the abdominal wall along the trocar tract is a real and legitimate concern (2,15), but given that this is never seen in the laparotomy scars of women who have had advanced disease and ascites, prompt chemotherapy, closure of the peritoneum below the trocar insertion sites, or coagulation of the trocar tracts alone or in combination should avert this problem.

Tumor Dissemination during Laparoscopy

▶ **Oophorectomy:** Although laparoscopic cystectomy almost always involves cyst rupture, oophorectomy does not, and it is not immediately obvious that laparoscopic oophorectomy carries a greater risk of cyst rupture than open oophorectomy. The greatest risk of rupture with laparoscopic oophorectomy is during removal of the specimen, but removal without rupture has been facilitated by the availability of an impermeable bag in which the ovary can be housed during removal as well as by better techniques for colpotomy. Moreover, even if the cyst does rupture, seeding of the peritoneal cavity is much less likely with the techniques of extraction currently being used than with rupture during laparotomy. What data are available, in fact, suggest that most adnexal masses that are removed by laparoscopic oophorectomy or salpingo-oophorectomy are not ruptured in the process (16–19). Common sense suggests that the likelihood of rupture during removal increases with the size of the cyst, but the larger the cyst, the more likely the tumor is to have already disseminated, in which case the issue of rupture becomes irrelevant. Most ovarian carcinomas occur in postmenopausal women, and postmenopausal women with adnexal masses are not candidates for ovarian cystectomy. Therefore, it is unclear to this author by what line of reasoning one arrives at a proscription of laparoscopic oophorectomy in postmenopausal women with suspicious adnexal masses.

▶ Ovarian Cystectomy: The risk of tumor dissemination during laparoscopic surgery is a serious issue only if ovarian cystectomy is contemplated, and this is appropriate only in premenopausal women. The incidence of ovarian carcinoma in premenopausal women is very low, and the risk of disseminating a localized malignancy is still lower than the incidence because (1) some of the malignancies will already have disseminated by the time the diagnosis is made, and (2) the use of appropriate criteria for oophorectomy will ensure that ovarian cystectomy will not be performed on most localized malignancies. For example, Nezhat et al. (20) report finding only 3 ovarian carcinomas and 1 borderline tumor in 1101 laparoscopies for adnexal masses, and in only one of these did management result in the rupture of a Stage I ovarian carcinoma. Hulka et al. (21) report a similar experience from a survey of the 1990 AAGL membership. Thus, the presence of ultrasonographic criteria suggestive of a malignancy should be used not so much as a proscription of laparoscopy but as indications for performing laparoscopic oophorectomy in women who would otherwise have been candidates for an ovarian cystectomy. The ultrasonographic criteria of malignancy used by Parker are the presence of solid areas, papillations, and thick septa (>2 mm) in the cyst (6).

CYST RUPTURE IN STAGE I OVARIAN CARCINOMA

The case we have made for the laparoscopic management of adnexal masses has so far tacitly assumed that cyst rupture is detrimental. However, evidence that, in fact, it is is not compelling and is based on a rather poorly analyzed retrospective study from the Mayo Clinic (22). The authors analyzed 271 patients with Stage I epithelial cancer of the ovary retrospectively and found that the 5-year survival rate dropped from 90% to 56% in patients whose cysts had been ruptured. However, cyst rupture was not corrected for many other factors that affect prognosis in early stage ovarian carcinoma, such as tumor grade and adherence, so it is unclear whether it was cyst rupture per se or the factors with which cyst rupture is associated that were the key adverse prognostic factor.

The detrimental effect of cyst rupture on survival in Stage I ovarian cancer could not be confirmed in more recent retrospective studies in which multivariate analysis was used to adjust survival rates for factors that are confounded with cyst rupture. In a very large study involving over 500 patients, Dembo (7) found that cyst rupture did not influence survival in patients with Stage I carcinoma of the ovary after adjusting for the effects of grade, adherence of the cyst to surrounding structures, and penetration of the ovarian capsule. His analysis is particularly persuasive because the data used for hypothesis generation and hypothesis testing were gathered at different institutions. Similar findings have been reported from Vienna (23).

The view that cyst rupture is not in itself a significant factor in tumor dissemination is supported by the work of Poste and Fidler (24) on the metastatic process. These investigators showed that cells capable of forming metastases are phenotypically quite different from most of the cells that make up a primary tumor by virtue of having the biochemical wherewithal necessary to enter blood vessels, arrest in the capillary bed of the would-be metastatic site, egress from those blood vessels, and stimulate neovascularization as the cells replicate and organize at that site. On this view, simple mechanical dispersion of tumor cells would not in itself be sufficient to ensure the development of metastases. In experimental animals, for example, only about 0.01% of cells from a primary tumor have the capacity to form metastases following vascular dissemination. In other words, if cells possessing the metastatic phenotype are absent, mechanical dissemination of fluid within an encapsulated ovarian carcinoma will not result in dissemination of those cells within the peritoneal cavity. *Per contra*, if cells capable of forming metastases are already present, then they will metastasize even without rupture of the cyst.

SUMMARY

The fear of adversely affecting the prognosis of women whose adnexal masses prove to be malignant has raised concern over the laparoscopic management of these masses, particularly in postmenopausal women. Most protocols for the laparoscopic management of adnexal masses are based on the premise that ovarian carcinoma cannot be properly managed laparoscopically and focus on trying to identify masses that are likely to be malignant with a view to avoiding laparoscopy in these patients. However, if careful consideration is given to what the purpose of surgery in the management of ovarian carcinoma is, it becomes readily apparent that much of what has to be done surgically can be carried out just as well laparoscopically as via a laparotomy. Careful preoperative evaluation should identify women who have masses that are too large to be extracted without rupture and large, fixed pelvic or upper abdominal masses that cannot be removed laparoscopically. Unless the cyst is extremely large or there is a large fixed pelvic mass or omental cake, a diagnostic laparoscopy is warranted if the surgeon is experienced at laparoscopic surgery and can complete therapy laparoscopically.

REFERENCES

1. Maiman M, Seltzer V, Boyce J. Laparoscopic excision of ovarian neoplasms subsequently found to be malignant. Obstet Gynecol 1991;77:563–565.

2. Gleeson NC, Nicosia SV, Mark JE, Hofman MS, Cavanagh D. Abdominal wall metastases from ovarian cancer after laparoscopy. Am J Obstet Gynecol 1993;169:522–523.

3. Moore DH. Laparoscopic management of persistent ovarian masses: reasons against. In: Hulka J, Reich H, eds. Textbook of Laparoscopy, Philadelphia: WB Saunders, 1994, pp 256-258.

4. Nezhat C, Winder WK, Nezhat F. Laparoscopic removal of dermoid cysts. Obstet Gynecol 1989; 73:278–281.

5. Reich H, McGlynn F, Sekel L, Taylor P. Laparoscopic management of ovarian dermoid cysts. J Reprod Med 1992; 37:640–644.

6. Parker WH. Management of adnexal masses by operative laparoscopy: selection criteria. J Reprod Med 1992; 37:603–606.

7. Dembo AJ, Davy M, Stenwig AE, Berle EJ, Bush RS, Kjorstad AK. Prognostic factors in patients with stage I epithelial ovarian cancer. Obstet Gynecol 1990;75; 263–273.

8. Parker WH, Nezhat F, Canis M. Laparoscopic ovarian surgery. J Am Assoc Gynecol Laparosc 1993;1:78–84.

9. Herrmann UJ, Locher GW, Goldhirsch AA. Sonographic patterns of ovarian tumors: prediction of malignancy. Obstet Gynecol 1987;69:77–81.

10. Luxman D, Bergman A, Sagi J, David MP. The postmenopausal adnexal mass: a correlation between ultrasonic and pathologic findings. Obstet Gynecol 1991; 77:726–728.

11. Weiner Z, Thaler I, Beck D, Rottem S, Deutsch M, Brandes JM. Differentiating malignant from benign ovarian tumors with transvaginal color flow imaging. Obstet Gynecol 1992;79:159–162.

12. Hata K, Hata T, Manabe A, Sugimura K, Kitao M. A critical evaluation of transvaginal Doppler studies, transvaginal sonography, magnetic resonance imaging, and CA 125 in detecting ovarian cancer. Obstet Gynecol 1992;80:922–926.

13. Jacob JH, Gershenson DM, Morris M, Copeland LJ, Burke TW, Wharton JT. Neoadjuvant chemotherapy and interval debulking for advanced epithelial ovarian cancer. Gynecol Oncol 1991;42:146–150.

14. Burghardt E, Pickel H, Labousen M, Stettner H. Pelvic lymphadenectomy in operative treatment of ovarian cancer. Am J Obstet Gynecol 1986;155:2:315–319.

15. Hsiu J, Given FT, Kemp GM. Tumor implantation after diagnostic laparoscopic biopsy of serous ovarian tumors of low malignant potential. Obstet Gynecol 1986; 68:90–93.

16. Bratschi HU, Heiz B. Video laparoscopy in total removal of ovarian tumors of uncertain origin in a bag through posterior colpotomy. (Abstract) Presented at 2nd European Congress in Gynecological Endoscopy and New Surgical Techniques, Heidelberg, October 21–23, 1993. Gynaecol Endosc 1994;3:23.

17. Hettenbach A, Possover M, Morawski A. Laparoscopic surgery of ovarian tumors in post menopausal women. (Abstract) Presented at 2nd European Congress in Gynecological Endoscopy and New Surgical Techniques, Heidelberg, October 21–23, 1993;60. Gynaecol Endosc 1994;3:34.

18. Ottersen T. Laparoscopic (plastic bag) surgery: What are the benefits? (Abstract) Presented at 2nd European Congress in Gynecological Endoscopy and New Surgical Techniques, Heidelberg, October 21–23, 1993;93. Gynaecol Endosc 1994;3:43.

19. Ulrich U. The use of endobags in operative laparoscopy. (Abstract) Presented at 2nd European Congress in Gynecological Endoscopy and New Surgical Techniques, Heidelberg, October 21–23, 1993;158. Gynaecol Endosc 1994;3:59.

20. Nezhat F, Nezhat C, Welander CE, Benigno B. Four ovarian cancers diagnosed during laparoscopic management of 1011 women with adnexal masses. Am J Obstet Gynecol 1992;167:790–796.

21. Hulka JF, Parker WH, Surrey MW, Phillips JM. Management of ovarian masses. AAGL 1990 Survey. J Reprod Med 1992; 37:599–602.

22. Webb MJ, Decker D, Mussey E, Williams TJ. Factors influencing survival in stage I ovarian cancer. Am J Obstet Gynecol 1973;116:222–226.

23. Sevelda P, Dittrich C, Salzer H. Prognostic value of the rupture of the capsule in stage I epithelial ovarian carcinoma. Gynecol Oncol 1989;35:321–322.

24. Poste G, Fidler I. The pathogenesis of cancer metastasis. Science 1980;283:139–146.

Chapter 15
Ectopic Pregnancy and Linear Salpingostomy, Salpingectomy

What is now proved was once only imagined.
—*Blake*

The diagnosis and treatment of extrauterine pregnancies has undergone truly remarkable, indeed, revolutionary, changes over the last 10–15 years. The diagnosis can now be made nonsurgically in most patients by the combined use of ultrasound and serum hCG measurements (either single or serial), and many patients can be managed nonsurgically, either with parenteral methotrexate or expectantly. These developments have served to wed diagnosis and therapy because if the diagnosis can be made without laparoscopy, nonsurgical therapy becomes much more attractive. Only some aspects of these developments can be discussed here, and a more detailed discussion is available elsewhere (1).

DIAGNOSIS

A nonsurgical approach to the diagnosis of ectopic pregnancy was first described by the author in 1981 (2). Many minor variations of the original algorithm have been devised, but all involve the combined use of ultrasound and a sensitive hCG assay and serial hCG testing in some patients. The value of serial hCG testing as originally described, although questioned by some, has been repeatedly validated (3–5) and extended to cases with falling hCG value (6). Valid estimates and fiducial limits for the discriminatory zone have also been made for vaginal sonography (7). The diagnostic workup that remains valid to this day is summarized below.

Briefly, women of childbearing age complaining of abdominal pain and/or abnormal vaginal bleeding are examined and a urinary pregnancy test is performed. Urinary (ELISA) pregnancy tests are now sensitive enough for a negative result to exclude the diagnosis for practical purposes. If the pregnancy test is positive, a vaginal ultrasound is performed, which will allow a definitive diagnosis of ectopic or intrauterine pregnancy to be made in 50–70% of cases. If the ultrasound findings are nondiagnostic and the patient clinically stable, the serum hCG concentration is measured by radioimmunoassay, and if the concentration is >3000 mlU/ml, a presumptive diagnosis of ectopic pregnancy is made. If the serum hCG concentration is <3000 mlU/ml, the serum hCG concentration is measured 48 hours later, and the doubling time or half-life of hCG calculated. Fortunately, there is now only one hCG standard available, and all hCG assays are standardized against it. The standard, formerly called the International Reference Preparation (IRP or 1st-IRP) has been renamed by the World Health Organization the Third International Standard (3rd IS).

Some have advocated algorithms based on a serum progesterone measurements instead (8). The use of serum progesterone measurements had its origins in the observation by Radwanska et al. (9) that the serum progesterone increased little during the first trimester of normal pregnancy and that serum progesterone concentrations were lower in ectopic and aborting pregnancies than in normal intrauterine ones. Thus, it appeared that an age-independent measurement was available in the first trimester that might be useful in differentiating normal and abnormal pregnancies. Rather implausibly, Mathews et al. (10) and

Yeko et al. (11) subsequently claimed that ectopic and nonectopic gestations could be differentiated with 100% reliability on the basis of a single serum progesterone determination, an observation that has, of course, not withstood the test of time (12–14). Although Stovall and colleagues still favor a diagnostic algorithm centered on a serum progesterone concentration (9,15), in agreement with others (16), we have not found this to be at all useful in practice (14).

Although it is true that normal intrauterine pregnancies have progesterone concentrations >5 ng/ml, and ectopic pregnancies are rarely associated with serum progesterone concentrations >25 ng/ml, most women with suspected ectopic pregnancies will have values in between these extremes, and the progesterone level will add nothing but cost to the diagnostic workup. Moreover, if the serum progesterone concentration is >25 ng/ml, the serum hCG is almost always >3000 mIU/ml and vaginal ultrasound will be diagnostic of either an intrauterine or an ectopic pregnancy, and the progesterone concentration adds nothing here either. Finally, although a serum progesterone concentration <5 ng/ml establishes that a pregnancy is nonviable, failure to detect villi in a curettage specimen from these cases does not necessarily mean that an ectopic pregnancy is present, as has been suggested by the Tennessee group, nor do falling hCG levels necessarily signify that an aborting intrauterine rather than a tubal pregnancy is present (3). Thus, only a very small proportion of women with suspected ectopic pregnancies and nondiagnostic sonar findings will, in fact, have missed abortions associated with progesterone levels below 5 ng/ml and positive curettage specimens, and a correct diagnosis can be made in these patients without the serum progesterone value.

SELECTION OF THERAPY

The optimal surgical management of tubal pregnancies has been a matter for debate since the turn of this century, and remains so today. The debate originally centered on whether to save or remove the affected tube, and subsequently on what type of operation to perform both if the tube was to be removed or conserved. The advent of laparoscopic surgery did little to resolve these questions because each type of operation could be performed laparoscopically just as well as by laparotomy. Rather, it increased controversy because added questions were raised first about the safety and then about the efficacy of these laparoscopic operations. Even before published data clearly established the advantages of laparoscopic surgery, however, the debate moved on to where it is today, focused on the place of nonsurgical therapy.

Compounding the plethora of treatment options available has been the inability to interpret the results obtained with different operations because pregnancy rates after surgery (both tubal and intrauterine) have rarely been adjusted for the many other factors besides treatment that affect outcome following the treatment of a tubal pregnancy. It is, therefore, hardly surprising that identical operations yielded statistics as disparate as, for example, live birth rates of 100% and 50%, and recurrent ectopic pregnancy rates of 0% and 20% (17,18).

Despite these uncertainties, a number of procedures were, with justification, consigned to the dustbin of surgical history, namely, resection of the ampulla, cornual resection at the time of salpingectomy, and, under almost all circumstances, "milking" of the tube and salpingo-oophorectomy. It also became apparent, doubtless to the silent relief of laparoscopists, that salpingostomy incisions did not require closure and that salpingostomy yielded results comparable to segmental tubal resection, except perhaps in the case of isthmic pregnancies. Thus, one was essentially left with a choice between salpingectomy and salpingostomy, a choice that simply took one back to the original debate over the relative merits of conservative and ablative operations.

Salpingostomy Versus Salpingectomy

Whether we like it or not, and despite little conclusive support from published data, it is now widely accepted that a conservative operation is almost always to be preferred over an ablative one for women who are desirous of future childbearing. It is not our intention here to try to resolve this controversy, which has been with us for almost a century, not the least because it is impossible to settle it dispassionately with the evidence at hand. Suffice it to say that despite incontrovertible evidence that salpingostomy can restore the reproductive function of an oviduct after a tubal pregnancy and that repeat ectopic pregnancies are distributed with equal frequency between the conserved tubes and the contralateral ones, it does not follow that preservation of the tube, when the patient has another functional one, will increase her chance of bearing a living child without increasing her risk of having another ectopic pregnancy (19). In fact, most case series show no indication that tubal conservation increases subsequent live birth rates (20–23), and many show it to be associated with a trend toward higher recurrent ectopic pregnancy rates. It is also incontestable that complications (hemorrhage, persistent trophoblast), however few, are more frequent after salpingostomy than after salpingectomy, which makes salpingostomy contraindicated in women who do not wish to bear more children. Despite these uncertainties, however, solid indications for salpingostomy can be identified, as discussed more fully elsewhere (19).

Tubal conservation is clearly indicated if the pregnancy is located in a woman's only remaining tube, or if the contralateral tube is blocked. The procedure is about three times more likely to result in a live birth than in vitro fertilization, and if conception occurs, a term pregnancy is at least twice as likely as an ectopic pregnancy. Tubal conservation is contraindicated if the contralateral tube and ovary appear to be normal and patent on intraoperative chromotubation, but the gravid tube shows evidence of preexisting disease or has been operated on before either for a previous ectopic pregnancy or blockage, although these circumstances are not common. When both tubes show evidence of prior disease, the decision to conserve the gravid tube when it has been operated upon previously or when it appears to have been damaged much more than the opposite one is not an easy one and has to be made on an individual basis, using as one's guide the extent to which the gravid tube has been damaged both in absolute terms (amount of scarring, mobility, and length) and relative to the other side.

If the contralateral adnexum appears to be completely normal and patent at intraoperative chromotubation, the case for tubal conservation is not very compelling. Those who favor salpingostomy argue that if a salpingectomy is performed and an ectopic pregnancy recurs, the opportunity to save what is then the only remaining tube may not present itself. This is the strongest argument justifying salpingostomy under these circumstances, but it is a weak one, since this eventuality is likely to occur in <5% of cases after salpingectomy. It has also been argued that intraoperative chromotubation is unreliable and that a normal appearing tube may nonetheless be diseased. However, the problem with chromotubation is that a patent tube may appear blocked (usually because blood and/or decidua occlude the cornua), and patency on intraoperative chromotubation is clearly a valid finding. The case against salpingostomy is that when the contralateral tube and ovary are normal, even the most favorable results obtained show no increase in the sub-

sequent live birth rate, but tubal conservation probably does increase the recurrent tubal pregnancy rate even if only by about 5%, and the risk of early and late postoperative hemorrhage is also greater.

Based on the available information, therefore, one can legitimately adopt either a conservative or an ablative operation in the presence of a normal contralateral adnexa. For example, if the pregnancy in the tube is small and unruptured and shells out easily at salpingostomy without bleeding, the tube should almost certainly be conserved. However, if there is a large ruptured tubal pregnancy present or, after attempting a salpingostomy, there is persistent bleeding from the tube, one should have a much lower "threshold" for removing the gravid tube if the contralateral adnexa are normal than if the affected tube is the patient's only oviduct or if the contralateral adnexa are severely diseased.

Salpingostomy Versus Segmental Resection

Segmental tubal resection or partial salpingectomy is the procedure of choice whenever a gravid oviduct is to be conserved but its wall is ruptured or there is persistent or uncontrollable bleeding from the tube following salpingostomy. Although segmental resection with primary or delayed anastomosis has been advocated for the treatment of all tubal pregnancies on the grounds that salpingostomy conserves what is an abnormal implantation site, there is no evidence that better results are obtained by resecting the implantation site than by salpingostomy. Salpingostomy, therefore, remains the conservative operation of choice for tubal pregnancies.

There is persuasive evidence that the reproductive performance of women following conservative surgery for a tubal pregnancy is less good if the pregnancy is located in the isthmus rather than the ampulla. Hallatt (24) stated, without giving figures, that the intrauterine-to-ectopic pregnancy ratio after conservative surgery was about four times higher when the pregnancy was located in the ampulla as opposed to the isthmus. Pouly et al. (25) reported that intrauterine pregnancy rates following laparoscopic salpingostomy were 64/96 (67%) for ampullary pregnancies and 12/22 (55%) for isthmic pregnancies; the recurrent tubal pregnancy rates were 18/96 (19%) and 8/22 (36%), respectively.

Whether the reproductive performance of women with isthmic pregnancies is any better following segmental tubal resection than after salpingostomy remains, however, far from clear. DeCherney and Boyes

(26) have argued strongly that it is, but their argument is based on rather meager evidence. In a retrospective audit, they found that 3 of 4 women with unruptured isthmic pregnancies who were treated by salpingostomy had tubal occlusion on hysterosalpingography and none conceived, whereas 3/6 women who were treated by segmental resection and delayed anastomosis delivered live infants and 1/6 women so treated had a recurrent tubal pregnancy. However, these authors' dismal experience with salpingostomy in isthmic pregnancies was reflected neither in the results obtained by Pouly et al. (25) with laparoscopic salpingostomy nor in a subsequent, randomized, prospective clinical study reported by Smith et al. (27).

These authors randomly allocated the treatment of women with unruptured isthmic pregnancies to segmental resection and anastomosis (four cases) or to salpingostomy (nine cases). [Some cases randomized to segmental resection, in fact, had a salpingostomy if a tubal surgeon was not available, and cases of ruptured isthmic pregnancies were treated by segmental tubal resection alone (seven cases)]. All four tubes that were primarily anastomosed following segmental resection were patent on subsequent hysterosalpingogram (HSG), and one of the two women who were actively trying to conceive had an intrauterine pregnancy (IUP). Four of the nine women treated with salpingostomy subsequently had IUPs (two having delivered at the time of the report), while five were using contraception. Because the number of patients studied was so small, no meaning can be attached to the lack of statistical significance between the differences in outcome in the different treatment groups. Nonetheless, inasmuch as all women who tried to become pregnant after salpingostomy conceived IUPs, the results provide a striking contrast to those reported by DeCherney and Boyes (26).

The optimal treatment of unruptured isthmic pregnancies must, therefore, be considered *sub judice* because the available data do not provide compelling evidence for treating women with isthmic and ampullary pregnancies differently. Because salpingostomy is a much simpler operation, it should still be regarded as the operation of choice, certainly as far as the general gynecologist is concerned.

Laparoscopic Versus Abdominal Salpingostomy

The credit for pioneering the laparoscopic treatment of ectopic pregnancy belongs to Professor Bruhat and his colleagues in France, who were the first to perform laparoscopic salpingostomy and fimbrial expression, and who, during the 10-year period 1974–1984, treated 321 cases of tubal pregnancy endoscopically (26) and currently treat over 90% of tubal gestations in this way. Despite early skepticism, there are abundant data, including some from randomized trials, to show that compared with the open operation, laparoscopic salpingostomy is associated with shorter hospital stay, a shorter postoperative convalescence, and a reduced requirement for analgesia after surgery as well as less postoperative adhesion formation (28–31). Live birth rates are similar, but the recurrent ectopic pregnancy rate, surprisingly enough, tends to be lower for reasons that are unclear (19,29).

The only absolute contraindication to laparoscopy is a hemodynamically unstable patient. Initially, the procedure was considered applicable only to a very select group of patients (unruptured ampullary pregnancies <3 cm in size, otherwise normal pelvis and contralateral tube), but Reich et al. (32) were among the first to show that virtually all tubal pregnancies could be managed endoscopically unless the patient was hemodynamically unstable.

Laparoscopic Versus Nonsurgical Therapy

Although the nonsurgical management of ectopic pregnancies has been shown to be feasible and safe, the selection criteria used for medical management have been ill-defined and variable. Two aspects of nonsurgical therapy have become fairly well established: (1) conservative therapy is ill-advised if a heart beat is detected ultrasonographically, and (2) intratubal injection of chemotherapeutic agents is associated with an unacceptably high failure rate. It has been known for a long time that some tubal pregnancies resorb spontaneously without treatment, and we would consider observation alone with no active intervention to be an appropriate way to manage women with ectopic pregnancies who have minimal symptoms, hCG concentrations <1000 mIU/ml, and falling hCG levels (half-life <1.5 days) (33). The type of patient who goes on to have a chronic ectopic pregnancy needs to be better defined, however. Women who have relatively small (<3 cm) unruptured pregnancies can also be managed with a single, intramuscular dose of methotrexate 50 mg/m² provided a heart beat cannot be detected on ultrasound, a hemoperitoneum (fluid) is not present, and serum hCG levels are increasing subnormally (doubling time >2.7 days) and, preferably, plateauing (33). Carson and Buster (8) recently compiled published statistics pertaining to the medical management of tubal pregnancies and found that the tubal patency rate among those tested (about a third of the total treated) was 81%, the live birth rate was 71% and 11% had recurrent ectopic pregnancies. Inasmuch as women treated nonsurgically are highly selected, the temptation to compare these figures with those obtained by surgery should be resisted.

OPERATIVE TECHNIQUES

Linear Salpingostomy

The pneumoperitoneum is obtained with the usual direct trocar insertion technique, and the usual trocar arrangement is used except that the lateral trocar on side contralateral to the pregnancy is often not required. Also, a 10-mm trocar is placed suprapubically and the specimen extracted through it. If the pregnancy is too large, the trocar site can be easily enlarged using the gall bladder extractor, as described in Chapter 8, and/or the specimen can be morcellated in the cul-de-sac.

The pelvis is evaluated carefully to determine if a laparoscopic approach is feasible. Special attention is paid to the amount of active bleeding, the size and site of the pregnancy, and the contralateral adnexa. If there is any doubt about contralateral tubal patency, we use intraoperative chromopertubation. If laparoscopic salpingostomy is felt to be feasible, the tube is stabilized and put on stretch, if possible without actually grasping the tube. A dilute vasopressin solution (20 U in 100 ml normal saline) is injected into the antimesenteric border of the tube along the line of the proposed incision, which should be about two-thirds or three-quarters of the length of the swelling in the tube. (The mesosalpinx is no longer infiltrated because it is easy to cause both bleeding and intravascular injection of the vasopressin, which will cause hypertension and bradycardia.) The tube is then incised using a needle electrode and a nonmodulated current (Figures 15.1A,B). Clot and tissue in the tube is then removed gently with grasping forceps, but tissue that will not separate easily is left behind (Figure 15.1C). Attempts to strip this tissue off the decidual bed in the tube will cause uncontrollable bleeding. The tube is then irrigated copiously to remove additional debris, and the area just beyond the proximal and distal end of the tube is gently explored with grasping forceps to ensure that all material has been removed (Figure 15.1D).

There will usually be some bleeding points. These can be controlled with point cautery using a blended current or by simple pressure with nontraumatic for-

ceps. Occasionally, coagulation of the mesosalpinx below the site of the pregnancy will help stop bleeding from the implantation site, but continued bleeding may necessitate partial salpingectomy (see below).

All tissue removed from the tube must also be removed from the peritoneal cavity; otherwise, some of the retained fragments can implant secondarily on the peritoneal surfaces of the pelvis, bowel, omentum, etc. If the tubal pregnancy is large, it may need to be cut into small pieces in the cul-de-sac before it is removed through the suprapubic trocar.

Salpingectomy

Laparoscopic salpingectomy is a very straightforward procedure. The proximal part of the fallopian tube and the underlying mesosalpinx are coagulated with Kleppinger forceps and divided. The mesosalpinx is then successively coagulated and divided and the tube removed (Figures 15.2A,B). Some prefer to place a Roeder loop around the distal part of the tube before dividing it (Figure 15.2C). The specimen is removed through a 10-mm suprapubic trocar after prior morcellation, if necessary, as previously described.

Partial Salpingectomy

The segment of tube containing the pregnancy can be removed if there is persistent bleeding after salpingostomy or there is tubal rupture. The oviduct is coagulated with Kleppinger forceps on either side of the distention caused by the pregnancy and then divided. The mesosalpinx is then coagulated and divided, and the involved segment excised (Figures 15.3A,B). Alternatively, a Roeder-type loop can be placed around the proximal and distal limbs of the involved segment (Figure 15.3C). It is important to make sure that the proximal segment is occluded at the end of the procedure unless a primary tubal reanastomosis is carried out. The specimen is then removed as previously described.

PERSISTENT ECTOPIC PREGNANCY

In at least 40% of tubal pregnancies, the trophoblast penetrates the tubal wall and some trophoblastic tissue is, therefore, left behind if the implantation site is not removed, as is the case with a salpingostomy. Usually, however, this tissue degenerates, but in about 5% of cases, instead of resorbing, the residual trophoblastic tissue persists and resumes growing, until the patient eventually develops symptoms again from intraperitoneal hemorrhage or a pelvic mass. The fre-

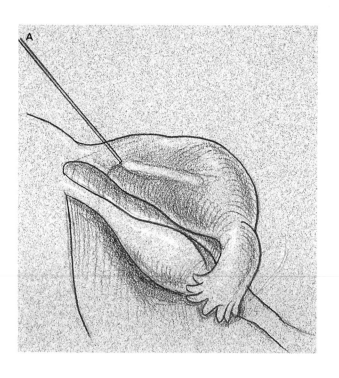

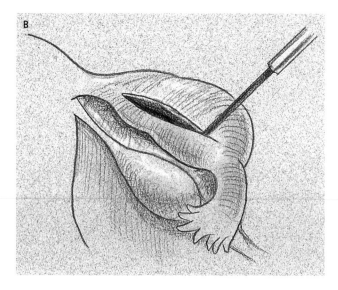

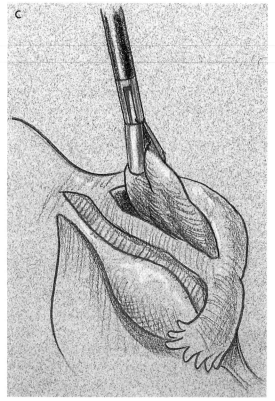

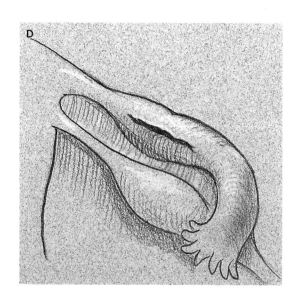

Figures 15.1A–D Linear salpingostomy.

quency of this complication is ill-defined, probably subject to considerable publication bias, and depends on how "persistence" is defined. It is also slightly more common after laparoscopic salpingostomy than ab-dominal salpingostomy. Stock (35), however, attrib-utes the problem to incomplete evacuation of the tro-phoblastic tissue, and, intuitively, the author feels he is probably correct.

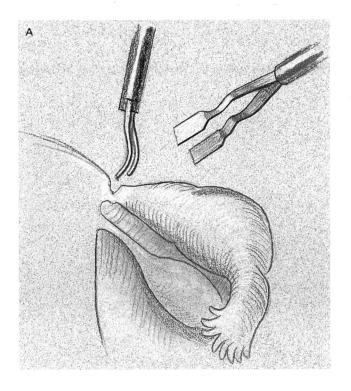

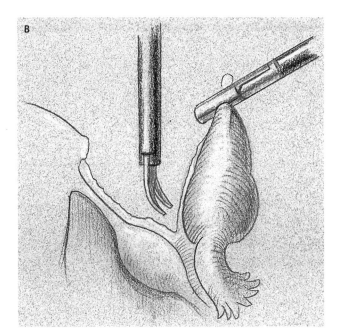

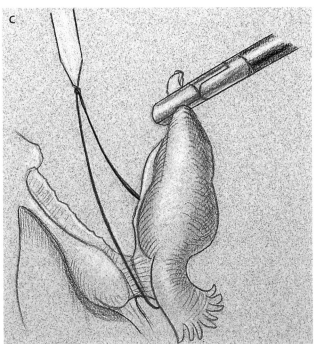

Figures 15.2A–C Salpingectomy.

Symptomatically, persistent ectopic pregnancies present with signs of intraperitoneal hemorrhage or pain referable to a pelvic mass usually 10 days or more after the original surgery and, occasionally, as early as a week later (36). Serial hCG monitoring after conservative operations has been instituted in the hope of forestalling this problem by identifying persistent trophoblastic activity at an asymptomatic stage.

hCG Monitoring Following Conservative Surgery

Several tacit assumptions underlie the policy of screening for residual trophoblastic activity follow-

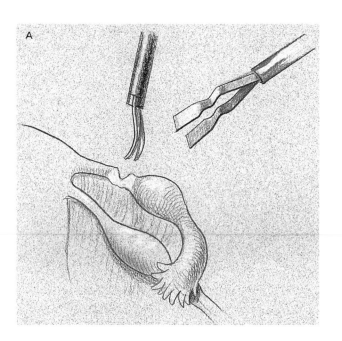

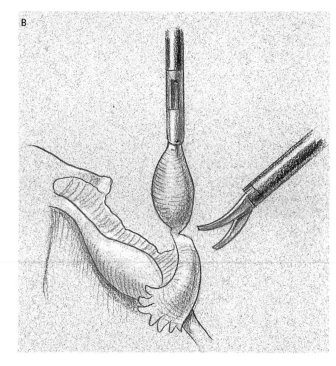

Figures 15.3A–C Partial salpingectomy.

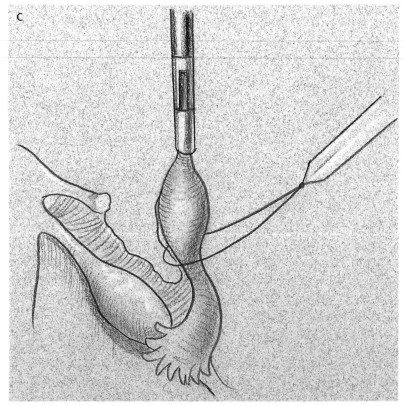

ing conservative surgery for tubal pregnancy. The first assumption is that in the absence of residual functioning trophoblast, the serum hCG will fall unabatedly and in a predictable manner. The second assumption is that a period of renewed trophoblastic growth is required for symptoms to develop. The third assumption is that during this preclinical stage, renewed trophoblastic growth will manifest itself first by a delayed rate of fall in the serum hCG levels and, eventually, by rising serum hCG values.

Vermesh et al. (36) described the use of serial postoperative hCG and progesterone measurements following the conservative operative treatment of tubal pregnancies. They found that even in patients with persistent trophoblastic activity, hCG levels fell precipitously in the early postoperative period, reaching 13–25% of the baseline value by 3 days after surgery and 6–25% by 6 days. Thereafter, the serum hCG between the "persistent ectopic" and the "resolved ectopic" groups diverged, there being no overlap at all between the groups by the 12th postoperative day. However, the definition of persistent trophoblastic activity was not made totally clear in the paper inasmuch as 2/6 patients with this diagnosis had continually decreasing hCG values and were managed by simple observation.

"Normal" limits for the rate of hCG clearance are difficult to define because the dynamics of hCG clearance are rather complex, involving at least two half-lives (an initial half-life of 5–6 hours, and a second, slower one of 11–38 hours). The between patient variation in the rate of hCG clearance is also large. Part of the reason may be that, unless a pregnancy is terminated by salpingectomy or hysterectomy, some trophoblast is always disseminated into the circulation and will continue to secrete hCG. In tubal pregnancies, the presence or absence of trophoblastic tissue within the tubal wall is an added factor that complicates and increases the variability of hCG clearance rates. Consequently, no hCG pattern invariably presages continued trophoblastic growth or predicts resolution of the pregnancy.

Because the bulk of the trophoblast is always removed during surgery (barring gross technical errors), hCG levels invariably fall precipitously during the first few days after surgery, even in patients destined to develop symptoms from continued trophoblastic growth. There is, therefore, no merit in measuring the hCG concentration earlier than a week after surgery because hCG levels in women with persistent and resolving trophoblastic activity overlap before this time (36). hCG measurements should, therefore, commence a week following conservative surgery, but the optimal method of monitoring patients has not been defined, and few studies have been undertaken to identify those at particular risk for developing this problem. Those who have an hCG concentration >1000 mIU/ml a week after surgery are probably at greater risk (37), and hCG titers should be monitored every 3 days. If the level is less than 1000 mIU/ml a week after surgery, titers can be obtained at weekly intervals until they become negative or at least <100 mIU/ml.

In the absence of symptoms, intervention is not indicated so long as hCG levels continue to fall, however slowly. Rising values are more ominous but do not by any means invariably presage continued trophoblastic growth. A reasonable compromise between overtreatment and undertreatment is to intervene if the rate of increase is "normal," i.e., doubling time <2.7 days, or to follow subnormally increasing titers for a few days with repeat measurements to ensure that the rising pattern persists (because it often does not) before intervening. We intervene with chemotherapy and have always used methotrexate 50 mg/m² intramuscularly, which we know works in uncomplicated trophoblastic disease.

REFERENCES

1. Kadar N. Diagnosis and treatment of extrauterine pregnancies. New York: Raven Press, 1990.

2. Kadar N, Caldwell BV, Romero R. A method of screening for ectopic pregnancy and its indications. Obstet Gynecol 1981;58:162–165.

3. Kadar N, Romero R. Further observations on serial hCG patterns in ectopic pregnancy and abortions. Fertil Steril 1988;50:367-370.

4. Dàya S. Human chorionic gonadotropin increase in normal early pregnancy. Am J Obstet Gynecol 1987;156:286-290.

5. Fritz MA, Guo S. Doubling time of human chorionic gonadotropin (hCG) in early normal pregnancy: relationship to hCG concentration and gestational age. Fertil Steril 1987;47:584-589.

6. Kadar N, Bohrer M, Kemman E, Sheldon R. The hCG-time relationship in early gestation: a prospective randomized study. Fertil Steril 1993;60:409-412.

7. Kadar N, Bohrer M, Kemman E, Shelden R. The discriminatory hCG zone for endovaginal sonography: a prospective, randomized study. Fertil Steril 1994;61:1016:1020.

8. Carson SA, Buster JE. Ectopic pregnancy. N Engl J Med 1993;329:1174–1181.

9. Radwanska E, Frankenberg J, Allen E. Plasma progesterone levels in normal and abnormal early human pregnancy. Fertil Steril 1978;30:398-402.

10. Mathews CP, Coulson PB, Wild RA. Serum progesterone levels as an aid in the diagnosis of ectopic pregnancy. Obstet Gynecol 1986;68:390-394.

11. Yeko TR, Gorrill MJ, Hughes LH, et al. Timely diagnosis of early ectopic pregnancy using a single blood progesterone measurement. Fertil Steril 1987;48:1048-1050.

12. Buck RH, Joubert SM, Norman RJ. Serum progesterone in the diagnosis of ectopic pregnancy: a valuable diagnostic test. Fertil Steril 1988;50:752-755.

13. Hubinont CJ, Thomas C, Schwers JF. Luteal function in ectopic pregnancy. Am J Obstet Gynecol 1987;156:669-674.

14. Kadar N, Blumenthal S. Serum progesterone levels in ectopic pregnancy. Infertility 1992;15:7–17.

15. Stovall TG, Ling FW, Cope BJ, et al. Preventing ruptured ectopic pregnancy with a single serum progesterone. Am J Obstet Gynecol 1989;160:1425-1431.

16. Cunningham GA, MacDonald PC, Gant NF. Ectopic pregnancy. Williams Obstetrics. 19th Ed. Norwalk, CT: Appleton & Lange, 1994.

17. Valle JA, Lifchez AS. Reproductive outcome following conservative surgery for tubal pregnancy in women with a single fallopian tube. Fertil Steril 1983;39:316.

18. DeCherney AH, Maheaux R, Naftolin F. Salpingostomy for ectopic pregnancy in the sole patent oviduct. Fertil Steril 1982;37:619-622.

19. Kadar N. Ablative versus conservative operations. In: Diagnosis and Treatment of Extrauterine Pregnancies. New York: Raven Press, 1990:107-111.

20. DeCherney AH, Kase N. The conservative surgical management of unruptured ectopic pregnancy. Obstet Gynecol 1979;54:451-455.

21. Toumivara L, Kauppila A. Radical or conservative surgery for ectopic pregnancy? A follow-up study of fertility of 323 patients. Fertil Steril 1988;50:580-583.

22. Thorburn J, Philipson M, Lindblom B. Fertility after ectopic pregnancy in relation to background factors and surgical treatment. Fertil Steril 1988;49:595-601.

23. Sultana CJ, Easley K, Collins, RL. Outcome of laparoscopic versus traditional surgery for ectopic pregnancies. Fertil Steril 1992;57:285–289.

24. Hallatt JG. Tubal conservatism in ectopic pregnancy: a study of 200 cases. Am J Obstet Gynecol 1986;154:1216–1221.

25. Pouly JL, Mahnes H, Canis M, et al. Conservative laparoscopic treatment of 321 ectopic pregnancies. Fertil Steril 1986;46:1093-1097.

26. DeCherney AH, Boyes SP. Isthmic ectopic pregnancy: segmental resection as the treatment of choice. Fertil Steril 1985;44:307-312.

27. Smith HO, Toledo AA, Thompson JD. Conservative surgical management of isthmic cornual pregnancies. Am J Obstet Gynecol 1987;157:604–610.

28. Brumsted J, Kessler C, Gibson C, Nakajima S, Riddick DH, Gibson M. A comparison of laparoscopy and laparotomy for the treatment of ectopic pregnancy. Obstet Gynecol 1988;71:889-892.

29. Vermesh M, Silva PD, Rosen GF, et al. Management of unruptured ectopic gestation by linear salpingostomy: a prospective, randomized clinical trial of laparoscopy versus laparotomy. Obstet Gynecol 1989;73:400-403.

30. Murphy AA, Nager CW, Wujek JJ, Kettel LM, Torp VA, Chin HG. Operative laparoscopy versus laparotomy for the management of ectopic pregnancy: a prospective trial. Fertil Steril 1992;57:1180–1185.

31. Lundorff P, Hahlin M, Kallfelt B, Thorburn J, Lindblom B. Adhesion formation after laparoscopic surgery in tubal pregnancy: a randomized trial versus laparotomy. Fertil Steril 1991;55:911–915.

32. Reich H, Johns DA, DeCaprio J, McGlynn F, Reich E. Laparoscopic treatment of 109 consecutive ectopic pregnancies. J Reprod Med 1988;33:885–888.

33. Kadar N. Treatment of ectopic pregnancy after pelvic inflammatory disease. In: Berger GS, Westrom LV, eds. Pelvic Inflammatory Disease. New York: Raven Press, 1992;139–162.

34. Stock RJ. Persistent tubal pregnancy. Obstet Gynecol 1991;77:267–270.

35. Kadar N. Conservative operations. In: Diagnosis and Treatment of Extrauterine Pregnancies. Raven Press, New York: 1990;112–128.

36. Vermesh M, Silva PD, Sauer MV, et al. Persistent tubal ectopic gestation: patterns of circulating beta-human chorionic gonadotropin and progesterone and managements options. Fertil Steril 1988;50:584-588.

37. Lundorrf P, Hahlin M, Sjoblom P, Lindblom B. Persistent trophoblast after conservative treatment of tubal pregnancy: prediction and detection. Obstet Gynecol 1991;77:129–133.

Chapter 16
Endometriosis, Infection, and Infertility

*Age cannot wither her nor custom stale
her infinite variety.*
—Anthony and Cleopatra, William Shakespeare

The topics covered in this chapter have been themselves the subjects of entire books and only some aspects of their management can be discussed here. The surgical management of these conditions has two features in common. First, laparoscopy is required to make a definitive diagnosis, and it can be used to treat the disease that is found at the same time that the diagnosis is made. Second, operative treatment consists of delicate dissection and excision of diseased tissues rather than the extirpation of diseased organs or structures.

Critics of operative laparoscopy see in this ability to diagnose and simultaneously to treat any abnormality that is found an opportunity to overtreat minimal abnormalities whose relationship to the patient's main complaint may be less than certain. However, as we shall see in Chapter 19, there is evidence that the treatment of pelvic adhesions and minimal endometriosis is, in fact, beneficial to patients with pelvic pain. Whether the same therapy enhances fertility is somewhat less certain but it is the subject of ongoing randomized trials.

Nonrandomized trials have suggested that the treatment of minimal endometriosis does not significantly enhance fertility when compared to no treatment, but it is important to bear in mind that this conclusion applies mostly to medical therapy and that the studies were all small and had limited power to detect significant differences between treatments. In as much as mild endometriosis does not severely impair fertility, pregnancy rates can be expected to be quite high in the absence of therapy. Therefore, even if it is

effective, treatment is likely to have only a small benefit, and studies large enough to detect small differences between treatment and no therapy have not been carried out.

ENDOMETRIOSIS

Endometriosis has a varied gross appearance, and in up to 6% of women, normal-appearing peritoneum may contain microscopic evidence of endometriosis, although it is obviously difficult to be certain that the peritoneum did, in fact, look normal in these cases (1). There is little doubt that endometriosis causes pain. Pain appears to be correlated with deeply infiltrating implants, and it is very effectively relieved by medical therapy, although recurrence rates are also very high (2). There is a clearcut relationship between endometriosis and infertility if adhesions are present or the disease otherwise distorts the pelvis and the fallopian tubes. However, in the absence of adhesions, it is far from clear that endometriosis impairs fertility (3). Not surprisingly, therefore, medical therapy is not effective for the treatment of infertility associated with endometriosis because it obviously cannot correct mechanical abnormalities.

Conservative surgery, although not curative in this disease, is associated with much lower recurrence rates than medical therapy (4). It is effective in relieving pain (see Chapter 19), and improves fertility rates associated with moderate to severe disease. There has been considerable controversy over whether the surgical treatment of minimal disease enhances fertility. Recent retrospective studies involving laparoscopic surgery have yielded apparently conflicting results (5,6), but Adamson et al. (6) point out that their study lacked power to detect differences in pregnancy rates after laparoscopic surgery and no treatment. The only prospective randomized trial reported to date showed that ablation of endometriosis enhanced fertility among women with minimal endometriosis if they had not conceived after 8 months of expectant management (7). Other randomized trials are in progress in England. It is also worth pointing out that the laparoscopic treatment of minimal endometriosis has not had any detrimental effect on fertility or the therapy of endometriosis.

LAPAROSCOPIC SURGERY

Laparoscopic surgery has become the treatment of choice for endometriosis. Diagnostic laparoscopy is required to make the diagnosis, and if a diagnosis of endometriosis is made, the disease can be treated at the same time and the patient discharged on the day of surgery or the day after. Medical therapy that is effective only for treating pain has no advantages, given that diagnostic laparoscopy is still required and that it is expensive and has a higher recurrence rate.

Implants on the peritoneum should be excised using a needle electrode and an unmodulated current, or 3-mm scissors (Figure 16.1). Normal-appearing peritoneum around the lesion is elevated and incised and the lesion dissected from the underlying tissue (Figure 16.2). Implants on the uterus, fallopian tube, or ovary are vaporized directly using the needle electrode until healthy tissue is seen at the base of the crater created. Ovarian endometriomas are excised as described in

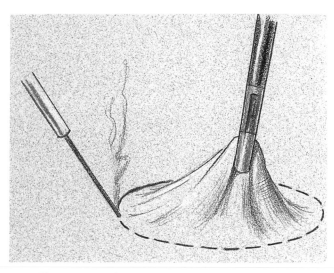

Figure 16.2 Electrosurgical excision of peritoneal endometriotic implants.

Chapter 14. The capsule is incised if it has not ruptured during elevation of the ovary, and the cavity irrigated. The capsule is then identified, grasped, and peeled off the inner aspect of the ovary working away from the utero-ovarian ligament (Figure 16.3A–C).

Endometriosis that obliterates the cul-de-sac partly or totally is usually deeply infiltrating and involves the uterosacral ligaments and the anterior rectal and posterior vaginal walls. This kind of disease requires en bloc excision and may, occasionally, require excision of part of the anterior rectal wall, although full thickness excision of the rectum is rarely necessary. It is helpful to try to identify which structures make up what appears to be the cul-de-sac. The rectal probe developed by Reich (Reznick Instruments) and the uterine mobilizer designed by Pelosi (Nova Endoscopy), which allows the uterus to be sharply anteflexed, are most helpful, and the illuminator attachment to the uterine mobilizer is also sometimes useful (see Chapter 8). If there is uncertainty as to what is vagina and what is rectum, a sponge held by ring forceps should be inserted into the vagina to help identification, and a digital examination can also be carried out if need be.

Endometriosis, like ovarian cancer, is mostly a peritoneal disease and does not obliterate the extraperitoneal tissue planes. Therefore, we use Redwine's classical approach of en bloc resection using sharp-scissor dissection (8). Incisions are made in normal peritoneum just above the uterosacral ligaments, and the incision carried forward toward the cervix, which is incised just above the attachment of the bowel to the back of the cervix after dissecting it off from the back

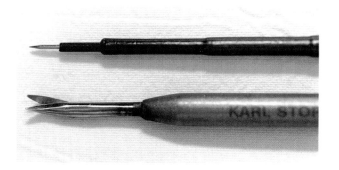

Figure 16.1 3-mm electrosurgical scissors and needle electrode used for lysis of adhesions and excision of endometriotic implants.

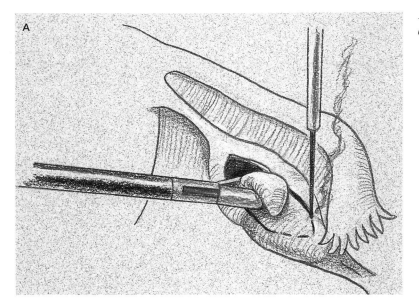

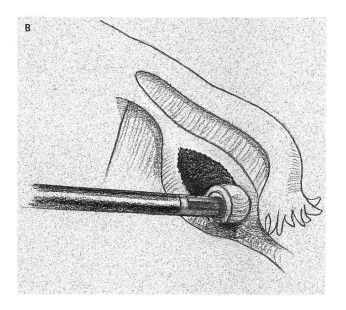

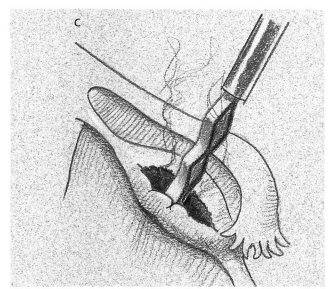

Figures 16.3A–C Excision of
endometriomas of the ovary.

of the uterus if necessary. A plane is then developed between the cervix, posterior vagina, and rectum until the rectovaginal space is entered and loose fatty tissue encountered (Figure 16.4A). The lateral border of the uterosacral ligaments is freed by blunt dissection in the pararectal space to ensure that the ureter is lateral and well away from the dissection. If there is a great deal of distortion, we like to identify the ureter at the pelvic brim and reflect it off the medial border of the broad ligament (see Chapter 7). The uterosacral ligaments are then coagulated with bipolar forceps near their attachments to the back of the cervix and transected (Figure 16.4B). They are dissected proximally toward the sacrum until the proximal edge of the rectal endometriotic nodule is reached. The incisions are

continued horizontally from the base of the broad ligament across the front of the rectum from either side, and the nodule is excised from the anterior rectal wall (Figure 16.4C).

Usually, a plane can be developed between this fibrotic nodule and one of the muscle layers of the rectum because endometriosis of the bowel wall rarely penetrates its mucosa, and the mucosa does not, therefore, usually have to be entered. If it does, wedge excision of the anterior rectal wall is usually all that is necessary, and full thickness excision of the rectum is rarely required. One or two interrupted sutures should be placed in the anterior rectal wall if the mucosa is intact, and if a wedge resection has been performed, a two-layered, horizontal closure should be used and

Endometriosis, Infection, and Infertility 159

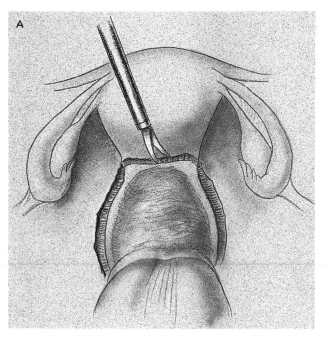

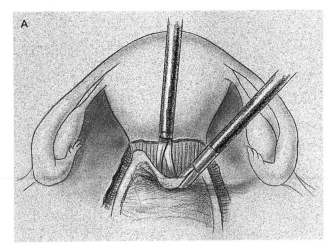

Figure 16.4A Peritoneum over the back of the uterus is incised and the rectovaginal space developed.

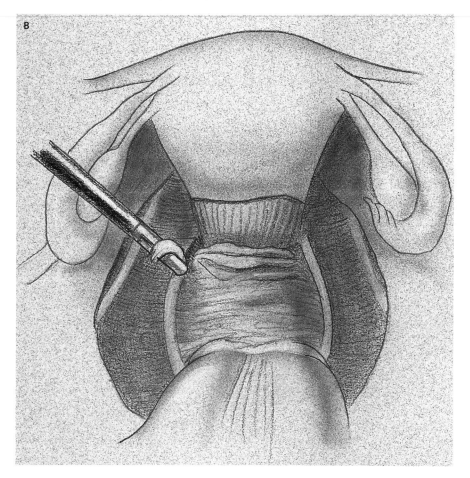

Figure 16.4B The peritoneum over the uterosacral ligament is incised, the pararectal space lateral to the ligament developed and the ureter identified, and the uterosacral ligament divided.

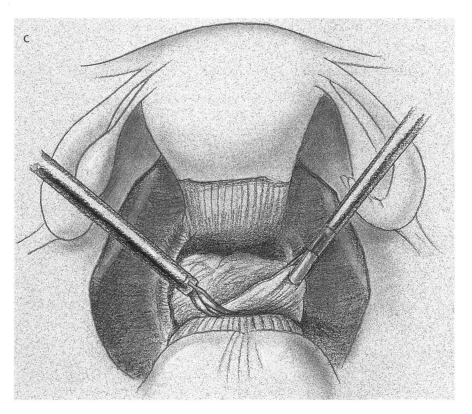

Figure 16.4C The dissection is carried proximally and then across the front of the rectum to meet a similar incision in the contralateral side, and the nodule is excised from the anterior rectal wall.

the closure tested by filling the pelvis with fluid and then instilling air into the rectum with a bulb syringe. Very low rectal incisions can also be closed through the vagina after making a colpotomy incision.

INFECTION

Laparoscopy is the only definitive means of making a diagnosis of pelvic inflammatory disease (PID), but the frequency with which laparoscopy should be used has become a subject of controversy. Westrom's classic study demonstrated that approximately one-third of women laparoscoped for a presumptive diagnosis of PID did not, in fact, have the disease (9). Major complications occurred in 1/1000 cases.

The disadvantage of diagnostic laparoscopy is that it is unnecessary for the treatment of patients, most of whom will be cured by antibiotics, and it is expensive and occasionally causes serious complications. Moreover, a visual diagnosis of PID will not change therapy, and it is a subjective diagnosis that may be in error in at least 25% of cases when compared with a fimbrial histopathologic diagnosis. In one study, the diagnostic sensitivity of laparoscopy for PID was only 50% and its specificity only 80% (10). The advantages claimed for diagnostic laparoscopy are that it

enables microbiologic specimens to be obtained and allows agglutinated tissues to be bluntly separated and the pelvis to be copiously irrigated, which may be therapeutic.

Reich (11) has made a cogent argument for using laparoscopy both diagnostically and therapeutically in the management of PID. Citing work that has shown that fibrin deposition in the abdomen serves to trap bacteria and reduce the frequency of septicemia, he pointed out that the process ultimately works to the detriment of the patient by forming thick fibrous bands that ultimately impair fertility and can prevent antibiotics from penetrating into the site of continuing bacterial growth and lead to abscess formation.

The weakness of the argument is, of course, that tubo-ovarian abscesses are uncommon today and medical therapy is nearly always successful. Moreover, it is difficult to believe that some of the acute adhesions that are lysed laparoscopically would not reform after surgery, although it is possible that adhesion formation might be less deleterious. Given the considerable adverse consequences of PID, which include not only infertility and tubal pregnancies, but also pelvic pain and polymenorrhagia, prospective studies comparing medical therapy with and without laparoscopic intervention are warranted but would face formidable problems with follow-up.

Tubo-Ovarian Abscess

Tubo-ovarian abscesses can be managed very satisfactorily laparoscopically provided the right approach is used, which, as Reich has put it, is largely an exercise in careful blunt dissection (11,12). Tissues should be separated gingerly using the suction irrigator probe and occasionally be peeled apart with grasping forceps. Irrigation is used constantly and copiously, and sometimes the force of the water jet helps to separate tissues ("aquadissection"). There is no place for sharp dissection in this setting.

Antibiotics should be started preoperatively if they have not been given already, and the abdomen should be entered using the open technique (see Chapter 2) because of the increased risk of adhesion formation. Once the abscess cavity is identified, it should be drained and irrigated copiously. All loculations must be broken down, and if there is any question of whether this has been achieved, the abscess cavity can be explored digitally with the index finger placed through the suprapubic trocar site once this has been enlarged with the gall bladder extractor. The goal should be to try to separate all adhesions and to irrigate the abscess cavity until the fluid is clear. A Jackson-Pratt drain is left in the pelvis for 1–2 days and antibiotics continued postoperatively.

INFERTILITY

The advent of operative laparoscopy had its first major impact on the management of women with tuboperitoneal causes of infertility. The diagnostic evaluation of patients with infertility is outside the scope of this chapter; suffice it to say that diagnostic laparoscopy plays an important part in that evaluation, and that definitive therapy can now be carried out at the same time in most patients rather than be deferred to a second anesthetic and laparotomy. As we have noted before, there is no place at the present time for laparoscopic tubotubal reanastomosis (13). Salpingo-ovariolysis, fimbrioplasty, and neosalpingostomy can, however, all be performed very satisfactorily via the laparoscope, and the same results can be achieved as with a laparotomy but with much less morbidity. There is also compelling evidence that postoperative adhesion reformation and de novo adhesion formation is less after laparoscopic surgery than after laparotomy (14,15).

Salpingo-Ovariolysis

Various energy sources can be used to cut adhesions. Our preferred method is to use either 3-mm scissors or the needle electrode (Figure 16.1). Adhesions are put on tension and divided close to the tube or ovary taking care not to damage the serosa of the tube and also not to leave straggly adhesions on the surface of the ovary. Vascular adhesions should be coagulated before they are divided. The adhesion is then picked up and its other attachment divided, and the entire tissue excised. Adhesions between omentum or bowel and the pelvic peritoneum are also freed using a sharp scissor dissection. If there is complete agglutination of the pelvic organs ("cohesive disease"), this is best managed by a combination of blunt and sharp dissection. The order of the surgery is to divide bowel adhesions first and free the pelvis and then to free and elevate the ovaries from the back of the broad ligament or the uterus. Tubal adhesions are divided last. Very filmy adhesions are best removed from the tube and ovary by covering these with fluid and letting the adhesions float free.

Fimbrioplasty

Fimbrioplasty can be very satisfactorily carried out laparoscopically by dividing the narrow fibrous bands that cover the distal portion of the tube or that are found between the fimbria. If there is phimosis of the tube, this can be released by placing an incision in the antimesosalpingeal border of the tube using a needle cautery. If the terminal ends of the fimbria are agglutinated, fine dissecting forceps can be introduced into the tube and then gently withdrawn as the instrument is opened. Agglutinated fimbriae are best freed by floating them under water. The adhesions between the fimbriae can be distinctly seen and divided with 3-mm scissors (Figure 16.4).

Terminal Neosalpingostomy

Before neosalpingostomy is performed, the tube is freed of any adhesions and then distended with methylene blue injected through a cervical cannula. The tube is stabilized indirectly by manipulating the ovary, and the punctum at the end of the tube is identified and incised. Linear incisions are made in the ampulla from the punctum along avascular lines so that tubal flaps are created (Figure 16.5A). The edges of these flaps are then everted by superficially desiccating the serosal surface of the terminal flaps (Figure 16.5B). Large series of laparoscopic distal tuboplas-

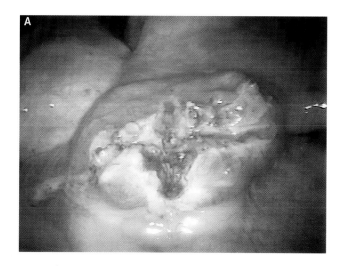

Figure 16.5A *Cruciate incision is made in the end of the tube along avascular lines with a needle cautery.*

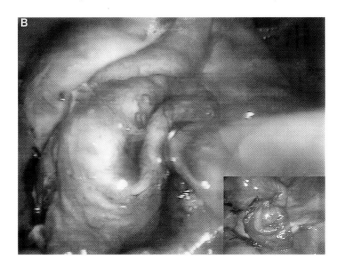

Figure 16.5B *The end of the tube is everted by slightly coagulating the serosa with bipolar forceps, which shrinks the tissues.*

ties have been reported from France by Canis et al. (16) and Dubuisson et al. (17). The intrauterine pregnancy rates were 27–33%, and the ectopic pregnancy rate was 6%.

Salpingo-Oophorectomy

Rarely, when there is gross discrepancy in the amount of damage to the two adnexa, fertility can be enhanced by unilateral salpingo-oophorectomy (18). Mature surgical judgment is required before performing this operation, but in select cases, fertility can be significantly enhanced. Salpingo-oophorectomy is carried out as previously described in Chapters 14 and 15.

REFERENCES

1. Murphy AA, Green WR, Bobbie D, de la Cruz ZC, Rock JA. Unsuspected endometriosis documented by scanning electron microscopy in visually normal peritoneum. Fertil Steril 1986;46:522–524.

2. Olive DL, Schwartz LB. Endometriosis. N Engl J Med 1993;328:1759–1769.

3. Dunphy BC, Kaye R, Barratt CLR, Cooke ID. Female age, and the length of involuntary infertility prior to investigation and fertility outcome. Human Reprod 1989; 4:527–530.

4. Redwine DB. Conservative laparoscopic excision of endometriosis by sharp dissection: life table analysis of reoperation in persistent or recurrent disease. Fertil Steril 1991;56:628–634.

5. Tulandi T, Mouchawar M. Treatment-dependent and treatment-independent pregnancy in women with minimal and mild endometriosis. Fertil Steril 1991;56:790–791.

6. Adamson GD, Heard SJ, Pastor DJ, Rodriguez BD. Laparoscopic endometriosis treatment. Is it better? Fertil Steril 1993;59:35–44.

7. Nowroozi K, Chase JS, Check JH, Wu CH. The importance of laparoscopic coagulation of mild endometriosis in infertile women. Int J Fertil 1987;32:442–444.

8. Redwine DB. Laparoscopic en bloc resection for the treatment of the obliterated cul-de-sac in endometriosis. J Reprod Med 1992;37:695–698.

9. Westrom L. Effects of acute pelvic inflammatory disease on fertility. Am J Obstet Gynecol 1975;121:707–713.

10. Sellors J, Mahoney J, Goldsmith C, et al. The accuracy of clinical findings in laparoscopy and pelvic inflammatory disease. Am J Obstet Gynecol 1991;164:113–120.

11. Reich H, McGlynn F. Laparoscopic treatment of tubo-ovarian and pelvic abscesses. J Reprod Med 1987; 32:747–752.

12. Reich H, McGlynn F, Parente C, Sekel L, Levie M. Laparoscopic tubal anastomosis. J Am Assoc Gynecol Laparosc 1993;1:16–19.

13. Heny-Suchet J, Soler A, Loffredo V. Laparoscopic treatment of tubo-ovarian abscesses. J Reprod Med 1984;29:579–582.

14. Filmar S, Gormel V, McComb P. Effectiveness of CO_2 laser and electromicrosurgery in adhesiolysis: a comparative study. Fertil Steril 1986;45:407–410.

15. Luciano AA, Maier DB, Koch EI, Mulsen JC, Whitman GF. A comparative study of postoperative

adhesions following laser surgery via laparoscopy vs laparotomy in the rabbit model. Obstet Gynecol 1989; 74:220–224.

16. Canis M, Mage G, Pouly JL, Manhes H, Wattiez A, Bruhat MA. Laparoscopic distal tuboplasty: report of 87 cases and a 4-year experience. Fertil Steril 1991; 56:616–621.

17. Dubuisson JB, Bouquet de Joliniere J, Aubriot FX, Darai E, Foulot H, Mandelbrot L. Terminal tuboplasties by laparoscopy: 65 consecutive cases. Fertil Steril 1990; 54:401–403.

18. Scott JS, Lynch EM, Anderson JA. Surgical treatment of female infertility: value of paradoxical oophorectomy. Br Med J 1976;1:631–634.

Chapter 17
Fibroids and Myomectomy

A wise man will make more opportunities than he finds. —Bacon

Leiomyomata or fibroids are the commonest solid pelvic tumors in women, and many aspects of their management are controversial. They are frequently asymptomatic, in which case no treatment is required (1), or they may be associated with a variety of complaints, which, with varying degrees of justification, warrant their removal by hysterectomy or myomectomy. Hysterectomy is always to be preferred, however, because it is easier, quicker, and associated with less morbidity, blood loss, and postoperative adhesions.

Clear indications for removing fibroids are menorrhagia associated with anemia, rapid growth, and a variety of pressure symptoms associated with very large myomata. "Rapid growth," which is almost never associated with sarcomatous change, and infertility and habitual miscarriages are less solid indications, and true pain is rare outside of pregnancy, unless a subserous myoma has protruded through the cervix or torsion of a pedunculated fibroid is suspected (a highly unusual event).

Habitual miscarriage should only be attributed to fibroids if there is demonstrable distortion of the uterine cavity, but if this is present, myomectomy halves the subsequent rate of pregnancy loss, from approximately 40% to 20% (2,3). Infertility should also not be attributed to fibroids without searching for other causes first because fibroids are rarely the only cause of infertility. On the other hand, fibroids are frequently associated with factors that are known to impair fertility, which obviously makes it difficult to determine whether myomectomy helps to correct infertility in

these women. Nonetheless, 40–60% of women complaining of infertility become pregnant after myomectomy, even if no other causes of infertility can be identified (2–5). The prophylactic removal of fibroids to avert some of the many pregnancy-related complications that may be associated with fibroids is almost never indicated.

USE OF PREOPERATIVE GnRH

Gonadotropin-releasing hormone (GnRH) agonists, whether administered intramuscularly in depot form or intranasally as a snuff, induce a reversible hypoestrogenic state and a reversible reduction in the volume of fibroid uteri (6). Not surprisingly, therefore, they have been used frequently as a presurgical adjunct to both myomectomy and hysterectomy (see Chapter 13). By inducing amenorrhea, they are of undeniable benefit to patients with severe anemia in that they allow blood counts to recover before surgery without transfusion and make autologous blood donation possible, where, otherwise, it would not have been feasible. Whether GnRH agonists are helpful in the many other ways in which they have been claimed to be is rather more questionable.

The proposition that GnRH agonists allow an abdominal hysterectomy to be "converted" into a vaginal hysterectomy is examined in Chapter 13. As for facilitating the removal of fibroids, our experience and those of others has been that if GnRH agonists have any impact on myomectomy, it is to make the surgery more difficult by blurring the tissue planes and, on occasions, even almost liquefying the fibroid. The ease or difficulty of a myomectomy is obviously a subjective matter, and a meaningful study to measure the effect of GnRH on the ease of surgery is precluded by the inability to blind any would-be study. Although many studies involving GnRH have claimed to be "double blinded," such a design is, in fact, impossible because, as pointed out in Chapter 13, the drug, unlike a placebo, induces amenorrhea. As we have said, we do not question that the drug can reduce uterine volumes by 30–40%. But, it follows from the formula for the volume of a sphere that it only takes a reduction in diameter of 7–15% to shrink volume by 30–40% (see Chapter 13), and normal myometrium contributes more to that shrinkage than the fibroids (7).

The use of GnRH has many disadvantages: (a) it is expensive, (b) it may shrink small myomas sufficiently to make them undetectable at myomectomy, and this may result in a higher and earlier myoma recurrence rate, (c) it produces menopausal symptoms, and (d) it can cause ascites (8). Bone mineral density is reduced, but this is not an issue with short-term use, and, rather esoterically, the treatment of an unsuspected leiomyosarcoma may be delayed.

PREOPERATIVE EVALUATION

The endometrium should always be sampled to exclude malignancy and an attempt made to determine the size, location, and number of fibroids present, and how deeply they penetrate the uterine wall. An ultrasound usually suffices for this. Although ultrasound will frequently miss small myomas and overestimate the size of larger ones, magnetic resonance imaging is expensive and not appropriate for routine preoperative use, even though it is superior to ultrasound in differentiating fibroids from other tumors and adenomyosis, in assessing degeneration within the fibroid and the degree to which it has penetrated the uterine wall.

Hysterosalpingography is useful in patients complaining of infertility and recurrent abortion. It helps to assess the relationship of the myomata to the endometrial cavity, to evaluate tubal patency and intratubal characteristics, and to identify mechanical distortion of the tube(s) by the fibroid(s). Hysteroscopy is very useful in establishing the presence of submucous or intrauterine pedunculated myomas.

Laparoscopic myomectomy is contraindicated if there are more than three to five myomas present, or if they are larger than 10–15 cm in size, unless they are pedunculated. If an intramural fibroid penetrates the myometrial wall by more than 50%, hysteroscopic resection is to be preferred. If there are both submucous and subserous fibroids, both hysteroscopic and laparoscopic resection may be required, but they should not be carried out at the same time.

Pedunculated, subserous fibroids are removed vaginally, and prolapsed myomas that have dilated the cervix are particularly simple to excise. The stalk of the myoma is identified, clamped, divided, and sutured. It must be kept in mind that, on occasions, the prolapsed myoma may be associated with uterine inversion, which may include the bladder and ureters. Prophylactic antibiotics should be used because necrosis of the fibroid can cause secondary systemic infection.

If the myoma is large, it may be necessary to advance the bladder and incise the cervix anteriorly in the midline to expose the myoma and the base of the pedicle. This is then transfixed as before and divided, and after the fibroid has been removed, the cervix is reapproximated. On rare occasions, the cervical incision has to be extended and a vaginal hysterotomy carried out in order to remove the myoma. It can be very useful to have dilated the cervix with a laminaria tent before a vaginal myomectomy.

LAPAROSCOPIC MYOMECTOMY

The usual four-trocar arrangement is used, but the trocar insertion sites may need to be adjusted to best suit the configuration of the uterus. As a general rule, the bigger the myoma, the higher the surgical ports need to be placed. Special care is needed during introduction of the trocars if the uterus is very large (see Chapter 13).

The well-established principles of myomectomy must be adhered to regardless of whether the fibroid is being removed laparoscopically or via a laparotomy. The incision in the uterine wall should be anterior and vertical whenever possible and as many fibroids as possible removed through a single incision (2,3). Compared with posterior incisions, anterior uterine incisions cause fewer adhesions to the adnexa and bowel (9), and incisions in the midline tend to bleed less than those made in the lateral uterine wall, and they are also less likely to damage the intramural part of the fallopian tube. By keeping the number of incisions to a minimum, the integrity of the myometrium is better preserved. If a lateral incision must be made, it should be transverse, parallel to the direction of the vasculature in the uterine wall.

It is of the utmost importance to achieve meticulous hemostasis during myomectomy. Unfortunately, none of the many methods used to reduce blood loss during abdominal myomectomy can be used laparoscopically because these make use of clamps and tourniquets. A vasopressin solution (20 U/100 ml saline) is, therefore, injected into the myoma, which serves as a very effective vasoconstrictor. The injection needs to be repeated approximately every half hour.

Laparoscopic myomectomy consists of three phases: excision of the myoma from the uterus, repair of the myometrium, and extraction of the myoma from the peritoneal cavity. The same methods of extraction are used regardless of the type of myoma present, but the method of excision used and the need for myometrial repair varies considerably.

Excision of the Myoma

A *pedunculated myoma* is easily removed laparoscopically by division of its stalk close to the uterus after it has been coagulated with bipolar forceps. The edge of the closed dissecting scissors and an unmodulated unipolar current are used to cut the pedicle. If the stalk is very thick, coagulation and division may need to proceed in stages. Some have used the Roeder loop (see Chapter 4).

Subserosal and *intramural fibroids* are somewhat more difficult to remove. Anterior and fundal fibroids are technically easier to resect than posterior ones, and a hinged uterine manipulator capable of providing maximal uterine anteversion is required to expose posterior fibroids adequately. It is helpful to instill a concentrated methylene blue solution into the uterine cavity through the cannula of the uterine manipulator to stain the endometrium because this will help to detect entry into the uterine cavity and facilitate layered closure of the uterine wall.

Using an 18-gauge spinal needle, the vasopressin solution is injected subserosally over the myoma along the path of the proposed incision, and the serosa incised with the closed tips of the dissecting scissors using an unmodulated current. The incision is made only large enough to allow extraction of the myoma. The incision is carried down through the serosa, myometrium, and pseudocapsule of the myoma until the white, whorly appearance of the subserosal myoma has been identified. The fibroid is grasped with claw-toothed forceps to stabilize it and placed on traction,

and a plane of dissection is developed between the fibroid and the myometrium using a combination of sharp and blunt dissection.

Blunt dissection is carried out with the suction-irrigator placed in the cleavage plane between the myoma and the surrounding myometrium (Figure 17.1A). The probe is pressed against the myoma or the uterine wall, and countertraction is provided by a grasper and/or the uterine manipulator. A mechanical leverage effect is thereby created (Figure 17.1B), but excessive force must not be used; otherwise, the tissue bridges between the fibroid and the myometrium will be ruptured. Sharp dissection is carried out with the dissecting scissors and an unmodulated current. The tissue bridges between the myoma and the myometrial wall must be coagulated before they are divided; otherwise, brisk bleeding from the vessels in these tissue bridges will complicate the dissection.

The surgical challenge in removing *intraligamentous fibroids* laparoscopically lies in defining the extraperitoneal anatomy because once the correct plane of dissection has been entered, it is surprisingly easy to develop a cleavage plane between the fibroid and the surrounding extraperitoneal tissues. These tumors frequently impinge on the ureter and distort the retroperitoneal anatomy, and because their size, shape, and location vary greatly, the method of removal must be individualized. Nonetheless, a common strategy is followed, which consists of entering the retroperitoneum as described in Chapter 6 (although the pelvic sidewall triangle may be distorted), and identifying the major blood vessels lateral to the myoma and the ureter, which usually lies medial or below. Once the retroperitoneal dissection is complete, the anterior leaf of the broad ligament is incised lateral to the bladder, which, on occasions, may need to be dissected from the myoma. The broad ligament incisions are left unsutured at the end.

After a fibroid is removed, it is placed in the cul-de-sac for later removal and its bed inspected for hemostasis. The area is irrigated thoroughly and bleeding points coagulated with bipolar forceps. Diffuse oozing is controlled with fulguration (coagulation in the noncontact mode), using the dissecting scissors held just off the tissues. This is one of the few occasions in which a high-voltage blended current may be useful. It is important to remove all significant fibroids, especially when they are intramural, to reduce the risk of recurrence, which occurs in approximately 15–27% of patients, although only about 10% require subsequent surgery.

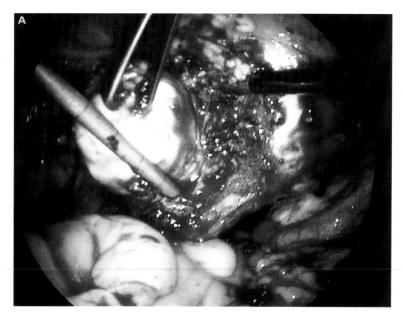

Figure 17.1A *Blunt dissection is used to develop a plane between the myoma and the uterine wall. The claw forceps stabilizes the fibroid, and the grasper and/or uterine manipulator provides countertraction.*

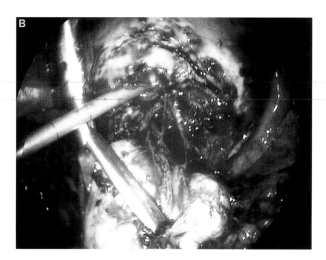

Figure 17.1B *The fibroid is further separated from its uterine bed by traction–countertraction.*

Repair of the Myometrium

The question of myometrial repair arises only with subserosal and intramural fibroids. Excision of subserosal fibroids results in relatively superficial damage to the uterine wall, and the myoma bed and the uterine serosa can be left open. Absolute hemostasis must, however, be achieved. The value of currently available adjuvant therapies to prevent adhesion formation remains unproven, and we rely on copious irrigation and meticulous hemostasis.

Removal of intramural myomas, especially when they are large, deep, and multiple, creates a significant defect in the uterine wall, which can lead to the for-

mation of uteroperitoneal fistulas (10) and rupture of the uterus in a subsequent pregnancy (11). Current techniques of laparoscopic suturing do not allow large defects to be closed adequately. For example, recent ultrasound studies of the uterus after laparoscopic myomectomy have shown that hematomas frequently form at the excision site, even after multiple-layered closure of the defect, although they generally disappear by 3–6 months after surgery (12). Although uteroperitoneal fistulas and rupture of the scar in a subsequent pregnancy have been reported (10,11), others have not observed these problems after layered endoscopic suture of the uterus (13,14).

Nonetheless, we close uterine defects through a transverse, suprapubic laparoscopically assisted minilaparotomy incision. The area of the uterus to be sutured is brought up to, and maintained at, the incision with the uterine manipulator. A traditional, two- or three-layer closure is then used to close the uterine defect. This approach works extremely well with anterior, fundal, and upper posterior tumors. In patients with large, deep, and posterior myomas, the defect can be repaired through the colpotomy incision. After closure of the uterus, the fibroids are removed suprapubically, or through a colpotomy incision.

Removal of the Myoma

The removal of large myomas from the abdominal cavity is frequently the most time-consuming part of laparoscopic myomectomy. Myomas can be removed either abdominally or vaginally, but tumors larger than 5 cm are best removed through a posterior colpo-

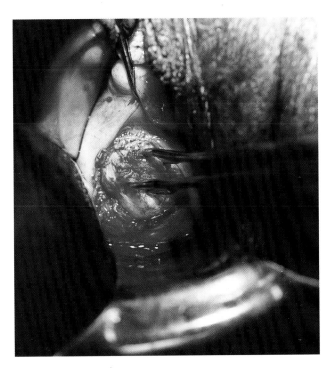

Figure 17.2 Fibroid being removed through a colpotomy incision.

tomy incision, which is made as described in Chapter 8. After the transverse colpotomy incision has been made, the myoma is placed in the cul-de-sac and guided towards the colpotomy incision, where it is grasped with a strong tenaculum and pulled out through the vagina (Figure 17.2). If the myoma is very large, it is either cut into three or more pieces inside the pelvis with scissors or extracted by vaginal morcellation. If multiple fibroids are being extracted, the pneumoperitoneum has to be reestablished after each one has been extracted, and the colpotomy incision temporarily sealed by holding its edges together. Following removal of the myomas, the colpotomy incision is closed vaginally with a running, nonlocking absorbable suture. The patient is advised to abstain from vaginal intercourse for at least a month after colpotomy.

Fibroids that are ≤5 cm in size are removed using Hasson's "orange peel" technique (5). This consists of converting the fibroid into a long strip with a spiral incision, which is then removed through the suprapubic trocar site.

SINGLE UMBILICAL PUNCTURE TECHNIQUES

The single-puncture technique of myomectomy is almost identical to the multiple-puncture technique. Most of the operation is carried out with three instru-

ments, a suction-irrigator, hook scissors, and bipolar forceps. Pedunculated fibroids are dealt with in an identical manner of bipolar coagulation followed by division of the stalk (Figure 17.3). Incisions in the uterus are also made in a similar way using subserosal injection of vasopressin at the site of the proposed incision (Figure 17.4A), followed by incision of the uterus with a needle electrode or hook scissors and an unblended current (Figures 17.4B,C). Once the correct plane of dissection has been entered, it is opened by a combination of blunt and sharp dissection with the suction-irrigator, hook scissors, and the bipolar forceps. The suction-irrigator is pressed against the fibroid, and countertraction is provided by the hinged uterine manipulator to create a mechanical leverage effect. Again, tissue bridges between the myoma and the myometrium are first coagulated with bipolar forceps and then divided with hook scissors. Once the fibroids are freed, they are removed from the peritoneal cavity either through a posterior colpotomy incision or through the umbilicus.

If the umbilicus is used to extract the fibroid, the incision is first enlarged to about 3 cm and the edges of the incision held together by Allis clamps to restore the pneumoperitoneum, which is lost once the incision is enlarged. The myoma is then grasped with a toothed grasping forceps through the operative channel of the laparoscope and brought to the umbilicus. The Allis clamp is released, and, as a single unit, the laparoscope, its cannula, and the grasping forceps are removed from the abdominal cavity. The protruding portion of the specimen is grasped with heavy, toothed clamps. The myoma is delivered by a combination of pulling and rotating as the shape and size of the structure allows. In the presence of large myomas, a tedious and time-consuming morcellation is performed through the extended umbilical incision (Figure 17.5). The incision must be closed with care in layers to incorporate the fascia in order to avoid the possibility of herniation.

If the uterine wall needs to be sutured this is done through the umbilical incision, or, if the myoma was extracted through the vagina, a suprapubic microceliotomy incision as previously described. The main point of difference between the single- and multiple-puncture techniques is the inability to stabilize the uterus with claw forceps or a myomectomy screw in the single-puncture approach. This creates fewer problems, however, than might be imagined because a hinged uterine manipulator specially designed for the purpose gives the surgeon great freedom to select

Figure 17.3 Excision of a
pedunculated fibroid.

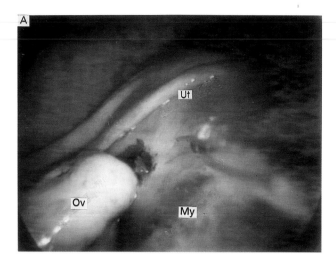

Figure 17.4A The serosa over the fibroid is infiltrated
with vasopressin.

a working position for the uterus and for fixing it in place.

Laparoscopic myomectomy using the single-puncture technique has been successfully performed for the removal of single and multiple subserosal myomas 10 cm or larger in 38 patients. Second-look laparoscopy was performed in 13 women. In these cases, a characteristic pale uterine indentation, with a depth that correlated with the size of the removed myoma(s), was encountered. A simultaneous hysteroscopic transillumination of the uterine cavity showed an appropriate uterine wall thickness in all cases. We found no adhesions in 5 patients, minimal adhesions in 4 patients, and moderate adhesions in 3 (Figure 17.6).

Laparoscopic Myoma Coagulation (Myolysis)

Myolysis is a relatively new technique for shrinking subserosal and intramural fibroids that attempts to destroy their blood supply by coagulating cylindrical areas of tissue every 5 mm with a fiber energy laser or a long bipolar needle electrode. The technique was first used by Mergui in France and Dequesne in Switzerland in 1990. Before surgery, patients are treated with a GnRH agonist to reduce the size of the fibroid as much as possible. A dilute vasopressin solution is injected intracervically and into the myoma(s) to improve hemostasis. The drilling sites are made in two planes. Drilling in the anterior plane is carried out through a suprapubic port; drilling in the horizontal plane is either through the operating channel of an operating laparoscope or an auxiliary puncture site placed high on the left- or right-hand side. A 50- to 70- watt current is needed for the bipolar needle electrode (Figure 17.7). Concurrent hysteroscopic resection of submucous fibroids or endometrial ablation in patients with abnormal bleeding may be indicated af-

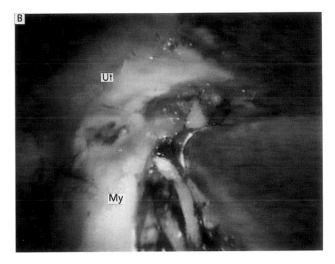

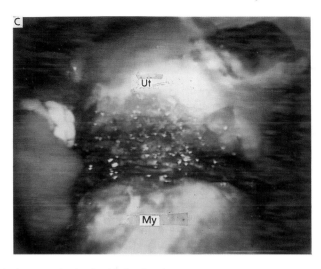

Figures 17.4B,C The serosa and myometrium are incised with hook scissors.

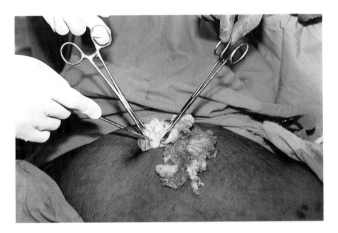

Figure 17.5 Morcellation of a myoma through an extended umbilical incision.

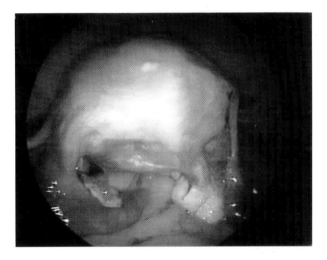

Figure 17.6 Second look laparoscopy following laparoscopic myomectomy, showing no adhesions.

ter malignancy has been excluded. The technique is most appropriate for perimenopausal women and is used to avoid a myomectomy or hysterectomy.

In a recent study, 75 symptomatic patients were treated with Nd:YAG laser laparoscopic myolysis, and myoma volumes were reduced by 50–70% over and above the shrinkage induced by a GnRH agonist. No myoma regrowth was observed, and the myomas in 20% of the patients have virtually disappeared. There were also no serious complications (15). This technique may become a useful alternative to myomectomy or hysterectomy in select patients, but further experience with the technique is required.

DISCUSSION

In general, myomectomy is a controversial operation. Most fibroids that unequivocally require removal are large and associated with bleeding and/or pressure symptoms, and in almost all women, a hysterectomy will be indicated. Thus, absolute indications for myomectomy are uncommon. Laparoscopic myomectomy is even more controversial than the open operation because the clearer the indications for the myomectomy, the less clear the advantages of a laparoscopic removal become. A number of women with good indications for myomectomy will have submucous fibroids that are far better removed hysteroscopically than laparoscopically, and in another significant group of women, fibroids will be deeply imbedded in the myometrium and multiple. Although the removal of these fibroids is technically almost always possible and it can even be accomplished with minimal blood loss if sufficient care is taken over their

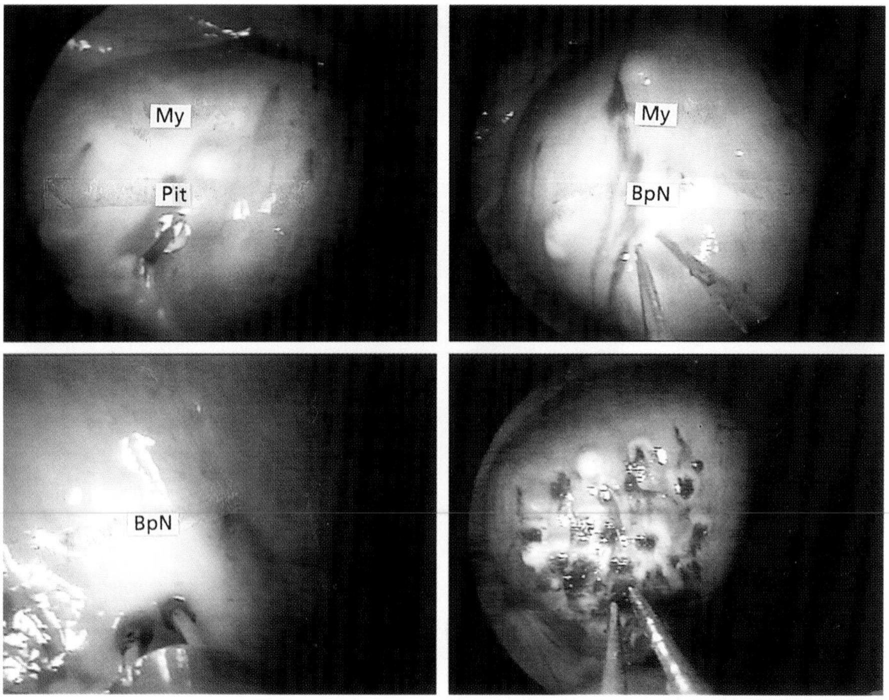

Figure 17.7 Myolysis using bipolar needle electrodes.

removal, there is justifiable concern over the adequacy of the laparoscopic repair of the myometrial wall. There is no question that hemostasis can be achieved, and there is also no question that the tissues can be approximated to some extent in almost all cases, but proper obliteration of dead space created by the removal of a deeply imbedded intramural fibroid can usually only be accomplished at laparotomy by manual compression of the area as the sutures are placed, many of which are on considerable tension. This same result cannot be achieved endoscopically regardless of how satisfactorily the surface appearance of the repaired myomectomy site may be. The sonographic appearances of these areas, as reported by Darwish et al. (12), undoubtedly represent postoperative seroma formation within the dead space. This is ultimately replaced by scar tissue, which corresponds to the disappearance of the sonolucency within the uterus by 3–6 months. Extensive scar formation within the myometrium is likely to weaken it perhaps sufficiently to cause uterine rupture in a subsequent pregnancy. Considerable judgment and common sense need to be exercised when deciding which myomata to remove laparoscopically and which are best left to a laparotomy. With that said, many fibroids that are currently being removed abdominally can be removed laparoscopically perfectly satisfactorily and with considerable reduction in morbidity and perhaps even blood loss. Comparisons are difficult, however, because only selected fibroids are removed laparoscopically.

We do not believe that the currently available evidence justifies the use of GnRH agonists preoperatively unless the patient is anemic. It must be said that our experience with fibroids is limited to rather extreme cases that are selectively referred to us. But, GnRH agonists have had virtually no impact on these large tumors, and in one or two instances, they have caused almost complete liquefaction of the lesions. However, there is little evidence that GnRH agonists are beneficial even for smaller fibroids. A multicenter randomized trial accrued only 18 cases in which the use of a GnRH agonist prior to myomectomy was compared with placebo (16). Although in women with "large" fibroids, pretreatment with GnRH agonist significantly reduced mean blood loss during myomectomy compared with controls, the difference (200 ml) was hardly of enough practical significance to warrant the use of such expensive therapy.

The value of second-look laparoscopy following laparoscopic myomectomy is a contentious issue. Myomectomy causes significant adhesions postoperatively, which are more marked if a posterior uterine incision is used rather than a fundal or an anterior one. It is uncertain whether adhesion formation after myomectomy is less if the operation is performed laparoscopically rather than via laparotomy, but this is true for almost all other operations (17,18). Nonetheless, adhesions do still occur, especially if a posterior uterine incision has been used, and second-look laparoscopy with lysis of new adhesions is probably worthwhile, although its effect on fertility has not been proven (13).

REFERENCES

1. Friedman AJ, Haas ST. Should uterine size be an indication for surgical intervention in women with myomas? Am J Obstet Gynecol 1993;168:751–755.

2. Buttram VC, Reiter RC. Uterine leiomyomata: etiology, symptomatology and management. Fertil Steril 1981;36:433–445.

3. Verkauf BS. Myomectomy for fertility enhancement and preservation. Fertil Steril 1992;58:1–15.

4. Rosenfeld DL. Abdominal myomectomy for otherwise unexplained infertility. Fertil Steril 1986;46:328–330.

5. Starks GC. CO_2 laser myomectomy in an infertile population. J Reprod Med 1988;33:184–186.

6. Friedman AJ, Hoffman DI, Comite F, Browneller RW, Miller JD. Treatment of leiomyomata uteri with leuprolide acetate depot: a double-blind, placebo-controlled, multicenter study. Obstet Gynecol 1991;77:720–725.

7. Schlaff WD, Zerhouni EA, Huth JA, Chen J, Damewood MD, Rock JA. A placebo-controlled trial of a depot gonadotropin-releasing hormone analogue (Leuprolide) in the treatment of uterine leiomyomata. Obstet Gynecol 1989;74:856–862.

8. Lee MJ, Kazer RR. Massive ascites after leuprolide acetate administration for the treatment of leiomyomata uteri. Fertil Steril 1992;58:416–418.

9. Tulandi T, Murray C, Guralnick M. Adhesion formation and reproductive outcome after myomectomy and second-look laparoscopy. Obstet Gynecol 1993;82:213–215.

10. Nezhat C, Nezhat F, Silfen SL, Schaffer N, Evans D. Laparoscopic myomectomy. Int J Fertil 1991;36:275–280.

11. Harris WJ. Uterine dehiscence following laparoscopic myomectomy. Obstet Gynecol 1992;80:545–546.

12. Darwish A, Tuttlies F, Paulus DW, Grab DD, Keckstein J. Sonographic evaluation of laparoscopy myomectomy scars. 2nd European Congress in Gynecologic Endoscopy and New Surgical Techniques, Heidelberg, October 21–23, 1993:32.

13. Hasson HM, Rotman C, Rana N, Sistos F, Dmowski WP. Laparoscopic myomectomy. Obstet Gynecol 1992;80:884–888.

14. Dubuisson JB, Chapron C, Mouly H, Foulot H, Aubriot F. Laparoscopic myomectomy. Gynaecol Endosc 1993;2:171–174.

15. Goldfarb H. Nd:YAG laser laparoscopic coagulation of symptomatic myomas. J Reprod Med 1992;36:636–639.

16. Friedman AJ, Rein MS, Harrison-Atlas D, Garfield JM, Doubilet PM. A randomized, placebo-controlled, double-blind study evaluating leuprolide acetate depot treatment before myomectomy. Fertil Steril 1989;52:728–733.

17. Lundorff P, Hahlin M, Kallfelt B, Thornburn J, Lindblom B. Fertil Steril 1991;55:911–915.

18. Nezhat C, Metzger MD, Nezhat F, Luciano AA. Adhesion formation following reproductive surgery by videolaseroscopy. Fertil Steril 1990;53:1008–1011.

Chapter 18
Incontinence and Colposuspension

No man who is correctly informed
as to the past will be disposed to take a morose
or desponding view of the present.
—*History of England, Lord Macaulay*

Retropubic colposuspension was first described by Burch in 1961 and the operation was popularized for the treatment of stress urinary incontinence in women by Tanagho (1). It is a simple operation that entails suturing the vagina to the pectineal line (Cooper's ligament) with two to four sutures placed submucosally in the vagina at the level of the urethrovesical junction. The vagina thus forms a hammock or sling below the bladder neck and elevates it to a point behind the pubic bone. When abdominal pressure suddenly increases, as when the patient coughs, the urethra is compressed against the back of the pubis and urine loss is prevented (2). The operation does not, however, increase pressure at rest in the urethra (3).

The operation has three advantages over its forerunner, the Marshall-Marchetti-Krantz (MMK) procedure. First, all sutures in a colposuspension are placed in the plane of the urethrovesical junction, whereas in the MMK operation, only the most proximal of three sutures are placed at this level. The more distal sutures of the MMK operation contribute little to the restoration of continence and can predispose to voiding difficulties. Second, colposuspension will correct any coexistent cystocele, whereas the MMK procedure will not. Third, because the vagina is fixed to Cooper's ligament rather than to the back of the symphysis, the rare complication of osteitis pubis is avoided with a colposuspension.

Colposuspension does, however, have one disadvantage compared to the MMK procedure; it anteverts the axis of the vagina to a much greater extent and predisposes patients to enterocele formation. The operation also cannot be performed in everyone for the vagina must have adequate capacity to reach the pelvic sidewall. The occasional patient with a narrow vagina or one that is not sufficiently pliable may, therefore, still be a candidate for the MMK procedure.

Needle suspensions of the bladder neck have become popular alternatives to the Burch procedure in recent years because of their lower morbidity. Short-term results obtained with these operations appear to approximate those obtained with the Burch procedure. However, long-term results seem to be less good and the operation is also less effective for recurrent stress urinary incontinence. In a randomized study, the Burch procedure enjoyed a 19% higher cure rate (91%) than Stamey needle suspension of the bladder neck (72%) (4).

INCONTINENCE IN WOMEN: SOME NEW CONCEPTS

By far, the most common causes of incontinence in women are *stress urinary incontinence* (SUI) and *detrusor instability* (DI). It is still widely taught that these two conditions cannot be distinguished clinically and that preoperative cystometry must be performed in all incontinent women to avoid misdiagnosing DI as SUI. This great emphasis on the preoperative identification of DI stems from the belief that DI is never cured, but

Table 18.1 Proportion of women with mixed incontinence cured by surgery

Many Women with GSUI + DI Are Cured of Both Problems by Surgery

				Type of Operation
McGuire et al.	1980	67/101	(67%)	Miscellaneous
McGuire & Savastano	1985	148/172	(86%)	Miscellaneous
Beck & Lai	1982	10/13	(77%)	Sling procedure
Langer et al.	1986	17/29	(59%)	Colposuspension
Stanton et al.	1978	6/14	(43%)	Colposuspension
Steele et al.	1986	6/13	(46%)	Colposuspension
Sand et al.	1988	11/20	(55%)	Colposuspension
Karram and Bhatia	1989	16/27	(59%)	Colposuspension

Table 18.2 Frequency of de novo postoperative detrusor instability following operations for incontinence

Detrusor Instability (DI) Can Develop de Novo After Surgery

				Type of Surgery
Cardozo et al.	1979	17/92	(18.5%)	Colposuspension
McGuire et al.	1980	21/246	(8.5%)	Miscellaneous
Beck et al.	1982	4/55	(7.3%)	Sling procedure
Mundy	1983	2/26	(7.7%)	Colposuspension
Langer et al.	1986	17/61	(28.0%)	Colposuspension
Sand et al.	1988	5/66	(7.6%)	Colposuspension

is often made worse by surgery, that it can mimic genuine SUI clinically, and that the misdiagnosis of DI as SUI has been a major reason why operations for SUI fail. The high frequency of DI among women who remain incontinent after "continence" operations is cited as evidence for this view (5). Pioneering work by Dr. Edward McGuire has rendered this view of female incontinence both simplistic and anachronistic.

First, in a significant minority of women (15–30% in most reports), the two conditions coexist (*mixed incontinence*). When they do, the two conditions seem to be causally linked, at least in some women, because an operation that relieves the SUI will also often relieve the DI (6,8). Although urogynecologists were slow to learn of this finding and very skeptical of it when they did, it has been confirmed repeatedly in many centers (8–10). Debate over mixed incontinence now centers on how frequently, and not on whether, women are cured of both conditions by surgery and on whether management should be initially directed towards the DI or the SUI. Even the worst results reported show that in the presence of SUI, about 50% of women are cured of any coexistent DI by surgery, and most of the remaining patients experience marked clinical improvement (Table 18.1). This author is not aware of any evidence that suggests women with mixed incontinence are actually made worse by surgery.

Second, DI can develop for the first time after an operation that successfully relieves SUI, i.e., de novo after surgery (6-16), Table 18.2. That is a very important observation that clearly renders invalid the assumption that if DI is present postoperaticely, it must have been present preoperatively (5). Thus, a finding of DI in an incontinent woman after a "continence" operation does not permit one to infer that the DI was present before surgery and that failure to diagnose it led to an inappropriate operation as has been implied so often in the past (5).

Indeed, on the assumption that 10% of women with SUI have mixed incontinence, and 50% of them will be rendered continent by surgery, and that 10% of women with pure SUI will develop DI de novo after surgery, it can be shown that if all patients with genuine stress incontinence are subjected to surgery regardless of whether their bladder is stable or unstable, at least two-thirds of those with unstable bladders postoperatively will have had stable bladders preoperatively (17). One must, therefore, agree with McGuire's view that "emphasis on the preoperative diagnosis of detrusor instability urodynamically seems to be somewhat misdirected" (18).

Another question of considerable clinical interest is why appropriately performed operations, i.e., correctly carried out for a correct diagnosis, fail to relieve incontinence in some women. At one time, this was attributed in part to the use of vaginal rather than retropubic operations to suspend the bladder neck, a viewpoint that is now generally accepted. However, this explanation has become somewhat anachronistic with the widespread adoption of needle suspension procedures that retain all the advantages of colporrhaphy (very low morbidity) and have cure rates, at least in the short term, almost as good as retropubic urethropexy.

It was again McGuire who provided a completely new perspective on the problem when he demonstrated that, in a significant minority of women complaining of SUI, closing function in the proximal urethra was very deficient or even completely absent and that merely supporting the bladder neck would not relieve incontinence in these women (18-22). To be successful, the operation had to increase resting urethral pressure. Because retropubic operations for SUI, including colposuspension, only restore pressure transmission across the bladder neck and do not reliably increase resting closing pressures in the urethra, McGuire recommended sling operations rather than. colposuspension for incontinence associated with low closing proximal urethral pressures (Type III incontinence).

We confirmed the validity of McGuire's concepts about the treatment of incontinence due to sphincter failure in women made incontinent by radical pelvic surgery (23,24). Others have also confirmed the superiority of a sling operation to colposuspension in the treatment of incontinent women with low urethral pressures in the more common setting of simple SUI without, regrettably, acknowledging McGuire's pioneering work (24,25).

These three new concepts—mixed incontinence, de novo postoperative detrusor instability, low pressure urethra—have deepened our understanding of incontinence in women and have allowed us to recognize that many earlier views about why operations for incontinence fail, how incontinent women should be evaluated preoperatively, and who should be operated upon with which operation were very simplistic, if not misleading. We need to refocus our questions about the surgical management of incontinent women from whether or not their detrusors are stable to whether or not they have SUI of a sufficient severity to merit surgery and, if so, which operation is most likely to relieve their incontinence. In this respect, the urodynamic "workup" currently in vogue is not very helpful.

A careful history and clinical examination of the patient with a full bladder in the standing position as she coughs and strains will allow the surgeon to answer these questions much more reliably than urodynamic tests (26). In women who have recurrent SUI or minimal mobility of the anterior vaginal wall, it is also important to obtain closure pressure profiles to identify those who have abnormally low proximal urethral pressures (<10 cm/H_2O) because better results will be obtained in these women with a sling operation than with a colposuspension (27). Alternatively, a standing, oblique cystogram can be obtained with 200 ml of contrast in the bladder. If the bladder neck is open at rest,

i.e., without straining of coughing, after the filling catheter has been removed, this signals the need to augment resting urethral pressures with a sling operation (28). Whether the bladder is stable or unstable may be of some prognostic significance, but if there is a significant degree of SUI, it is unlikely that an extemporizing course of anticholinergic therapy will cure the patient's incontinence, and she will ultimately come to surgery.

LAPAROSCOPIC COLPOSUSPENSION

Laparoscopic colposuspension was first performed by Vancaille and Schussler (29), and the largest experience has been reported by C. Y. Liu (30). The technique is identical to that used for an open operation, and it is very straightforward, provided the surgeon can suture endoscopically with a curved needle.

Review of Anatomy

The retropubic space of Retzius is bounded anteriorly by the symphysis pubis, posteriorly by the anterior wall of the bladder, inferiorly by the pelvic diaphragm, and on either side by the obliterated hypogastric arteries. The urachus is much less prominent than the obliterated hypogastric arteries, and it lies under the peritoneum in the midline connecting the dome of the bladder to the umbilicus (Figure 18.1).

Cooper's ligament is simply the inferior reflection or continuation of the medial end of the inguinal ligament onto the superior surface of the superior pubic ramus. Just beyond to the lateral portion of the ligament and out of view lies the external iliac vein as it passes under the inguinal ligament on its way to the femoral triangle (Figure 18.1). It is not seen during colposuspension, but its location must be borne in mind as the sutures are placed into Cooper's ligament, and the tip of the needle must be controlled and not be allowed to wander laterally out of view.

The Operation

The usual four-trocar arrangement is used, and if the needle is to be introduced through the suprapubic trocar rather than directly, it has to be 10- or 12-mm (see Chapter 4). After the pneumoperitoneum has been established and the trocars inserted, the space of Retzius is opened by incising the parietal peritoneum just above the symphysis pubis, including the urachus, using the unopened jaws of the dissecting scissors and an unblended monopolar current. The symphysis pubis can usually be identified by gently tapping the area

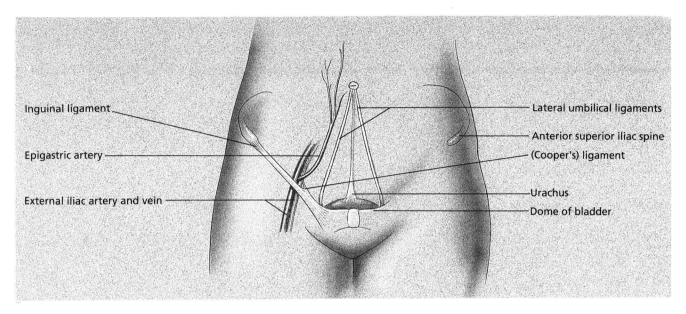

Figure 18.1 Anatomy of the lateral and medial umbilical ligaments and Cooper's ligament.

above the bladder with a probe, or the incision can be made 4–5 cm above the vesical fold, which is a constant landmark (Figure 18.2A). The urachus has to be coagulated with bipolar forceps. The peritoneum and bladder are peeled away from the symphysis pubis using blunt dissection, and the umbilical ligaments are swept laterally and upwards to expose the superior pubic ramus and the pectineal line (Cooper's ligament) (Figure 18.2B). These are cleaned of fatty tissue (Figure 18.2B, inset).

Sutures are then placed in the vaginal wall beneath the mucosa, at the level of the urethrovesical junction about two fingers' breadth from the urethra (Figure 18.3). The urethrovesical junction is identified with the help of the 30-cc balloon of a Foley catheter and the assistant's fingers in the vagina. A figure of eight suture is placed, using #2 Ethibond on a V37 needle, and the suture is tied down with two throws if there is any bleeding at the insertion site. The sutures are then stitched to the pectineal line, and tied down using the extracorporeal technique (Figure 18.3).

There are several noteworthy technical points about the operation. First, it is important to use permanent braided sutures as these will yield better long-term results than absorbable sutures, even though fibrosis also probably plays a significant role in the surgical result obtained. Second, it is important to avoid "air knots." When tying the sutures, an assistant should place a finger in the vagina and approximate it to Cooper's ligament. The assistant's finger is withdrawn momentarily as the knot is being tied down to allow the vagina to

approximate the Cooper's ligament, but pressure is reapplied as soon as the first hitch has been laid to relieve tension on it. The operating surgeon must also maintain tension on the suture after the first hitch has been laid, until the second throw has been tied down, to avoid slippage of the first hitch. If undue tension is likely to result, the needle can be inserted from the top of the pectineal line towards its inferior border rather than the other way around (Figure 18.3, inset).

Before placing the vaginal sutures in the open operation, the lateral border of the bladder has to be dissected off the vagina. This is the most unesthetic part

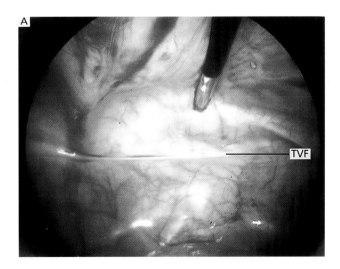

Figure 18.2A The transverse vesical fold provides a useful landmark for the peritoneal incision to enter the space of Retzius.

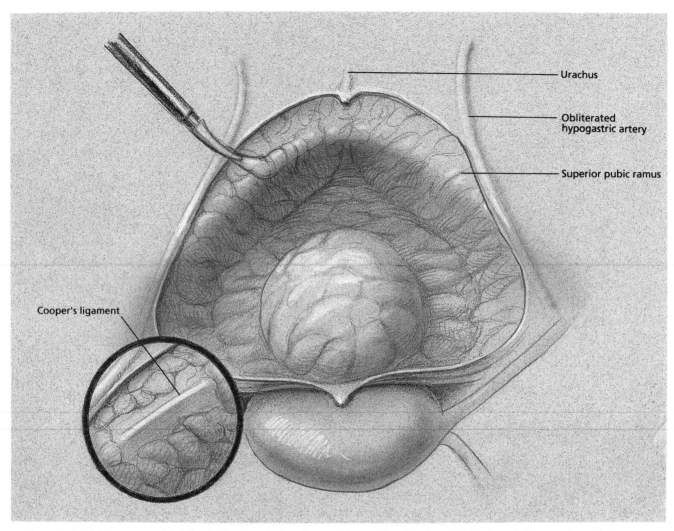

Urachus

Obliterated hypogastric artery

Superior pubic ramus

Cooper's ligament

Figure 18.2B The space of Retzius is developed bluntly after the urachus has been divided, and the superior pubic ramus cleaned of fatty tissue to expose Cooper's ligament (inset).

of the operation because there is no natural tissue plane between the lateral wall of the bladder and vagina beneath it. The "dissection," therefore, necessarily involves tearing the areolar fibrous attachments of the bladder to the vagina, usually bluntly with a "peanut." One of the advantages of performing the procedure laparoscopically is that a closeup view through the laparoscope provides a magnified view of the lateral borders of the bladder, which can usually be delineated well enough to allow the vaginal sutures to be placed without stripping the lateral wall of the bladder off the vagina. Therefore, dissection in this unnatural plane, which is felt by many to contribute to the voiding difficulties that can occur after the operation, is avoided.

Cooper's ligament should be cleaned of all fatty areolar tissue so that when the supporting sutures are tied down, the vaginal fascia is approximated to the liga-

ment without any intervening fat or fibrous tissue. We do not clamp the Foley during the procedure but check suture placement cystoscopically. This should be done before the sutures are tied down; otherwise, it can be difficult to see the lateral wall of the bladder.

Variations

A number of modified laparoscopic retropubic suspension operations have been devised and presented in abstract form at various international meetings. They differ from the parent operation in one of two respects, how the space of Retzius is entered and how the vagina is sutured to Cooper's ligament.

▶ **Retziuscopy:** It is possible to gain entrance to the space of Retzius by an extraperitoneal route by insufflating under the parietal peritoneum and then developing the space by blunt dissection. Various bags, or

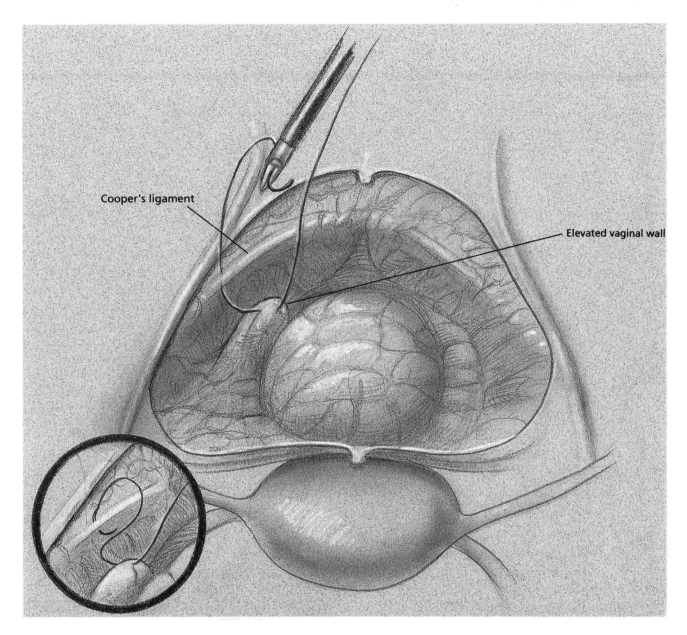

Cooper's ligament

Elevated vaginal wall

Figure 18.3 The vaginal wall is elevated by an assistant with a finger in the vagina, the vaginal wall transfixed, and sutured to Cooper's ligament. If there is limited vaginal mobility the needle can be inserted into the ligament from above downwards (inset).

even rubber gloves, insufflated with gas or saline have also been used by urologists to distend the space of Retzius. We have no experience of these approaches, but should they have any demonstrable advantage (which we doubt), we would anticipate no difficulty adopting them.

▶ **Alternative Methods of Suspension:** Because endoscopic suturing techniques are still far from ideal, a number of tactics have been used to facilitate suspension of the vagina from Cooper's ligament.

A technique we find attractive is Lyons' method of stapling the end of the suture to Cooper's ligament after the stitch has been placed into the vagina. Thus, as soon as the vagina has been stitched, one end of the suture is stapled to Cooper's ligament, and the stitch is ready to be tied. Davis uses a Stamey needle to pass a suture through the full thickness of the vagina and then to bring the suture through Cooper's ligament.

Numerous other methods of anchoring the vagina to Cooper's ligament have been preliminarily reported, but these all make use of some type of mesh, which is stapled or glued to the pectineal line and the vagina. We would not favor any technique that entails leaving foreign bodies in the space of Retzius.

Results

The results from laparoscopic retropubic urethropexy were discussed in Chapter 1. Short-term results show subjective cure rates in excess of 90%, an incidence of de novo postoperative instability of about 5%, and significant reduction in postoperative morbidity, blood loss, and recovery time compared with the open operation. Longer follow-up and further experience with the procedure will be required before a final assessment can be made of its relative merits, but initial experience with the operation clearly suggests that laparoscopic colposuspension is likely to join the growing list of pelvic operations that are better carried out laparoscopically than via a laparotomy.

SINGLE UMBILICAL PUNCTURE LAPAROSCOPIC TECHNIQUES FOR THE CORRECTION OF STRESS URINARY INCONTINENCE

Contributed by Marco Pelosi

Single umbilical puncture laparoscopic techniques make use of the same basic surgical principles that are traditionally used for the correction of stress urinary incontinence (31) and that also form the basis of the multiple-puncture techniques described above. Single- and multiple-puncture techniques for the Burch and MMK procedures differ in two relatively minor respects related to the methods used to (1) develop the space of Retzius and (2) place the sutures to suspend the vagina. Single-puncture laparoscopic needle suspension of the bladder neck and sling procedure differ even less from the open operations, the main point of difference being that a blind procedure is converted into one where the surgeon can actually see where the suspending sutures or the sling are being placed.

RETROPUBIC URETHROPEXY (BURCH OR MMK PROCEDURE)

The space of Retzius is entered transabdominally as in the multiple-puncture technique, but a much smaller incision is made in the peritoneum, just large enough to allow the operative laparoscope to be inserted into the retropubic space and to form a seal around the shaft of the laparoscope (Figure 18.4). Suture placement is a joint venture requiring cooperation between vaginal and endoscopic instruments that is the hallmark of single-puncture techniques.

Opening the Space of Retzius

The patient is positioned in the same way as for a multiple-puncture procedure, an 18-French, 30-ml balloon Foley catheter is placed in the bladder, which is then distended with 150 ml dilute methylene blue solution. The catheter helps us to identify the urethra and the urethrovesical junction, distension of the bladder to delineate its boundaries, and the dye to identify any injuries to the bladder.

The symphysis pubis and urachus are identified, and a 1-cm incision is made through the urachus about 1 cm *below* the symphysis with unipolar scissors, after the area has been coagulated with Kleppinger forceps. The area is dissected bluntly using the unopened jaws of the scissors or the end of the suction-irrigator until the end of the operating laparoscope can be slid past the opening in the peritoneum. Continued blunt dissection with the suction-irrigator, and aquadissection as needed, allows one to identify the back of the symphysis pubis. This is then cleaned of any fatty areolar tissue, and any blood vessels encountered are coagulated and divided. Continuous delivery of the CO_2 helps in the dissection of the retropubic space because the gas is trapped within the space by the tight peritoneal seal around the laparoscope. The bladder is also emptied at this stage to increase visibility, and blunt dissection is continued until the bladder neck, paravaginal tissues, and Cooper's ligament are all cleaned

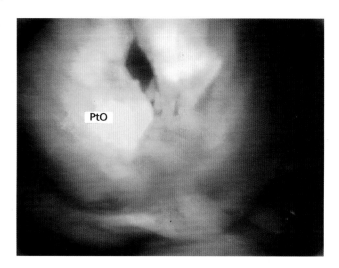

Figure 18.4 A small opening is made in the parietal peritoneum just large enough to fit snugly around the operating laparoscope.

of fatty areolar tissue. Identification of the bladder neck is facilitated by the assistant, who places a finger in the vagina on either side of the Foley catheter and balloon.

Placing Sutures

Permanent sutures (O Prolene or Novofil) are placed into Cooper's ligament or the symphysis pubis in exactly the same way as at laparotomy. Cooper's ligament is used if the vagina is capacious or if there is cystocele, and the symphysis pubis is used if the vagina is narrow and lacks mobility.

The needle is introduced into the space of Retzius from the vagina by an assistant at a point about 1 cm lateral to the urethrovesical junction (Figure 18.5A). The surgeon delineates the entry point for the assistant by pressing down on the vagina with the needle holder, which is introduced through the working channel of the operative laparoscope. A specially designed, 42-inch-long, angled Cook needle holder is used, which will lock the needle into the correct position unaided after the needle is picked up.

After the needle pierces the vaginal wall, the assistant can watch its progress on the video monitor with the surgeon. The needle is driven through the vaginal wall up to its hilt, whereupon the surgeon grasps it with the endoscopic needle holder. The assistant does not let go his grip on the needle until the surgeon has grasped the needle securely. The needle is then placed through Cooper's ligament or the back of the symphysis (Figure 18.5B), depending on whether a Burch or an MMK procedure is being carried out. Once well through the desired spot, the surgeon releases the nee-

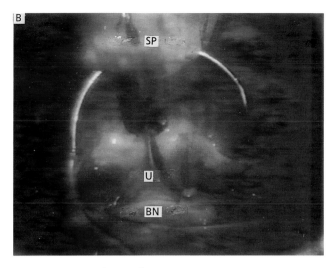

Figure 18.5B The needle is inserted into the periosteum of the symphysis pubis.

dle, picks it up again distally, and by grasping the needle at successively more proximal points, gradually brings the needle through the ligament or periosteum. Before completing the pass, the needle is grasped near its proximal end and the pass completed. The needle is now brought back out through the vaginal wall about 1 cm from where it was introduced into the space of Retzius, and the same process is repeated on the contralateral side.

Before the sutures are tied down, cystoscopy is performed to check that the sutures have not pierced the bladder. The sutures are then tied down through the vagina. A small nick is made in the vagina to create a furrow for the knot and the knot oversewn with fine suture.

NEEDLE SUSPENSION OF THE BLADDER NECK

The space of Retzius is opened in exactly the same way as for a Burch or MMK procedure. A 2-cm skin incision is then made on either side of the midline just above the symphysis pubis and the subcutaneous tissues dissected with a finger until the rectal fascia is identified. Before making each skin incision, the abdominal wall is transilluminated with the operative laparoscope, which not only helps to avoid injury to vessels in the abdominal wall, but facilitates finger dissection. Placement of the incision under direct vision also helps to prevent placing the incisions too high, or too laterally, errors that can cause postoperative pain.

A double-pronged ligature carrier is then passed through one of the abdominal incisions, and, under

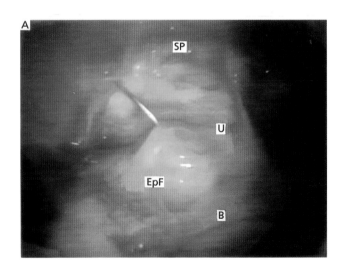

Figure 18.5A A needle is introduced into the space of Retzius through the vagina.

direct laparoscopic surveillance, the vaginal wall is pierced just lateral to the urethrovesical junction (Figure 18.6A). A nonabsorbable suture (O Prolene or Novofil) is then threaded onto the ligature carrier transvaginally (Figure 18.6B). The ligature carrier is then withdrawn through the abdominal incision, and a similar procedure is carried out on the opposite side (Figure 18.6C). If the paraurethral tissue is felt to be flimsy, three deep bites are taken of the paraurethral and vaginal tissues before the ends of the suture are threaded through the eye of the double-pronged ligature carrier, as in the Raz procedure. The ligature carrier is then withdrawn through the abdominal incision as before.

After sutures have been placed on either side, they are tied down over the rectus fascia as the assistant elevates the vagina. If adequate elevation has been

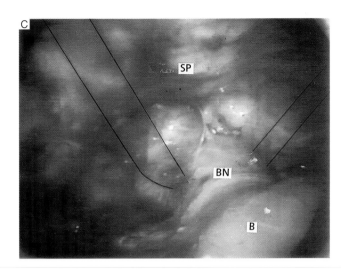

Figure 18.6C Suspension sutures are placed on either side of the bladder neck.

reached, the urethra, with the catheter in place, can be displaced laterally and a Q-tip placed in the urethra will make a 0–10° angle with the horizontal (32).

SLING-OPERATION

Placement of a suburethral sling, being a combined vaginal and suprapubic operation, lends itself naturally to single-puncture techniques. A sling is prepared from a large Marlex or Gortex mesh by cutting out a 25- × 1.5-cm strip of material, with a 3- × 2.5-cm elliptical portion in the center of the graft (33). The space of Retzius is opened as previously described, and the sling is introduced into the peritoneal cavity through the operating channel of the laparoscope and maneuvered into the space of Retzius with grasping forceps. A vertical incision is made in the anterior vaginal wall and the vaginal mucosa dissected off·the periurethral tissues to expose and mobilize the proximal urethra and urethrovesical junction. The endopelvic fascia is then perforated from the vaginal side with a pair of long forceps, and under laparoscopic guidance (Figure 18.7A), aided by laparoscopic grasping forceps, one end of the sling is grasped with the forceps and pulled through the opening in the endopelvic fascia into the vagina as far as the elliptical portion in the middle of the sling. The elliptical portion of the graft is then sutured to the fascia overlying the urethrovesical junction and proximal urethra with four nonabsorbable sutures (2-0 caliber Goretex) to create a hammock-like effect.

A small incision is now made in the endopelvic fascia and vagina on the right side of the endopelvic fas-

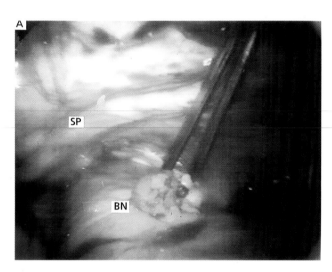

Figure 18.6A The vaginal wall is pierced lateral to the bladder neck with a double-pronged ligature carrier.

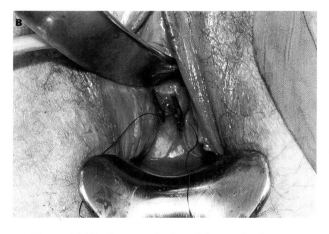

Figure 18.6B A suture is threaded onto the ligature carrier transvaginally.

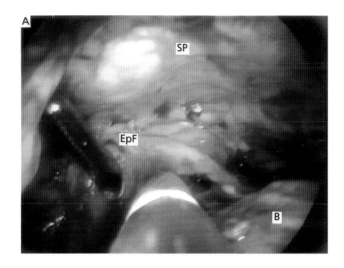

Figure 18.7A The endopelvic fascia is perforated with a clamp from the vagina under laparoscopic guidance.

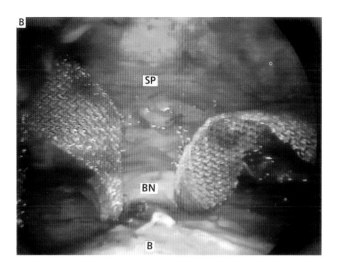

Figure 18.7B A Marlex sling has been passed around the proximal urethra to form a hammock.

cia with laparoscopic scissors inserted through the working channel of the operating laparoscope. The scissors are withdrawn and replaced by grasping forceps, which are used to grasp the free end of the sling in the vagina and bring it around the urethra back into the space of Retzius (Figure 18.7B). The vaginal incision is then closed with absorbable sutures.

The anterior abdominal wall is transilluminated with the operative laparoscope, and two incisions, about 2 cm in length, are made on either side of the midline, just above the symphysis pubis, and the underlying fascia dissected free of the overlying fatty tissue using blunt finger dissection. A small nick is made in the rectus fascia, and under laparoscopic guidance, a long Kelly clamp is introduced into the space of Retzius and used to grasp one end of the sling. The other end of the sling is grasped in the same way with a long Kelly clamp introduced through the contralateral incision in the anterior abdominal wall. Both clamps are then simultaneously pulled through the anterior abdominal wall, and the free ends of the graft are sutured with nonabsorbable sutures to the rectus fascia after suitably adjusting the sling tension. The skin is closed with absorbable subcuticular sutures.

REFERENCES

1. Tanagho E. Colposuspension: the way we do it. J Urol 1976;116:751–753.

2. Hertogs K, Stanton SL. Mechanism of urinary continence after colposuspension. Br J Obstet Gynaecol 1985;92:1184–1188.

3. Van Geelen JM, Theeuwes, Eskes TKAB. The clinical and urodynamic effects of anterior vaginal repair and Burch colposuspension. Am J Obstet Gynecol 1988;159: 137-144.

4. Bergman A, Ballard CA, Koonings PP. Comparison of three different surgical procedures for genuine stress incontinence: prospective randomized study. Am J Obstet Gynecol 1989;160:1102-1106.

5. Bates CP, Loose H, Stanton SL. The objective study of incontinence after repair operations. Surg Gynecol Obstet 1973;136:17–22.

6. McGuire EJ, Lytton B, Pepe V, et al. Stress urinary incontinence. Obstet Gynecol 1976;47:255-264.

7. McGuire EJ, Lytton B, Kohorn EI, Pepe V. The value of urodynamic testing in stress urinary incontinence. J Urol 1980;124:256-258.

8. McGuire EJ, Savastano JA. Stress incontinence and detrussor instability/urge incontinence. Neurourol Urodynam 1985;4:313-318.

9. Langer R, Ron-el R, Newman M, et al. Detrusor instability following colposuspension for urinary stress incontinence. Br J Obstet Gynaecol 1988;95:607-610.

10. Karram MM, Bhatia NN. Management of coexistent stress and urge urinary incontinence. Obstet Gynecol 1989;73:4-7.

11. Sand PK, Bowen LW, Ostergard DR, et al. The effect of retropubic urethropexy on detrusor stability. Obstet Gynecol 1988;71:818-822.

12. Beck RP, Arnusch D, King C. Results in treating 210 patients with detrusor overactivity incontinence of urine. Am J Obstet Gynecol 1976;125:593-596.

13. Stanton SL, Cardozo LD, Williams JE, Ritchie D, Allan V: Clinical and urodynamic features of failed incontinence surgery in the female. Obstet Gynecol 1978; 51:515-20.

14. Steel SA, Cox C, Stanton SL. Long term followup of detrusor instability following colposuspension operation. Br J Urol 1986;58:138-42.

15. Cardozo LD, Stanton SL, Williams JE. Detrusor instability following surgery for genuine stress incontinence. Br J Obstet Gynaecol 1979;51:204-207.

16. Mundy AR. A trial comparing the Stamey bladder-neck suspension procedure with colposuspension for the treatment of stress incontinence. Br J Urol 1983; 55:687-690.

17. Kadar N, Nelson JH. The place of pre-operative investigations in the management of stress urinary incontinence. In: Taymor M, Nelson JH, eds. Progress in gynecology, Volume VII. New York: Grune and Stratton, 1983:379–401.

18. McGuire EJ. Mechanisms of urethral continence and their clinical application. World J Urol 1984;2:272-279.

19. McGuire EJ. Urodynamic evaluation after the abdomino-perineal resection and lumbar intervertebral disk herniation. Urology 1975;6:63-70.

20. McGuire EJ, Wagner. The effects of sacral denervation on bladder and urethral function. Surg Obstet Gynecol 1977;144:343-346.

21. McGuire EJ. Experimental observations on the integration of bladder and urethral function. Invest Urol 1978;15:303-307.

22. McGuire EJ, Lytton B. The pubovaginal sling in stress urinary incontinence. J Urol 1978;119:82-84.

23. Kadar N, Nelson JH. Treatment of urinary incontinence after radical hysterectomy. Obstet Gynecol 1984;64:400-405.

24. Kadar N, Nelson JH. Sling operation for total incontinence following radical vulvectomy. Obstet Gynecol 1984;64:855-875.

25. Bowen LW, Sand PK, Ostergard DR, Franti CE. Unsuccessful Burch retropubic urethropexy: a case-controlled urodynamic study. Am J Obstet Gynecol 1989;160:452-858.

26. Horbach NS, Blanco JS, Ostergard DR, et al. A suburethral sling procedure with polytetrafluoroethylene for the treatment of genuine stress incontinence in patients with low urethral closure pressure. Obstet Gynecol 1988;71:648-657.

27. Kadar N. The value of bladder filling in the clinical detection of urine loss and selection of patients for urodynamic testing. Br J Obstet Gynaecol 1988;95:698.

28. McGuire EJ: Combined radiographic and manometric assessment of urethral function. J. Urol 1977;118:632-635.

29. Vancaillie T, Schussler W. Laparoscopic bladder neck suspension. J Laproend Surg 1991;1:169–173.

30. Liu CY, Paek W. Laparoscopic retropubic colposuspension (Burch procedure). J Am Assoc Gynecol Laparosc 1993;1:31–35.

31. Pelosi MA, Apuzzio J, Frattarola M, Li TS. The triple-bite single-suture technique for correction of urinary stress incontinence. J Med Soc New Jersey 1977; 74:753–756.

32. Pelosi MA, Apuzzio JJ, Frattarola M, Hung CT, Ctareini H. A diagnostic device for stress incontinence. Obstet Gynecol 1975;45:223–226.

33. Pelosi MA, Langer A, Sama J, Fricchione D, Devanesan M. The treatment of urinary stress incontinence: use of dermal graft in sling procedure. Obstet Gynecol 1976;47:377–380.

34. Beck RP, Arnush D, King C. Results in treating 210 patients with detrusor overactivity incontinence of urine. Am J Obstet Gynecol 1976;125:593-596.

Chapter 19
Pelvic Pain

Reason can ascertain the profound difficulties of our condition; it cannot remove them. —Newman

It has become fashionable to stigmatize the surgical treatment of chronic pelvic pain as an unthinking act (1,2), but the fact remains that the condition can be permanently cured by surgery much more often than by nonsurgical remedies (2–4). To be sure, not all women with pelvic pain need surgery, nor will they all be helped by surgery, but those who are not will rarely be cured by other means. It is also true that women with pelvic pain can and have been harmed by crude gynecologic care, of which haste to operate is frequently a symptom, but this is an indictment of the surgeon not of what surgical treatment, particularly laparoscopic therapy, can offer patients with chronic pelvic pain.

The laparoscope, in its diagnostic capacity, has revolutionized the management of pelvic pain by allowing women with pain to be separated into two fundamentally distinct categories, those with and those without identifiable pathology in the pelvis (5). This is an important distinction to make not only because it allows those with pathological findings to receive definitive therapy and those without to be spared ineffective medical treatment for a presumptive diagnosis that is incorrect, but also because the mechanism by which the pain is produced and the psychological makeup of women in these two categories may be different (6–10). The attempt to relive the past by predicting what the laparoscope is likely to show from the clinical findings is a probabilistic exercise that is of little benefit to individual patients (11).

To the extent that a one-to-one correspondence between the presence of pelvic pathology and pelvic pain does not exist and that treatment of the pathology found does not always relieve the pain, it may be argued that laparoscopy cannot determine the cause of pain but only uncover an associated condition, which may or may not be the cause of the pain in an individual patient. It is on these grounds that the routine treatment of pelvic abnormalities found at the time of diagnostic laparoscopy for pelvic pain, such as adhesions and endometriosis, has been questioned, especially when the changes are minimal (3,12). But, to seek such a one-to-one correspondence between pathology and pain is to take an altogether much too simplistic view of the mechanism by which pain in general is produced. Modern theories of pain seek to blur precisely the kind of clear demarcation between the psychological and the physical causes of pain that a cause-and-effect concept implies and prefer, instead, to attribute its genesis to a concatenation of physical, psychological, pathological, and cognitive factors (4). Put simply, if a woman has pelvic pain and adhesions, many factors besides the adhesions may be involved in producing her pain, but that is not to say that dividing the adhesions may not relieve the pain, nor indeed, that if it does, other factors were not involved in its genesis.

With that said, there is, in fact, good evidence that the treatment of adhesions relieves pelvic pain, including the "chronic pain syndrome," that is, pain associated with diminished physical activity, vegetative signs of depression, and substantial alteration of the patient's role in the family. Although women with pain who do not have these additional symptoms are twice as likely to obtain pain relief as those who do, 40% of women with the chronic pain syndrome are nonetheless helped by adhesiolysis (4). Preliminary data from a randomized, double-blind study has also been presented in abstract form to show that a significantly greater proportion of women who have minimal to moderate endometriosis associated with pelvic pain are relieved of their pain by laser ablation of their endometriosis than controls undergoing diagnostic laparoscopy alone (13). The balance of evidence, therefore, suggests that the ability to treat these minor abnormalities at the time of a diagnostic laparoscopy is a boon to the management of women with pelvic pain rather than the futile exercise it has sometimes been portrayed to be.

The same is true for hysterectomy, and at least 75% of women with no apparent cause for their chronic pelvic pain obtain pain relief from the operation (2,3). Moreover, Beard's detailed, prospective study further showed that even those who continued to have some pain nonetheless benefited considerably from the operation as judged by other parameters, such as resolution of marital discord and increase in sexual activity (3). Approximately 20% of these women did have endometriosis or adenomyosis that was not identified laparoscopically, but this is not surprising given that endometriosis can be detected in biopsies from normal-appearing peritoneum. However, hysterectomy was no more effective in women with occult pathology than in those without (2,3). This is not to deny that many women with pelvic pain who are subjected to a hysterectomy might have responded to more conservative measures, but to interpret these results as anything but salutary seems to us unjustified, especially as many of these women had been incapacitated by pain for years. Hasty surgery is most surely ill-advised, but to withhold therapy that is at least 75% effective in relieving an incapacitating condition seems equally misplaced.

PELVIC PAIN (CONGESTION) SYNDROME

Pelvic pain that is not associated with identifiable pathology in the pelvis has been attributed to pelvic venous congestion. Although pelvic varicosities can be identified laparoscopically in some of these women, this is a subjective finding, and a significant proportion of women without varicosities and pelvic pain may still have abnormal pelvic venous blood flow.

In a series of elegant and coherent clinical studies at St. Mary's Hospital, London, Beard and colleagues demonstrated that contrast material injected transcervically into the myometrium under anesthesia ("pelvic venography") took significantly longer to clear from the uterus in women who had the pelvic pain and normal laparoscopic findings than in normal volunteers undergoing sterilization (7). They then demonstrated that dihydroergotamine, a venoconstrictor, relieved acute pain when injected intravenously in these women, and that pain relief was associated with enhanced dye clearance on the pelvic venogram (8). The authors have tentatively attributed these changes to high circulating estrogen levels because many of their patients had multicystic changes in the ovaries demonstrable by vaginal ultrasound, which resembled those seen in polycystic ovarian disease. Ovarian suppression with medroxyprogesterone acetate lowered circulating estrogen levels in a randomized trial and also relieved pain more effectively than psychotherapy (9,10). The best results were obtained with a combination of psychotherapy and medroxyprogesterone acetate, but the effects were short-lived, and by 9 months after the end of therapy, there was no overall significant effect of either medroxyprogesterone acetate or psychotherapy compared with placebo.

The coherence of these studies has an irresistible intellectual appeal, but the findings need to be duplicated in other centers before the overall view can be accepted as valid. In addition, although the findings provide a logical basis for treatment, conservative therapy provided only temporary relief of pain in most women (10). By contrast, hysterectomy and oophorectomy, which the investigators were loathe to use, was almost uniformly effective (3).

Beard's theory clearly identifies the ovaries as the source of the pain, but the theory was not put to the test in the author's surgical series because all patients had a hysterectomy as well as bilateral oophorectomy (3). The implications for surgical therapy are, however, clear: presacral neurectomy (see below) cannot be expected to work, and if a hysterectomy is carried out, the ovaries must be removed as well.

Another important conclusion from this body of work is that the disruption of daily life and marital discord that accompanies pelvic pain in many women is the product rather than the cause of the pain (3). What remains unclear, however, is how many women with pain and no identifiable pelvic pathology have abnormal pelvic blood flow patterns and whether there is any relationship between abnormal blood flow and abnormalities on standardized psychological questionnaires.

This is both an important and an exciting area, and one must not be too surprised if the laparoscope will again provide important answers. Pelvic venography is far too invasive a procedure for general use, and despite a few detractors, laparoscopy remains the mainstay of diagnosis. Surely it must be possible to pass miniaturized sensors down an operative laparoscope or an auxiliary trocar to measure pelvic blood flow at different locations in the pelvis and enhance the diagnostic capabilities of our laparoscope.

PRESACRAL NEURECTOMY

Presacral neurectomy is a controversial operation in which afferent pain fibers from the uterus and cervix are divided at the level of the superior hypogastric plexus. These fibers mediate pain only from central structures, and pain from the ovary and distal fallopian tubes, as occurs in pelvic inflammatory disease, and, on the evidence presented by Beard and colleagues, the pelvic pain syndrome, will not be relieved by the operation. The operation has, however, been used with good effect to treat central pelvic pain associated with endometriosis and severe dysmenorrhea refractory to medical therapy. Approximately 60–70% of women with central pelvic pain treated by presacral neurectomy remain pain-free at 12 months (15,16).

ANATOMY

Pain from the cervix, uterus, and proximal fallopian tubes as well as the bladder and rectum is mediated by specialized visceral afferents that accompany the sympathetic nerves into the spinal cord at the level of T10-L1. These fibers reach the inferior hypogastric plexus, which lies extraperitoneally lateral to the rectum, cervix, vaginal fornix, and posterior part of the bladder, by traveling along the branches of the internal iliac artery. From here, they ascend in the left and right hypogastric plexus, which lie medial to each internal iliac artery, to reach the superior hypogastric plexus at the level of L5 and the sacral promontory. The superior hypogastric plexus lies between the common iliac arteries anterior to the aortic bifurcation and the left common iliac vein, below the posterior parietal peritoneum (Figure 19.1). Pain from the ovaries and distal fallopian tubes are mediated by nerve fibers that accompany the ovarian blood supply and join the inferior mesenteric plexus. It appears that in up to 30% of women, some pain fibers from midline structures also

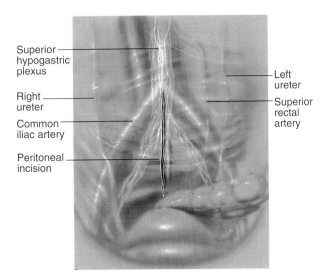

Figure 19.1 *The anatomic relations of the superior hypogastric plexus.*

take this pathway, a finding that may explain failure of the operation to relieve midline pain in some cases.

OPERATIVE TECHNIQUE

The standard four-puncture instrumentation of the abdomen is used, and either the umbilical or suprapubic trocar is used for the laparoscope. The uterus is anteverted and the sacral promontory identified, and its location verified by gently touching or "tapping" with the suction-irrigator. The posterior parietal peritoneum over the sacral promontory is picked up, desiccated, and incised with scissors. The incision is extended vertically for about 3 cm above and below the sacral promontory using scissor dissection with short bursts of unmodulated current to coagulate tiny vessels in the peritoneum. A plane is then developed between the peritoneum and the underlying fatty, nerve-bearing tissue (Figure 19.2A). It is important to clear all areolar tissue off the undersurface of the peritoneum because part of the plexus runs in this plane. The dissection is continued vertically about 1 cm above the aortic bifurcation and below the sacral promontory, where the presacral space is partly developed. The lateral limits of the dissection are the ureter on the right and the superior rectal or hemorrhoidal artery running in the base of the sigmoid mesentery on the left (Figure 19.2A).

A plane of dissection is developed between the right common iliac artery and the areolar tissue investing it, which contains nerve fibers and lymphatics. The incision is extended from the bifurcation of the common

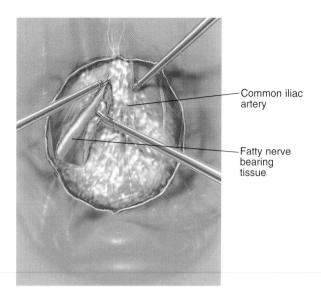

Figure 19.2A *The posterior parietal peritoneum has been incised, and a plane developed between the peritoneum and the underlying fatty nerve-bearing tissue. This tissue is incised along the medial border of the right common iliac artery and the incision extended 1–2 cm above the bifurcation of the aorta.*

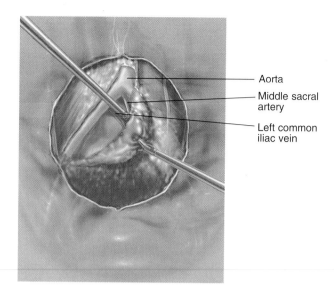

Figure 19.2B *The nerve-bearing tissue is transected at the superior limit of the dissection and dissected bluntly from the aorta, left common iliac vein, and sacral promontory.*

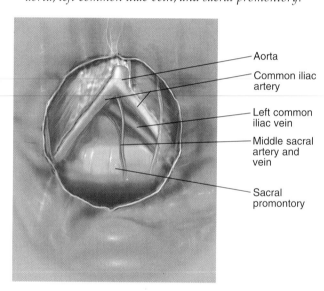

Figure 19.2C *The dissection is continued towards the left as far as the superior rectal artery, and inferiorly to the bifurcation of the left common iliac artery, at which point the specimen is transected and removed.*

iliac to just above the bifurcation of the aorta (Figure 19.2A). The tissue in front of the aorta is elevated at this point and transected with scissors using an unblended current (Figure 19.2B). The bundle of tissue is then picked up with forceps and dissected successively off the left common iliac vein and artery, and the periosteum in front of L5-S1, taking care not to injure the middle sacral artery and vein (Figure 19.2B). On the left, the areolar investment of the left common iliac artery is again incised and the incision is carried down to the bifurcation of the artery. The superior rectal artery marks the lateral limit of the dissection on the left, and the left ureter is usually not seen. Once the specimen has been freed distally, it is transected from right to left after the distal stump is coagulated with bipolar forceps (Figure 19.2C). The posterior parietal peritoneum is not closed and drains are not used.

LAPAROSCOPIC UTERINE NERVE ABLATION (LUNA)

Transection of the uterosacral ligament has also been used to interrupt the nerve fibers that mediate dysmenorrhea. The operation is straightforward, but the uterine arteries or veins and the ureters that lie lateral, but close by, can be injured. We rarely perform this operation, but our recommendation would be always to identify the lateral border of the uterosacral ligament before dividing it and to coagulate it with bipolar forceps before doing so. If the ureter can be seen on the medial leaf of the broad ligament, the medial approach for ureteric identification can be used (see Chapter 7). However, the ureter is frequently not visible through the broad ligament at this level. The peritoneum immediately above the uterosacral ligament is then divided and the pararectal space developed just lateral to the ligament (Figures 19.3A–C). The superior border of the uterosacral ligament can then be freed, followed by its lateral border, using a combination of blunt and sharp dissection. The ureter can often be identified on the lateral border of the space that is created (Figure 19.3C), but it may not be seen if it is mobilized laterally with the areolar tissue that invests it. Nonetheless, the ligament can be safely divided close to the uterus even if the ureter is not seen provided it has been clearly isolated.

DISCUSSION

Presacral neurectomy was used for many years in the treatment of incapacitating dysmenorrhea and midline pelvic pain, but from about the 1960s onwards, it fell into disuse, if not disrepute. There seem to be several reasons for this. First, the operation was frequently carried out improperly, and the specimen contained only fat without histologically identifiable nerve fibers. Second, patients were frequently poorly selected, and those with lateral pain, a sensation mediated by fibers running along the infundibulopelvic ligament, were also subjected to presacral neurectomy. Third, and perhaps most important, very effective medical therapy became available for what was once the most common indication for presacral neurectomy, primary dysmenorrhea. Nonetheless, in women who wish to retain their uterus, severe central pain refractory to medical therapy (nonsteroidal anti-inflammatory agents, birth control pills) remains an indication for this operation. The nature of the pain, that is, whether it is cyclical or acyclical, dysmenorrheic or dyspareunic, seems to be less important than the site of the pain. This is in keeping with the known fact that backache and pain from lateral pelvic structures are mediated by nerve fibers that do not run in the superior hypogastric plexus (17).

Perhaps the commonest indication for the operation is endometriosis associated with midline pain. Retrospective studies by Garcia and David (18) and Polan and DeCherney (19) indicated that 25–50% more women obtain pain relief if a presacral neurectomy is combined with excision of the endometriosis. These findings were confirmed in a randomized, double-blind clinical trial by Tjaden et al. (15), but they could not be verified in another randomized trial by Vercellini et al. (20). However, the Italian study, unlike that of Tjaden et al. (15), was not blinded, and although

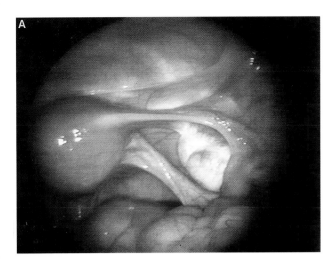

Figure 19.3A. The medial leaf of the broad ligament is inside, above the uterosacral ligament.

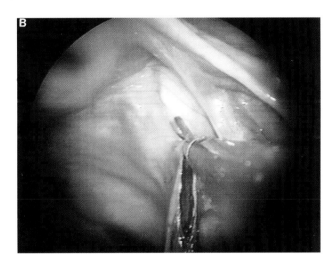

Figure 19.3B The pararectal space is developed medial to the ureter.

it yielded a null result, 17% more women who had a presacral neurectomy obtained relief from dyspareunia than those who did not. The study's lack of power explains why this trend failed to reach statistical significance because the study was designed to detect differences in pain relief of 40% or more (with 80% probability). Thus, the balance of evidence would support the use of presacral neurectomy to treat midline pain in women undergoing conservative surgical therapy for moderate to severe endometriosis.

Laparoscopic uterine nerve ablation (LUNA) has gained in popularity as an alternative to presacral neurectomy since the advent of lasers, and some, perhaps beguiled by the apparent simplicity and innocu-

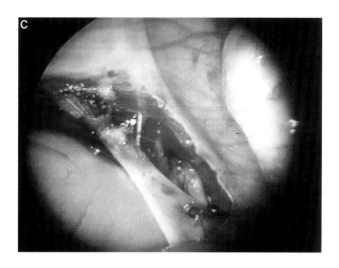

Figure 19.3C The ureter is identified and the uterosacral ligament prepared for division.

ousness of the procedure, offer it to all women with dysmenorrhea who are undergoing diagnostic laparoscopy. However, its simplicity is deceptive. From the accounts of the operation, it appears that the ureter is rarely identified other than perhaps when it can be readily seen through the broad ligament, which may partly explain why the procedure has been a more common cause of ureteric injury than any other laparoscopic operation (21). Two deaths have also apparently occurred as a result of bleeding from the uterosacral ligament. Division of the uterosacral ligament without removal of the cervix may also predispose women to future prolapse. The operation is probably overused, but, in all fairness, it has been shown to be beneficial in women with dysmenorrhea refractory to medical therapy by a carefully conducted randomized trial (22).

SUMMARY

Laparoscopic management is the cornerstone of therapy for women complaining of pelvic pain other than primary dysmenorrhea, unless this is refractory to medical therapy. Diagnostic laparoscopy simultaneously identifies the cause of the pain in many cases and allows it to be treated by adhesiolysis, resection of endometriosis, and/or presacral neurectomy, or LUNA. Presacral neurectomy is indicated in women with midline pain who have either moderate to severe endometriosis or dysmenorrhea refractory to medical therapy. Trials comparing its efficacy with that of LUNA are required. Although LUNA is a much simpler operation, it is not innocuous, and the

uterosacral ligament should always be dissected free before it is divided.

The management of women with pelvic pain who have no identifiable pathology in the pelvis and who have failed conservative measures is frustrating, but hysterectomy has been shown to cure the pain in many cases, and they would be ideal candidates for laparoscopic hysterectomy.

(This chapter was illustrated by Ed Jones.)

REFERENCES

1. Peters AAW, Dorst E, Jellis B, Zuuren E, Hermans J, Trimbos JB. A randomized clinical trial to compare two different approaches in women with chronic pelvic pain. Obstet Gynecol 1991;77;740–744.

2. Stovall TG, Ling FW, Crawford DA. Hysterectomy for chronic pelvic pain of presumed uterine etiology. Obstet Gynecol 1990;75:676–679.

3. Beard RW, Kennedy RG, Gangar KF, Stones RW, Rogers V, Reginald PW, Anderson M. Bilateral oophorectomy and hysterectomy and the treatment of intractable pelvic pain associated with pelvic congestion. Br J Obstet Gynaecol 1991;98:988–992.

4. Steege JF, Staut AL. Resolution of chronic pelvic pain after laparoscopic lysis of adhesions. Am J Obstet Gynecol 1991;165:278–283.

5. Kresch A, Seifer D, Sachs L, Barrese I. Laparoscopy in 100 women with chronic pelvic pain. Obstet Gynecol 1984;64:672–674.

6. Beard RW, Belsy E, Liebermann B. Pelvic pain in women. Am J Obstet Gynecol 1977;128:566–570.

7. Beard RW, Highman JW, Pearce S, Reginald PW. Diagnosis of pelvic varicosities in women with chronic pelvic pain. The Lancet 1984;ii:946–949.

8. Reginald PW, Beard RW, Kooner JS, Mathias CJ, Samatrage SU, Southerland I, Wadsworth J. Intravenous dihydroergotamine to relieve pelvic congestion and pain in young women. The Lancet 1987;ii:351–353.

9. Reginald PW, Adams J, Franks S, Wadsworth J, Beard RW. Medroxyprogesterone acetate in the treatment of pelvic pain due to venous congestion. Br J Obstet Gynaecol 1989;96:1148–1152.

10. Farquhar CM, Rogers V, Franks S, Pearce S, Wadsworth J, Beard RW. A randomized control trial of medroxyprogesterone acetate and psychotherapy for the treatment of pelvic congestion. Br J Obstet Gynaecol 1989;96:1153–1162.

11. Stovall TG, Elder RF, Ling FW. Predictors of pelvic adhesions. J Reprod Med 1989;34:345–348.

12. Rapkin AJ. Adhesions and pelvic pain: a retrospective study. Obstet Gynecol 1986;68:13–15.

13. Ewen SP, Sutton CJ, Whitelaw N, Haines P. Prospective randomized double blind controlled trial of the treatment of minimal to moderate endometriosis with laser laparoscopy. (Abstract) Presented at the 2nd European Congress in Gynaecologic Endoscopy and New Surgical Techniques, Heidelberg, October 21 –23, 1993. Gyneacol Endosc 1994;3:30.

14. Murphy AA, Green WR, Bobbie D, de la Cruz ZC, Rock JA. Unsuspected endometriosis documented by scanning electron microscopy in visually normal peritoneum. Fertil Steril 1986;46:522–524.

15. Tjaden B, Schlaff WD, Kambel A, Rock JA. The efficacy of presacral neurectomy for the relief of midline dysmennorhea. Obstet Gynecol 1990;76:89–91.

16. Lee RB, Stone K, Magelssen D, Belts RP, Benson WL. Presacral neurectomy for chronic pelvic pain. Obstet Gynecol 1986;68:517–521.

17. Ingersoll FM, Meigs JV. Presacral neurectomy for dysmenorrhea. N Engl J Med 1948;238:357–360.

18. Garcia CR, David SS. Pelvic endometriosis: infertility and pelvic pain. Obstet Gynecol 1977;129:740–747.

19. Polan ML, DeCherney A. Presacral neurectomy for pelvic pain and infertility. Fertil Steril 1980;34:557–560.

20. Candiani GB, Fedele L, Vercellini P, Bianchi S, Di Nola G. Presacral neurectomy for the treatment of pelvic pain associated with endometriosis: a controlled study. Am J Obstet Gynecol 1991;67:100–103.

21. Grainger DA, Sonderstrom RM, Schiff SF, Glickman M, DeCherney AH, Diamond MP. Ureteral injury at laparoscopy: insights into diagnosis, management and prevention. Obstet Gynecol 1990;75:839–843.

22. Lichten EM, Bombard J. Surgical treatment of primary dysmenorrhea with laparoscopic uterine nerve ablation. J Reprod Med 1987;32:37–41.

Part D
Oncologic Procedures

Chapter 20
Laparoscopic Management of Gynecological Malignancies: An Overview

Belief in truth begins with doubting all that has hitherto been believed to be true. —Nietzsche

Surgery plays an important role in the management of almost all gynecological malignancies, but many aspects of its use are controversial. Although complete discussion of these controversies is not possible here, it is essential to know at least what the controversies are if the laparoscopic management of these malignancies is to be placed in proper perspective. As we have said before, a laparoscopic operation cannot be expected to deliver therapeutically more than its open counterpart or be free from the unresolved controversies surrounding the open operation. All that one is aiming at with a laparoscopic approach is to achieve the same surgical result as with a laparotomy but with less morbidity to the patient. It follows immediately that the indications for a particular laparoscopic operation should be the same as those for its open counterpart, and if these indications are controversial, they will be just as controversial if the operation is performed laparoscopically. The controversy surrounding the routine use of surgical staging in cervix cancer, for example, is no argument against performing aortic lymphadenectomy laparoscopically.

The treatment of malignant disease, however, is usually accompanied by significant side effects and complications. In some circumstances, the side effects to be expected may sway one to withhold treatment, especially if the therapeutic gain to be expected is small. However, if the side effects can be reduced by laparoscopic management, this may tilt the risk-benefit ratio sufficiently for therapy to be recommended where otherwise it might have been withheld. What has changed here is not really the indication for treat-

ment, but the conclusion about where the risk-benefit ratio lies. Inasmuch as the goal of laparoscopic surgery is to reduce morbidity, and morbidity is generally higher after radical surgery than after operations for benign disease, laparoscopic surgery is potentially used to greatest advantage in our discipline in the treatment of gynecological malignancies.

USE OF LYMPHADENECTOMY

The most controversial aspects of surgical management in gynecologic oncology involve the use of lymphadenectomy. The passage of time has served only to increase these controversies because the indications for lymphadenectomy and the type of lymphadenectomy to be performed have changed with time and have become the subject of intense scrutiny and much disagreement.

For many years, the gynecologic indications for lymphadenectomy were considered to be early invasive carcinoma of the cervix and vulvar carcinoma metastatic to the inguinofemoral lymph nodes. Lymphadenectomy meant pelvic lymphadenectomy, excision of the external, internal, and common iliac and obturator nodes, and complete excision at that. From the early 1970s onward, however, not only were the indications for lymphadenectomy broadened to include endometrial and ovarian carcinoma, but the limits of the lymphadenectomy were extended to encompass the "para-aortic" lymph nodes to varying degrees.

At the same time, exact indications for lymphadenectomy were not defined, and the concept of a lymphadenectomy seemed to change. Curiously enough, lymphadenectomies became both more radical and less complete. Aortic lymphadenectomy, for example, not only crept into the classic Meigs-Bonney operation for carcinoma of the cervix, and did so for no very good reason, it also became a routine part of a "staging" operation for endometrial cancer. Yet, the concept of a therapeutic lymphadenectomy was discarded. Lymphadenectomy was looked upon merely as a diagnostic procedure and engendered the notion of lymph node sampling, a process that means different things to different people, but finds no real parallel in the traditional staging lymphadenectomies of our surgical or urological colleagues.

LYMPH NODE SAMPLING VERSUS LYMPHADENECTOMY

Lymph node sampling is a confusing term that crept unnoticed into the gynecologic oncologist's vocabulary coincidently, it would seem, with the adoption of surgical staging for endometrial cancer. When applied to the selective removal of clinically enlarged lymph nodes, as practiced, for example, by Wertheim, the term was both accurate and descriptive. But, we now know that at least 50–70% of lymph node metastases are clinically silent and cannot be detected by simply inspecting the lymph nodes at surgery. It follows a priori that lymph node sampling will be insensitive at identifying nodal disease. It is accepted that a lymphadenectomy is never complete in the sense that every lymph node in the targeted area will be removed, but clearly, this is a weak argument for purposefully not attempting a complete excision.

Arguments favoring the use of lymph node sampling, however defined, seem to rely on the proposition that there should be a difference between a staging and a therapeutic operation, but this is a proposition we do not accept. Patients with lymph node metastases may or may not benefit from adjunctive radiation or chemotherapy, but even if they do, that does not mean that the lymphadenectomy contributed nothing to their survival. More to the point, however, is that even if by identifying the presence of nodal metastases, lymphadenectomy served only to signal the need for additional therapy to achieve cure, this would still not justify a deliberately incomplete procedure because a selective operation might miss nodal metastases in some patients, who would thereby

be denied potentially curative therapy. It is for this reason that Donohue (1), commenting on retroperitoneal lymphadenectomy in testicular tumors, wrote, "Our position is that the more thorough the lymphadenectomy, the more accurate the staging," a view that would certainly be shared by Austrian gynecologic oncologists (2). Breast cancer is the classic example of a malignancy that disseminates early in its natural history, and, therefore, lymphadenectomy is not curative in its treatment. Nonetheless, no one, to this author's knowledge, has argued for selective removal of the primary lymph nodes in breast cancer just because an axillary dissection is not therapeutic and serves only to direct further therapy.

We also do not recognize a distinction between a therapeutic and a staging lymphadenectomy. Obviously, surgeons must always consider the circumstances of individual patients and may, at times, have to content themselves with an operation that was less complete than they might have wished or had originally intended, but if pelvic lymphadenectomy is felt to be indicated, we would advocate complete excision of the nodes, including mobilization of the iliac vessels to clear the proximal obturator fossa, regardless of what primary malignancy was being treated. In our view, sweeping nodes off the top of the external iliac artery and plucking out what tissue is in the distal part of the obturator fossa is not a lymphadenectomy. To substitute this type of procedure for a lymphadenectomy on the grounds that the patient is old, has a sarcoma, or any other reason is, in our view, born of an ambivalence towards the indication for the procedure, not of a valid pathophysiological or surgical argument. If the patient is felt to be a poor surgical candidate, we favor not doing the lymphadenectomy at all rather than doing it by half measures.

Every surgical undertaking must be tempered by considerations of morbidity, and our "all or none" approach to pelvic lymphadenectomy cannot be applied to the aortocaval region. Complete lymphadenectomy would necessitate a posterior aortocaval dissection, which, requiring as it does, the ligation of the lumbar and frequently the inferior mesenteric arteries, carries, quite apart from anything else, the prospect of paralysis and diarrhea, if not bowel ischemia, in elderly women even if fit young men tolerate the procedure surprisingly well. But, extending the anterolateral aortocaval dissection beyond the inferior mesenteric artery to the renal vessels, like mobilizing the iliac vessels to obtain better clearance of the obturator fossa at pelvic lymphadenectomy, is not a step that connotes this type of morbidity. Therefore, this is the kind of procedure we favor if aortic lymphadenectomy is considered indicated, regardless of the nature of the primary lesion. Few patients benefit from an aortic lymphadenectomy, and we favor a more selective and thorough operation rather than the liberal use of "sampling" procedures that come up empty-handed in virtually all cases.

With that said, there is, in fact, suggestive, if not persuasive, evidence that at least in some gynecological malignancies, pelvic lymphadenectomy and, perhaps, even aortic lymphadenectomy can be curative or at least contribute to survival. First, 40–60% of patients with Stage IB carcinoma of the cervix and positive pelvic nodes treated by surgery alone enjoy long-term survival (3). Unless one wishes to argue that had the nodes not been removed the disease in them might have remained dormant for many years, it can be assumed that the lymphadenectomy contributed to long-term survival in these women. Second, Downey and colleagues (4) have shown that the removal of clinically enlarged lymph nodes confers a survival advantage to patients with cervix cancer treated by primary radiation. The contribution that pelvic lymphadenectomy makes to the survival of patients with endometrial carcinoma is less certain. Nonetheless, it is clear from the GOG data reported by Morrow et al. (5) that some women with aortic lymph node metas-

tases who did not receive extended field radiation have remained disease free for extended periods after aortic lymph node "sampling" alone.

CERVIX CANCER

The author's approach to the laparoscopic management of cervix cancer is outlined in Figure 20.1. Compared with the alternative, laparoscopic aortic lymphadenectomy is arguably the most cost-effective laparoscopic procedure in gynecology. Patients go home in 1–2 days, start radiation in 10–12 days, and have virtually no pain or morbidity. The advent of a laparoscopic approach has, therefore, made surgical staging much more attractive. Before aortic lymphadenectomy is carried out, a search is made for metastatic disease using computerized tomography of the chest, abdomen, and pelvis, but we no longer use scalene node biopsy (6). We restrict primary aortic lymphadenectomy to patients with advanced stage disease or very bulky, nonoperable Stage IB lesions and to those with early lesions who are found to have clinically suspicious nodes, confirmed to be positive by frozen section. We do not routinely perform *pelvic* lymphadenectomy as part of the staging of advanced disease unless computerized tomography or clinical inspection reveals enlarged pelvic lymph nodes. There is no evidence that the removal of pelvic lymph nodes prior to lymphadenectomy enhances survival (4) unless

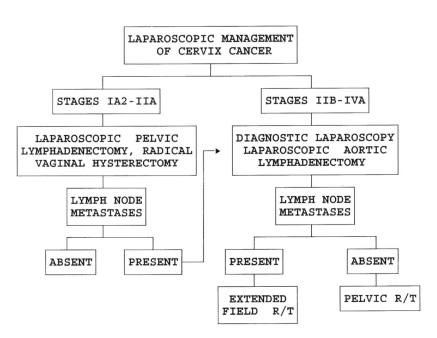

Figure 20.1 Laparoscopic management of carcinoma of the cervix.

the lymph nodes are clinically enlarged, and combined therapy has the potential to increase complications.

Women with Stage IA2-IIA carcinoma of the cervix, who are surgical candidates, undergo laparoscopic-vaginal radical hysterectomy and bilateral pelvic lymphadenectomy. In our view, the routine use of aortic lymphadenectomy at the time of radical hysterectomy for early stage disease finds no justification in the frequency of aortic nodal disease in Stage IB and IIA carcinoma of the cervix (7). Therefore, aortic lymphadenectomy is only carried out in early stage carcinoma of the cervix if the pelvic lymph nodes are positive. Only clinically suspicious nodes are examined intraoperatively by frozen section examination (8), and, in most cases, pelvic lymph node metastases are detected on the permanent sections. Laparoscopic aortic lymphadenectomy is, therefore, carried out as a second operation. However, as the probability of aortic lymph node metastases is, at most, 5% (9) and the probability of pelvic lymph node metastases about 10%, we believe it is preferable to subject about 10 women to two laparoscopic operations than to subject 95 or more to an unnecessary aortic lymphadenectomy. We do not treat all women with pelvic lymph node metastases further, and those with a single microscopic focus of cancer in one lymph node, especially if this is from the distal nodal chain, receive no further therapy (3).

CARCINOMA OF THE ENDOMETRIUM

Our approach to the management of endometrial carcinoma is outlined in Figures 20.2 and 20.3. The mainstay of therapy of carcinoma of the endometrium is simple hysterectomy, which can, of course, be carried out laparoscopically. Ignoring for the moment the unusual situations when gross disease is seen outside the uterus or on the cervix, the most important management decisions to be made are whom to subject to a lymphadenectomy, what kind of a lymphadenectomy to carry out, and how to use the results of the lymphadenectomy to select subsequent therapy. These issues have been considered in detail elsewhere (10), and only the main threads of the argument can be summarized here.

First, we take it as axiomatic that in routine practice, as opposed to clinical trials, a procedure that carries some morbidity cannot be justified unless it alters ther-

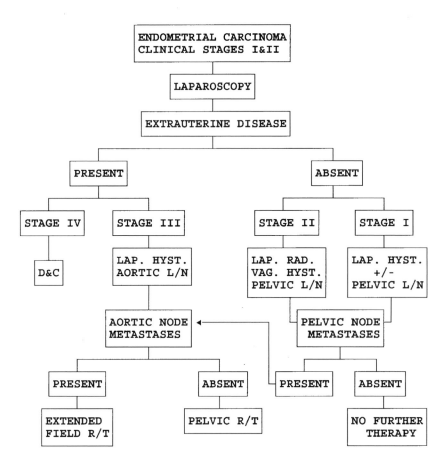

Figure 20.2 Management of clinical Stage I & II endometrial carcinoma.

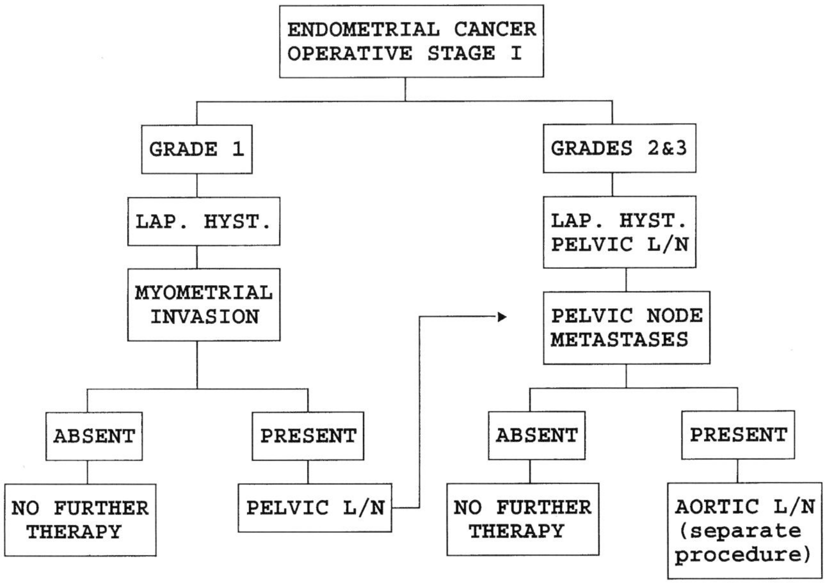

Figure 20.3 *Management of Stage I carcinoma of the endometrium.*

```
                    ENDOMETRIAL CANCER
                    OPERATIVE STAGE I

           GRADE 1                    GRADES 2&3

          LAP. HYST.                  LAP. HYST.
                                      PELVIC L/N

         MYOMETRIAL                   PELVIC NODE
         INVASION                     METASTASES

    ABSENT        PRESENT        ABSENT        PRESENT

  NO FURTHER    PELVIC L/N    NO FURTHER    AORTIC L/N
  THERAPY                     THERAPY       (separate
                                            procedure)
```

apy and/or potentially benefits patients in itself. Therefore, to justify its routine use, lymphadenectomy must either be carried out with a curative intent or lead to different treatment in patients who have positive and negative nodes, or both. We manage the pelvic lymph nodes in endometrial cancer in exactly the same way as we do in cervix cancer; that is, we carry out the same kind of lymphadenectomy, and we irradiate the pelvis if the nodes are positive unless only minimal microscopic lymph node metastases are present.

Using a decision-theoretic approach, we reanalyzed data published from the GOG (11,12) as well as our own data (13) in an attempt to quantify the therapeutic index of pelvic and aortic lymphadenectomy. The kernel of the analysis is as follows.

Using various combinations of tumor grade and depth of myometrial invasion as the selection criteria for lymphadenectomy, the proportion of women with pelvic and aortic lymph node metastases was first determined (sensitivity) for each potential criterion, and then the number of lymphadenectomies that had to be performed to identify one patient with pelvic or aortic node metastases was calculated. Based on the assumption that 60% of women with positive pelvic nodes and 40% of women with positive aortic nodes could be cured of their disease (5), we also calculated, for each criterion: (a) the number of lymphadenectomies required to prevent one death from pelvic and aortic lymph node metastases and (b) the number of lymphadenectomies required to prevent one additional death from pelvic and aortic lymph node metastases over and above that required to prevent one

death for the next less sensitive criterion. The results are shown in Tables 20.1 and 20.2 for selected criteria. These figures actually exaggerate the therapeutic value of lymphadenectomy in women with disease confined to the corpus and cervix because the analysis was based on data pertaining to women with *clinical* Stage 1 disease, some of whom actually had extrauterine disease, and they accounted for 50% (29/58) of the cases with positive pelvic nodes and 44% of the cases (15/34) with positive aortic nodes (11). In other words, the criteria would be less sensitive in women who did not have gross extrauterine disease, and more lymphadenectomies would be required to salvage one patient than these tables indicate. Nonetheless, the following conclusions were drawn.

Pelvic Nodes

Table 20.1 indicates that if pelvic lymphadenectomy is carried out in all women with endometrial carcinoma except those who have grade 1 lesions and no myometrial invasion (line 5), 93% of women would be subjected to pelvic lymphadenectomy, all those with positive pelvic nodes would be identified (column A), 17 pelvic lymphadenectomies would be required to salvage one patient with pelvic lymph node metastasis (column D), mortality would be reduced by almost 6% (column C, line 1 minus line 5), and approximately 30 lymphadenectomies would be required to cure one additional patient with positive pelvic nodes who was not salvaged by adopting a less sensitive criterion (column E). It seems to us justifiable to carry out a pelvic lymphadenectomy in these cases because pelvic

Table 20.1 Therapeutic index of selective pelvic lymphadenectomy

Criteria	A	B	C	D	E
None	0%	0%	9.3%	—	—
D3	60%	22%	6.0%	6.6	—
G2–3	91%	71%	4.2%	13.9	28
G2–3 and D3	95%	74%	4.0%	13.9	27
G2–3 and D1–3	100%	93%	3.7%	16.6	32

A = Proportion of patients with positive pelvic nodes identified

B = Proportion of patients subjected to pelvic lymphadenectomy

C = Death rate from pelvic nodal disease

D = Number of lymphadenectomies required to prevent one death from pelvic nodal disease

E = Number of lymphadenectomies required to prevent one additional death from pelvic nodal disease

G1–3 = Tumor Grade 1–3

D1–3 = Depth of myometrial invasion to:
    1 = inner third
    2 = middle third
    3 = outer third

Table 20.2 Therapeutic index of selective aortic lymphadenectomy

Criteria	A	B	C	D	E
None	0%	0%	5.4%	—	—
D3	71%	22%	3.9%	14	—
G3 and D3	76%	37%	3.8%	22	111
G2–3	91%	71%	3.5%	36	108
G2–3 and D2–3	97%	77%	3.3%	36	95
G2–3 and D1–3	100%	93%	3.3%	44	118

A = Proportion of patients with positive aortic nodes identified

B = Proportion of patients subjected to aortic lymphadenectomy

C = Death rate from aortic nodal disease

D = Number of lymphadenectomies required to prevent one death from aortic nodal disease

E = Number of lymphadenectomies required to prevent one additional death from aortic nodal disease

G1–3 = Tumor Grade 1–3

D1–3 = Depth of myometrial invasion to:
    1 = inner third
    2 = middle third
    3 = outer third

lymphadenectomy is not associated with a 3% mortality or a 3% serious morbidity rate (14). It also seems worthwhile extending the indications somewhat to simplify therapy and eliminate the need to assess myometrial invasion by intraoperative frozen sections and/or preoperative imaging studies. Thus, we carry out pelvic lymphadenectomy in all women except those with grade 1 lesions and no identifiable tumor in the opened uterus (Figures 20.2, 20.3).

Aortic Nodes

From the results shown in Table 20.2, we believe it would be difficult to justify aortic lymphadenectomy in the same group of patients who are candidates for pelvic lymphadenectomy. Although the death rate could be reduced by 2% at a "cost" of 44 aortic lymphadenectomies per patient saved (column C, line 1 minus line 6), which could questionably be justified, the more telling statistics appear in column E. This column shows that it takes 100 or more lymphadenec-

tomies to salvage a patient with aortic lymph node metastases who would not be salvaged by using deep myometrial invasion as the indication for aortic lymphadenectomy, and as we noted at the outset, these are optimistic figures. Thus, in our view, aortic lymphadenectomy cannot be justified in women who have endometrial cancer grossly confined to the uterus unless they have deep myometrial invasion.

We took the analysis one step further and compared deep myometrial invasion with pelvic lymph node metastases as a criterion for aortic lymphadenectomy. Obviously, if deep myometrial invasion is used as the criterion, the aortic lymphadenectomy can be carried out at the time of the primary operation, but if pelvic lymph node metastasis is used as the criterion, this must be deferred to a second operation. Approximately 5–7% of women with endometrial carcinoma who do not have gross extrauterine or cervical disease can be expected to have pelvic lymph node metastases,

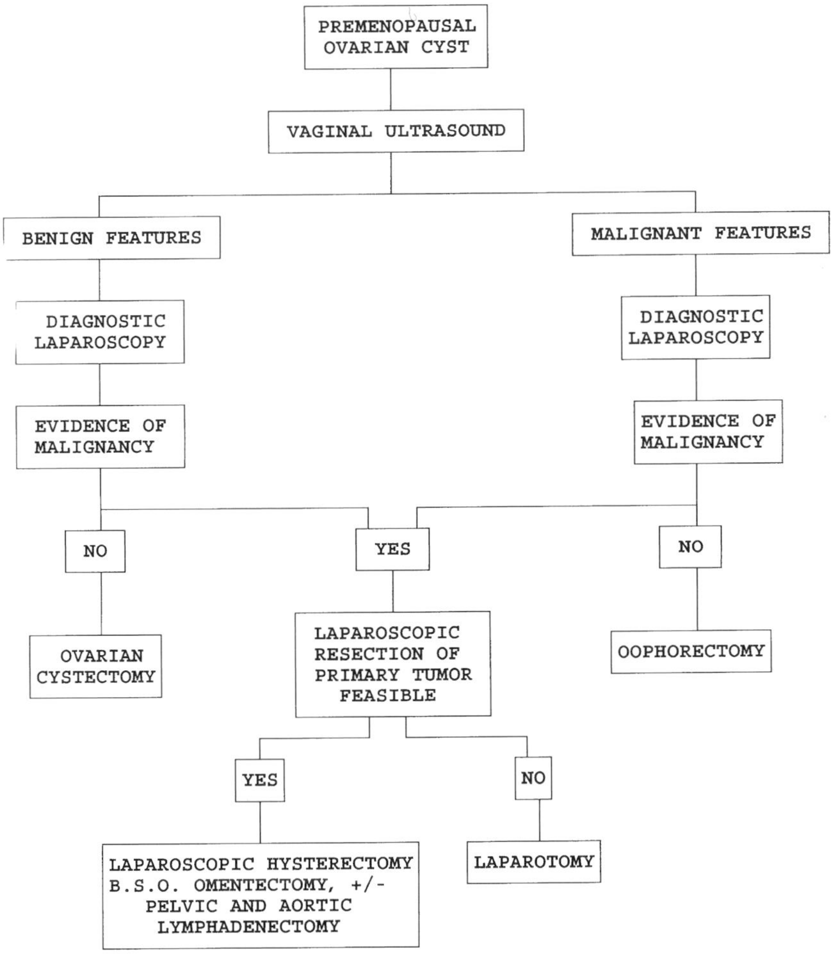

PREMENOPAUSAL OVARIAN CYST

VAGINAL ULTRASOUND

BENIGN FEATURES → DIAGNOSTIC LAPAROSCOPY → EVIDENCE OF MALIGNANCY → NO → OVARIAN CYSTECTOMY

EVIDENCE OF MALIGNANCY → YES → LAPAROSCOPIC RESECTION OF PRIMARY TUMOR FEASIBLE

MALIGNANT FEATURES → DIAGNOSTIC LAPAROSCOPY → EVIDENCE OF MALIGNANCY → NO → OOPHORECTOMY

LAPAROSCOPIC RESECTION OF PRIMARY TUMOR FEASIBLE → YES → LAPAROSCOPIC HYSTERECTOMY B.S.O. OMENTECTOMY, +/- PELVIC AND AORTIC LYMPHADENECTOMY

LAPAROSCOPIC RESECTION OF PRIMARY TUMOR FEASIBLE → NO → LAPAROTOMY

Figure 20.4 Management of ovarian cysts in pre-menopausal women.

and this proportion of women would be subjected to two operations if pelvic lymph node metastases were used as the indication for aortic lymphadenectomy. But, using this criterion, 23% more women with aortic lymph node metastases would be identified and 35% fewer primary aortic lymphadenectomies would need to be performed. Put another way, for every 100 aortic lymphadenectomies performed as a second procedure, 7 more women would be salvaged and 157 primary aortic lymphadenectomies would be avoided. Aortic lymphadenectomy does not carry a 7% mortality rate [14]; therefore, we believe this approach to be preferable even if the complications eliminated by avoiding 157 primary aortic lymphadenectomies are ignored. Moreover, the disadvantages of a two-stage approach are minimized if the operations are performed laparoscopically.

Thus, although it has been inferred from the 1988 FIGO staging for endometrial carcinoma and the surgical protocols of collaborative groups such as the GOG that aortic lymphadenectomy should be performed whenever pelvic lymphadenectomy is carried out, this cannot be justified in clinical practice, in our view. Many women require only pelvic lymphadenectomy or only aortic lymphadenectomy, e.g., those who have gross extrauterine or cervical disease, not both.

Rigid adherence to the unsupported view that lymphadenectomy in endometrial cancer necessarily means both pelvic and aortic lymph lymphadenectomy has also needlessly disqualified obese women from laparoscopic lymphadenectomy, precisely the ones most likely to benefit from avoidance of a laparotomy incision. Laparoscopic aortic lymphadenectomy has proved to be difficult to perform in women weighing more than 180 pounds [15], but the same restrictions do not apply to pelvic lymphadenectomy [16]. Therefore, if aortic lymphadenectomy were restricted to women who had pelvic lymph node metastases, most women could be satisfactorily managed laparoscopically because most do not need an aortic

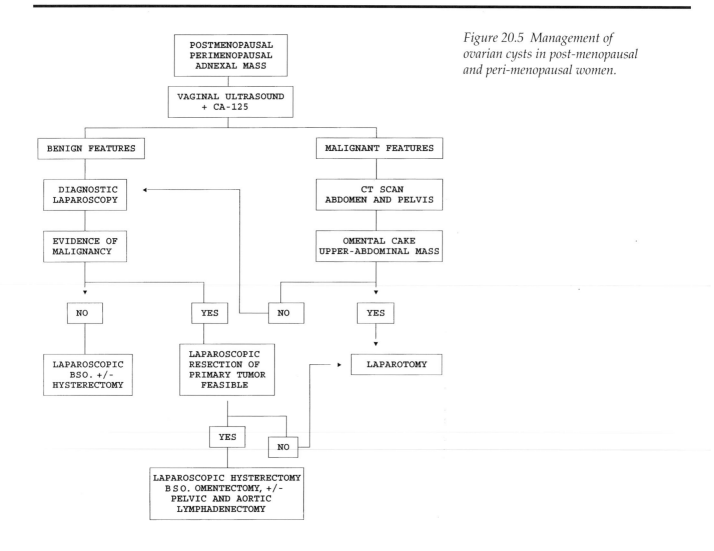

Figure 20.5 Management of ovarian cysts in post-menopausal and peri-menopausal women.

lymphadenectomy, especially not obese women who tend to have more favorable tumors.

CARCINOMA OF THE OVARY

The role of laparoscopic surgery in the management of ovarian carcinoma remains to be defined, the concepts are still evolving, and the whole area, to say the least, is controversial. The issues are intimately related to the management of adnexal masses and were discussed in Chapter 14. There we pointed out that it has been generally assumed that any suspicion of ovarian malignancy is a contraindication to laparoscopy, but that once the initial impulse to agree with this sentiment is resisted, it become less and less clear what the basis for this proscription is.

It must also be said that progress in this area has been hampered by the quality of scientific reporting pertaining to this area. For example, a study that has been widely quoted to condemn the use of laparo-

scopy in this malignancy consisted of a survey of select physicians (gynecologic oncologists), had a poor response rate (50%), and established no denominators for the outcome of interest (17). Other than document that patients with ovarian cancer are sometimes mismanaged, a fact we might have surmised without the survey, it provided no information that helped in any other way to define the indications for laparoscopy in this disease or to design protocols that might determine its role. All it did was to invite the conclusion that because someone had misused the laparoscope in some cases of ovarian cancer, any use of the laparoscope in this disease could be regarded *ipso facto* as misuse, a line of reasoning hardly conducive to clear thought in an area already rife with high emotion and patent bias.

The implantation of tumor in the trocar tracts used during laparoscopy is an undeniable possibility that must be considered when protocols involving the laparoscopic management of ovarian carcinoma are being designed (18,19). However, without knowing how frequently this occurs, it is impossible to assess whether this is a disadvantage that will offset all the many advantages of laparoscopy over a laparotomy or will be offset by them. Tumor implants are rarely, if ever, seen in a laparotomy scar following surgery for advanced ovarian cancer and ascites. It should, therefore, be possible to prevent implants in trocar tracts by closing the peritoneum beneath them and irrigating or fulgurating the tract (20).

With that said, we accept that large bulky tumors are unlikely ever to be amenable to laparoscopic treatment, but the majority of women with minimal upper abdominal disease almost certainly will eventually be treated in this way, as will those with primary peritoneal carcinomatosis. Nonetheless, the laparoscope may have a role in selecting patients with bulky unresectable tumors for neoadjuvant therapy, if that proves to be worthwhile. Patients with Stage III borderline tumors are also potential candidates for a laparoscopic approach because the treatment of these indolent malignancies relies much more on repeated surgical resection than on adjunctive chemotherapy or radiation therapy. Clearly, the advantages of a laparoscopic approach compound if therapy involves multiple surgeries.

Laparoscopic restaging following open ovarian cystectomy or oophorectomy is obviously a feasible undertaking because concerns over tumor bulk or cyst rupture do not arise, but this indication will vanish along with the use of laparotomy for ovarian cystectomy. In the long run, Stage I ovarian carcinoma will also almost certainly be managed laparoscopically because all the component parts of a surgical staging procedure (hysterectomy, lymphadenectomy, omentectomy) can already be carried out laparoscopically. Although the ability to inspect peritoneal surfaces adequately in these situations may have been questioned, this concern applies more to another era than to modern laparoscopic techniques, provided they are used properly and patiently. Indeed, the laparoscope may allow tumor in some reaches of the abdomen, e.g., the diaphragm, to be better detected and biopsied than a laparotomy. Finally, whatever the detrimental effect of cyst rupture, which is probably real but marginal, the incidence of ovarian carcinoma under the circumstances in which ovarian cystectomy is indicated and cyst rupture a concern is so low that it is almost certainly outweighed by the beneficial effects of laparoscopy in the vast majority of women who do not have a malignancy.

Possibilities for the management of ovarian cancer are shown in Figures 20.4 and 20.5.

REFERENCES

1. Donohue JP. Retroperitoneal lymphadenectomy. Urol Clin North Am 1977;4:509–521.

2. Burghardt E, Pickel H, Lahousen M, Stettner H. Pelvic lymphadenectomy in operative treatment of ovarian cancer. Am J Obstet Gynecol 1986;155:315–319.

3. Kinney WK, Alvarez RD, Reid GC, et al. Value of adjuvant whole pelvic irradiation after Wertheim hysterectomy for early stage squamous carcinoma of the cervix with pelvic nodal metastasis: a matched-control study. Gynecol Oncol 1989;34:258–262.

4. Downey GO, Potish RA, Adock LL, Prem KA, Twiggs LB. Pretreatment surgical staging in cervical carcinoma: therapeutic efficacy of pelvic lymph node resection. Am J Obstet Gynecol 1989;160:1056–1061.

5. Morrow CP, Bundy BB, Kurman RJ, et al. Relationship between surgical-pathological risk factors and outcome in clinical stage I and II carcinoma of the endometrium. A Gynecologic Oncology Group study. Gynecol Oncol 1991;40:55–65.

6. Stehman FB, Bundy BN, Hanjani P, et al. Biopsy of the scalene fat pad in carcinoma of the cervix metastatic to the periaortic lymph nodes. Surg Gynecol Obstet 1987; 165:503–506.

7. Patsner B, Sedlacek TV, Lovecchio JL. Para-aortic node sampling in small (3-cm or less) stage IB invasive cervical cancer. Gynecol Oncol 1992;44:53–54.

8. Bjornsson BL, Nelson BE, Reale FR, Rose PG. Accuracy of frozen section for lymph node metastasis in patients undergoing radical hysterectomy for carcinoma of the cervix. Gynecol Oncol 1993;51:50–53.

9. Jones WB. Surgical management for advanced or recurrent cancer of the cervix. Cancer 1987;60:2094–2103.

10. Kadar N, Homesley HD, Malfetano J. Some new perspectives on the indications for pelvic and para-aortic lymphadenectomy in the management of endometrial carcinoma. Gynaecol Endosc (in press).

11. Creasman WT, Morrow CP, Bundy BN, et al. Surgical pathologic spread pattern of endometrial cancer. Cancer 1987;60:2035-2041.

12. Boronow RC, Morrow CP, Creasman WT, et al. Surgical staging in endometrial cancer: clinical-pathologic findings of a prospective study. Obstet Gynecol 1984; 63:825-832.

13. Kadar N, Malfetano JH, Homesley HD. Determinants of survival of surgically staged patients with endometrial

carcinoma histologically confined to the uterus. Obstet Gynecol 1992;80:655–659.

14. Homesley HD, Kadar N, Lentz S, Barrett R. Selective pelvic and periaortic lymphadenectomy does not increase morbidity in surgical staging of endometrial carcinoma. Am J Obstet Gynecol 1992;167:1225–1230.

15. Childers JA, Hatch KD, Tran AN, Surwit EA. Laparoscopic para-aortic lymphadenectomy in gynecologic malignancies. Obstet Gynecol 1993;82:741–747.

16. Kadar N, Pelosi MA. Laparoscopically assisted hysterectomy in women weighing 200 pounds or more. Gynaecol Endosc 1994;3:159-169.

17. Maiman M, Seltzer V, Boyce J. Laparoscopic excision of ovarian neoplasms subsequently found to be malignant. Obstet Gynecol 1991;77:563–565.

18. Gleeson NC, Nicosia SV, Mark JE, Hoffman MS, Cavanagh D. Abdominal wall metastases from ovarian cancer after laparoscopy. Am J Obstet Gynecol 1993;169:522–523.

19. Hsiu J, Given FT, Kemp GM. Tumor implantation after diagnostic laparoscopic biopsy of serous ovarian tumors of low malignant potential. Obstet Gynecol 1986;68:90–93.

20. Kadar N. Numerators without denominators, again? Am J Obstet Gynecol 1994;170:1479.

Chapter 21
Laparoscopic Pelvic Lymphadenectomy

But in science the credit goes to the man who convinces the world, not to the man to whom the idea first occurs. —Osler

BACKGROUND

Dargent and Salvat (1) were the first to remove pelvic lymph nodes laparoscopically, but theirs was a limited (interiliac), extraperitoneal procedure, partly carried out by finger dissection with a finger inserted through the abdominal wall, and a technique has been abandoned by the authors in favor of a transperitoneal approach. Nonetheless, the credit for the concept of a laparoscopic pelvic lymphadenectomy belongs to them.

Transperitoneal laparoscopic pelvic lymphadenectomy was first performed almost simultaneously by Reich (2) and Querleu (3). Although Reich pipped Querleu to the post by a week, his real contribution to the development of laparoscopic lymphadenectomy was to have embraced the concept early and to have stimulated and helped others, including urologists, to undertake the procedure (4). The history of this operation in the U.S.A. can, in fact, be traced through him to Tucson because Childers was introduced to laparoscopic lymphadenectomy by Thierry Vancaillie, a coauthor with Reich on the first paper describing the urological application of laparoscopic pelvic lymphadenectomy (Childers, personal communication).

Querleu and colleagues were the first to systematically incorporate pelvic lymphadenectomy into the management of cervix cancer, but their procedure, although slightly more extensive than Reich's, was, and remains, a limited, "interiliac" dissection with which

the authors harvest only 8–12 nodes per case (3,5). The iliac vessels are neither mobilized nor skeletonized, which, at least in this author's opinion, is the *sine qua non* of a true pelvic lymphadenectomy. Pelvic lymphadenectomy was also not used for definitive therapy but rather to select patients for either an abdominal or radical vaginal hysterectomy, which was initially done as a separate operation (an approach that has since been abandoned).

Although a year later, Nezhat et al. (6) also performed bilateral pelvic lymphadenectomy as part of a laparoscopic radical hysterectomy for Stage IA2 carcinoma of the cervix, theirs too was a sampling procedure rather than a complete lymphadenectomy. In 1991, in the U.S.A., pelvic lymphadenectomy began to be used systematically in the management of gynecological malignancies independently by Childers et al. (7,8), Kadar (9-11), and Fowler et al. (12). However, Kadar was the first to use it for definitive treatment rather than selection of therapy in cervix cancer (9-11) and to perform a complete lymphadenectomy that included mobilization of the iliac vessels from the psoas muscle and separation and skeletonization of the artery and vein (9).

OPERATIVE TECHNIQUE

The technique used for laparoscopic pelvic lymphadenectomy is essentially the same as that used at laparotomy except that the pelvic sidewall dissection

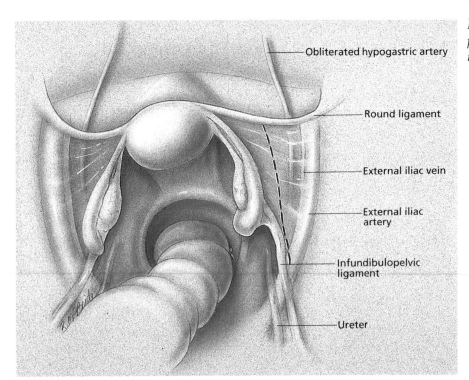

Figure 21.1 *The incision in the pelvic sidewall triangle peritoneum is made along the dotted line.*

Labels on figure:
Obliterated hypogastric artery
Round ligament
External iliac vein
External iliac artery
Infundibulopelvic ligament
Ureter

is carried out differently, as already described in Chapters 6 and 10. The key to a successful operation is (1) correct development of the pararectal and paravesical spaces and (2) systematic delineation of the surgical limits of the intended dissection.

Pelvic Sidewall Dissection

The technique for opening the pelvic sidewall and developing the paravesical and pararectal spaces was described in detail in Chapters 6 and 10, and the sequence of steps will only be summarized here.

The pelvic peritoneum is incised in the middle of the pelvic sidewall triangle (Figure 21.1), and the incision is extended to above the pelvic brim lateral to the infundibulopelvic ligament, and then to the round ligament, but the round ligament is *not* divided at this time. The broad ligament is opened with blunt dissection, and the dissection is continued under the round ligament until the umbilical ligament (obliterated hypogastric artery) is identified extraperitoneally. At the proximal end of the incision, the infundibulopelvic ligament is retracted medially and the ureter identified at the pelvic brim (Figures 21.2, 21.3). As this dissection is being carried out, it is important to coagulate all the vessels encountered running along the peritoneum and in the retroperitoneal tissues, however small; otherwise, they will bleed sufficiently to stain the tissues and impair visibility.

The paravesical space proper is next developed by placing the closed tips of the dissecting scissors lateral to the umbilical ligament and pulling it medially. The blunt dissection is assisted with the suction-irrigator, and the dissection is continued inferiorly as far as the pelvic floor. The medial part of the paravesical space between the umbilical ligament and the bladder is next opened by blunt dissection against the umbilical ligament in the opposite direction (Figures 21.4, 21.5). Finally, the umbilical ligament is traced retrogradely to the origin of the uterine artery and the pararectal space is opened by blunt dissection proximal and medial to the uterine artery and cardinal ligament. The dissection is then continued proximally to the sacrum and inferiorly to the pelvic floor, so that the entire pelvic course of the ureter is seen on the medial leaf of the broad ligament (Figure 21.6).

SURGICAL LIMITS OF THE DISSECTION

The surgical limits of the dissection are the *common iliac artery* proximally, i.e., cephalad, the *psoas muscle* laterally, the *circumflex iliac vein* and pubic bone distally, i.e., caudad, the *umbilical ligament* medially, and the *obturator fossa* inferiorly, i.e., ventrally. The circumflex iliac vein drains the lateral part of the anterior abdominal wall, and courses obliquely downwards from the inguinal ligament, crosses the lower part of

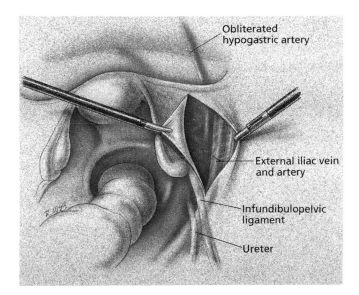

Obliterated
hypogastric artery

External iliac vein
and artery

Infundibulopelvic
ligament

Ureter

Figure 21.2 The broad ligament is opened.

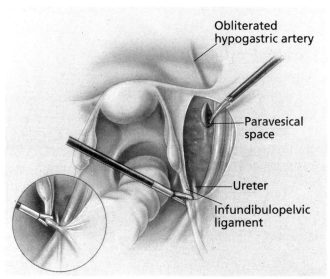

Obliterated
hypogastric artery

Paravesical
space

Ureter

Infundibulopelvic
ligament

Figure 21.3 The infundibulopelvic ligament has been pulled medially to expose the ureter at the pelvic brim.

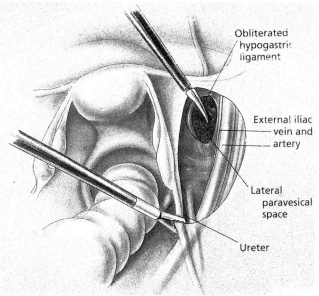

Obliterated
hypogastric
ligament

External iliac
vein and
artery

Lateral
paravesical
space

Ureter

Figure 21.4 The lateral paravesical space is opened.

the external iliac artery from lateral to medial, and drains into the external iliac vein below the artery (Figure 21.7). The proximal, distal, medial, and inferior limits of the dissection are delineated as the paravesical and pararectal spaces are developed, and all that remains is to separate the external iliac vessels from the psoas muscle.

Using sharp scissor dissection, the dense areolar tissue that attaches the external iliac artery and vein to the psoas muscle is scored very superficially from the proximal to the distal limits of the dissection, namely, the common iliac artery and the circumflex iliac vein, respectively. The initial incision must be kept very superficial to avoid injury to the external iliac vein, which lies just below the artery (Figure 21.8). If there is a great deal of fatty nodal tissue lying in front of the psoas muscle obscuring the lateral border of the artery, this tissue may need to be removed first with spoon forceps to expose the artery. Once an opening has been made in this areolar tissue, blunt dissection with the suction-irrigator or the back of the closed dissecting scissors is used to peel the external iliac artery and then the vein lying under it off the psoas muscle. Once the vein is freed, progressively deeper dissection will gain entry into the obturator fossa, which is identified by the bright yellow fatty nodal tissue that will come into view. By continuing the plane of dissection lateral to this tissue, the nodal bundle of the obturator fossa

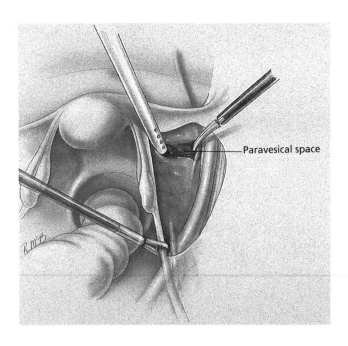

Figure 21.5 *The medial paravesical space is opened.*

will be mobilized medially (Figure 21.9). There are no branches lateral to the external iliac artery or vein, but very occasionally, nutrient muscular branches can be encountered that can be safely coagulated or clipped.

PELVIC LYMPHADENECTOMY

▶STEP 1. *Freeing the external iliac artery and vein from their aerolar sheaths and separating them.*

The external iliac artery and vein are next freed from their areolar investments. Each vessel is completely surrounded by its own distinct areolar sheath, and the two sheaths are fused along the entire course of the vessels. The sheath of the external iliac artery is incised with scissor along its dorsal surface from the level of the common iliac artery all the way down to the circumflex iliac vein (Figure 21.10). There are no branches of the external iliac artery in this region, but a hair-like vessel usually crosses the artery obliquely at its midportion superficial to its sheath, and it should be coagulated by touching it with the closed point of the dissecting scissors using an unmodulated current.

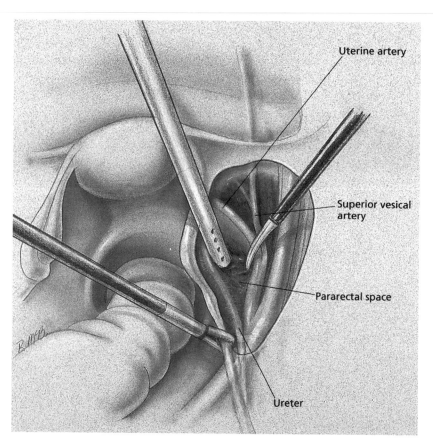

Figure 21.6 *The pararectal space is developed.*

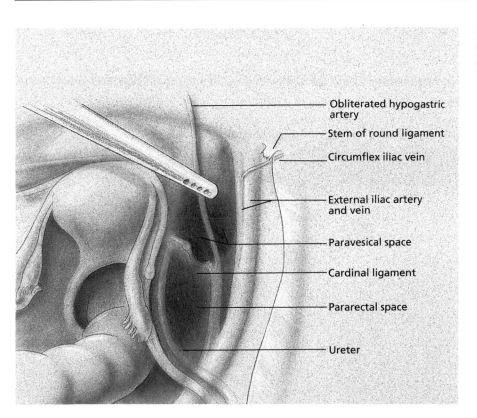

Figure 21.7 Pelvic lympha-denectomy: surgical limits of the dissection.

Obliterated hypogastric artery

Stem of round ligament

Circumflex iliac vein

External iliac artery and vein

Paravesical space

Cardinal ligament

Pararectal space

Ureter

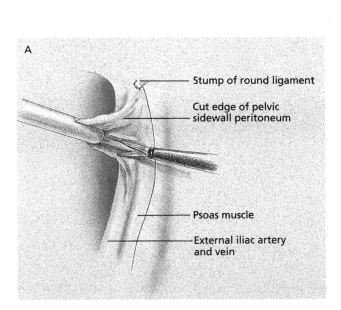

A

Stump of round ligament

Cut edge of pelvic sidewall peritoneum

Psoas muscle

External iliac artery and vein

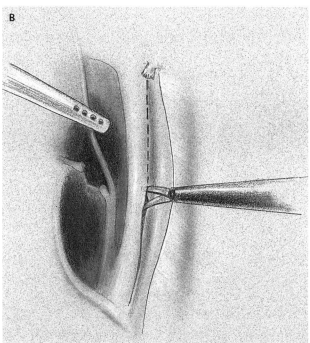

B

Figure 21.8 Fatty nodal tissue is removed from in front of the psoas muscle (A), and the attachments of the external iliac vessels to the psoas is divided (B).

Once it has been opened, the medial border of the sheath around the artery is grasped with the dissecting forceps and the artery is peeled off the inferior surface of its sheath using mostly blunt dissection with the suction-irrigator or the back of the scissors, cutting areolar attachments as needed (Figure 21.10). The same process is repeated on the lateral surface of the artery, and this will free it completely from the

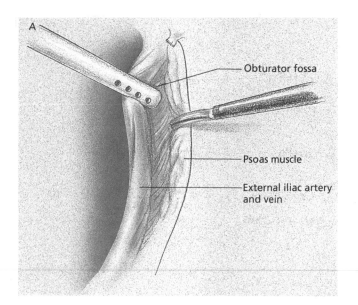

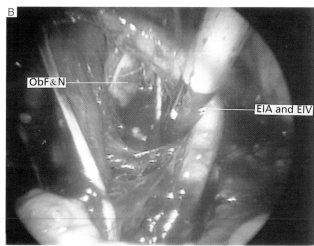

Obturator fossa

Psoas muscle

External iliac artery and vein

ObF & N

EIA and EIV

Figure 21.9 *The iliac vessels are separated from the psoas muscle, and the obturator fossa entered lateral to the vessels.*

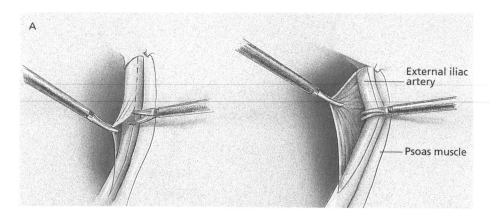

External iliac artery

Psoas muscle

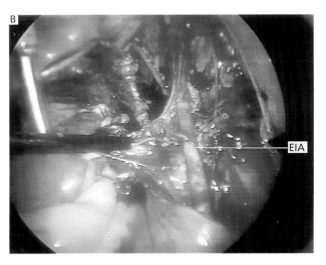

EIA

Figure 21.10 *The external iliac artery is dissected free of its areolar sheath.*

underlying vein. At this point, the sheaths of the external iliac artery and vein are still joined along the undersurface of the artery, and the next step is to cautiously incise the sheath of the external iliac vein. It is this step that requires the greatest care in the entire dissection as the edge of the vessel can easily be compressed and merge imperceptibly with the areolar sheath that covers it. However, once a nick has been made in the sheath, the glistening surface of the vein becomes unmistakably clear and distinct from its areolar covering (Figure 21.11). The same technique of sharp and blunt dissection can then be used to free the vein circumferentially from its sheath as is used to free the artery. The final step in this part of the dissection is to free the inferior border of the vein, which is tethered by loose areolar tissue to the pelvic sidewall and obturator fossa (Figure 21.11). Occasionally, an aberrant obturator vein is encountered at this point, coursing upwards from the obturator fossa to join the external iliac vein on its inferior aspect rather than the internal iliac vein, as is usually the case (Figure 21.11). An aberrant obturator vein usually has to be divided after it has been coagulated with bipolar forceps, or clipped.

▶STEP 2. Removal of node-bearing tissue from the front of the psoas muscle and external iliac vessels.

The external iliac nodes are distributed along the course of the external iliac artery in a cephalad-caudad or "north-south" direction and are attached laterally to the psoas muscle and medially to the sheath of the external iliac artery by loose areolar tissue. Distally, at the level of the circumflex iliac vein, there are quite prominent nodes lying in a lateral-medial or "east-west" direction across the lower part of the external iliac artery. The lateral-most part of this nodal bundle is about 2–3 cm from the artery itself, and there is usually a nutrient branch that has to be coagulated as these nodes are freed from the inferolateral part of the psoas muscle (Figure 21.12).

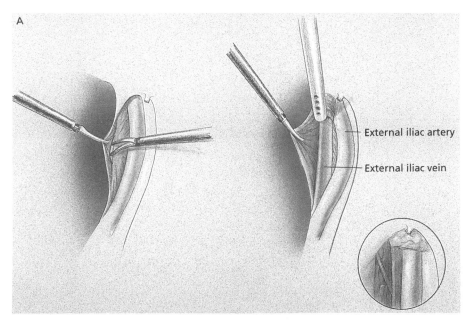

A

External iliac artery

External iliac vein

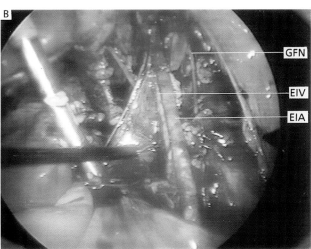

B

GFN

EIV

EIA

Figure 21.11A,B The external iliac vein is dissected free of its areolar sheath.

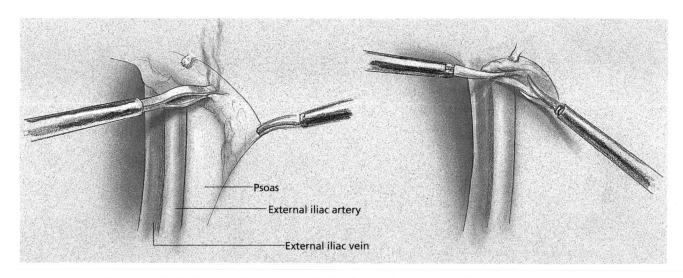

Psoas
External iliac artery
External iliac vein

Figure 21.12 Nodal tissue lying across the distal part of the external iliac vessels is removed.

The medial attachments of these nodes are freed when the external iliac vessels are dissected from their sheaths; all that remains, then, is to free their lateral attachments to the psoas muscle. As this is done, the ileofemoral and genitofemoral nerves are encountered but can easily be pushed laterally. Sometimes the fatty nodal tissue lying in front of the psoas muscle is removed at the start of the dissection, before the vessels are skeletonized. The nodal tissue and the areolar sheaths of the external iliac vessels to which they are attached can be removed at this point and sent as a separate specimen, or be allowed to fall away from the vessels into the obturator fossa and removed later en bloc with the remainder of the pelvic nodal tissue.

▶STEP 3. Dissection of the obturator nerve and fossa.

The obturator fossa and internal iliac vessels are next freed. This is done by retracting the external iliac vessels upwards and laterally and teasing out the obturator nerve from the inferior-most part of the obturator nodal bundle using the unopened tips of the dissecting scissors (Figure 21.13A). Once the nerve is freed, the distal attachments of the nodal bundle to the pubic bone are divided with the closed tips of the dissecting scissors using an unmodulated current to seal the lymphatics (Figure 21.13B). The nodal bundle is then grasped with the spoon forceps, elevated and placed on tension, and teased off its ventral-most attachments below the obturator nerve using a gentle pushing motion with the partly opened scissors. As this nodal tissue is freed in a cephalic direction, residual attachments to the external iliac vein

usually need to be freed. Eventually, the internal iliac artery is reached, and the nodal tissue lying anterior, lateral, and medial to it is freed in continuity with the obturator fossa nodal mass. The nodal tissue can be quite adherent in this region because the internal iliac artery does not have an areolar sheath as do the external iliac vessels. With further dissection cephalad, the crura or bifurcation of the iliac arteries is reached, and this region must be cleaned with care, ever mindful of the fact that the external and internal iliac veins lie just lateral to these structures (Figure 21.13C). Once the attachments of the nodal bundle in this region are divided, the bulk of the specimen is removed.

STEP 4. Dissection of the common iliac artery.

At this point, the dissection has reached the bifurcation of the common iliac artery, and the nodal tissue lying on top of the psoas muscle lateral to the distal part of the common iliac artery is next removed and sent as a separate specimen (Figure 21.14). The inferior aspect of this nodal bundle insinuates itself between the psoas and the lateral wall of the common iliac artery, and it is pierced by a constant nutrient artery that runs from the lateral wall of the artery and the psoas muscle. Brisk bleeding results if this artery is cut, but it can be controlled by pressure and then bipolar coagulation. If there is difficulty controlling the bleeding, the surgeon should not hesitate to insert a small gauze sponge into the peritoneal cavity through the 10-mm trocar as this will help compress the artery. Medial to the common iliac vessels lie the sacral nodes, which are also removed at this time (Figure 21.15).

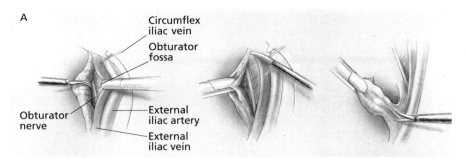

A

Circumflex
iliac vein

Obturator
fossa

Obturator
nerve

External
iliac artery

External
iliac vein

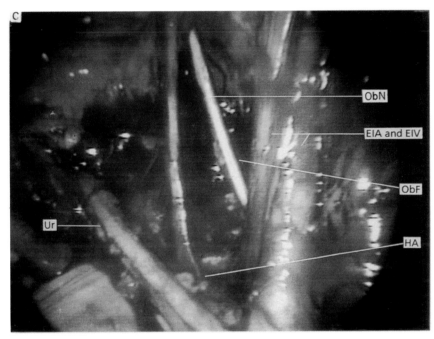

ObN

EIA and EIV

ObF

Ur

HA

Figure 21.13 The obturator nodes are dissected medially (A), detached from the pubic bone (B), and dissected cephalad along the hypogastric artery (C).

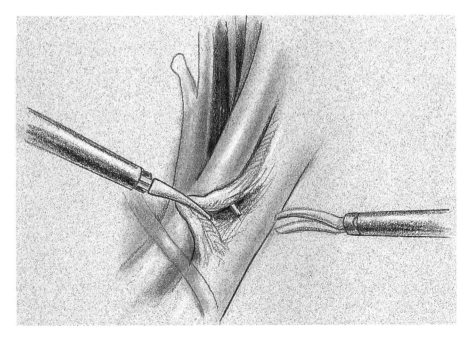

Figure 21.14 Nodal tissue lying lateral to the common iliac artery is removed and sent as separate specimen.

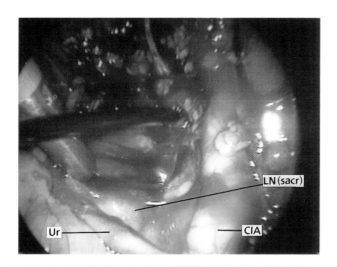

Figure 21.15 Presacral nodes lying medial to the common iliac vessels are removed.

Finally, we retract the proximal-most part of the external iliac artery and vein medially and remove residual nodes lying in the proximal-most part of the obturator fossa and between the obturator nerve and the psoas muscle (Figure 21.16). Once these nodes have been removed, the dissection is complete (Figure 21.17).

It is essential to use spoon forceps to remove the fatty nodal tissue as this instrument will compress tissue into the hollow of its jaws, enabling large chunks of nodal tissue to be removed without fragmenting. The author has used a surgical glove and the LapSac in the abdomen to store nodes prior to their extraction but has not found this to offer any advantages.

DISCUSSION

Preliminary results reported from a number of centers indicate that laparoscopic pelvic lymphadenectomy is a remarkably safe operation. In a recent paper, Querleu (5) makes reference to having performed 140 pelvic lymphadenectomies without serious complications. Childers et al. (7,8) report no significant complications in a total of at least 51 pelvic lymphadenectomies, and this author has had no significant complications in his first 25 cases (9-11). (In one of the author's recent cases, a small split developed in the medial edge of the right obturator nerve as nodal tissue was being removed from the proximal-most part of the obturator fossa, lateral to the nerve. The patient noted transient weakness with adduction in the affected leg, which disappeared after a week).

Although many factors besides the adequacy of the lymphadenectomy can affect node counts, the

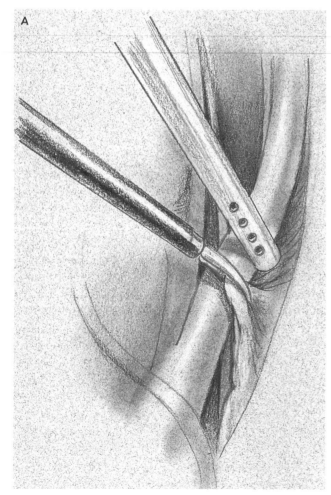

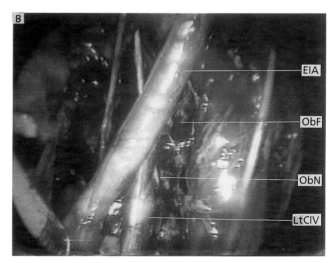

Figure 21.16 The iliac vessels are retracted medially, and nodes lying in the proximal obturator fossa are removed.

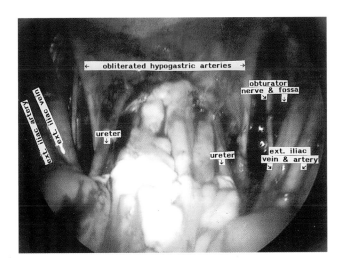

Figure 21.17 Bilateral laparoscopic pelvic lymphadenectomy: the completed operation.

Table 21.1 Average number of lymph nodes and proportion of positive nodes obtained by laparoscopic pelvic lymphadenectomy in women with carcinoma of the cervix

	Mean Node Count	Proportion of Positive Nodes
Kadar*	30.9	2/10 (20%)
Fowler et al.	23.5	2/12 (17%)
Childers et al.	28.4**	5/18 (28%)

*All patients had concurrent laparoscopic vaginal radical hysterectomies.

**Estimate because number of aortic and pelvic nodes not reported separately. Includes patients with advanced disease.

node counts and proportion of positive pelvic nodes obtained by laparoscopic pelvic lymphadenectomy has been similar to than usually obtained with an open technique. Querleu (3,5) has consistently reported much lower node counts that are usually obtained with an open technique, but this is a reflection of the type of lymphadenectomy the author feels is required to manage cervix cancer (interiliac lymphadenectomy) rather than of what can be achieved by the laparoscopic approach per se (Table 21.1). If the iliac vessels are not mobilized, it is not possible to clear the proximal part of the obturator fossa, especially the nodes lying below the vessels and lateral to the obturator nerve.

Fowler et al. (12) assessed the adequacy of laparoscopic pelvic lymphadenectomy by performing a laparotomy after completion of the laparoscopic lymphadenectomy. They recovered an average of 23.5 nodes laparoscopically, and the count was higher in their second six (29.2) than in their first six (17.8) cases, indicating rapid acquisition of proficiency with the technique. They recovered additional lymph nodes at subsequent laparotomy, but 75% of all the nodes removed were recovered laparoscopically, including all (albeit only two) positive nodes. However, the iliac vessels did not appear to have been mobilized.

The GOG has initiated a limited access study with a similar design. This design can be criticized, however, for not having a control group, which makes it impossible to interpret the major end-point used in the study, the proportion of nodes recovered laparoscopically. It is entirely possible, indeed likely, that if at the conclusion of a traditional pelvic lymphadenectomy, a different surgeon explored the pelvis to try to extract additional material, more lymph nodes could, in fact, be recovered. Without knowing how many additional nodes could be recovered after an open pelvic lymphadenectomy, it is impossible to interpret the number obtained after a laparoscopic pelvic lymphadenectomy. The overall frequency of positive nodes is much too low to use the number of positive lymph nodes missed at laparoscopy as an indicator of the potential inadequacy of the procedure. Thus, it is unrealistic to expect this study to add significantly to the information already available about laparoscopic pelvic lymphadenectomy from the node counts that have been obtained, the frequency of positive nodes harvested, and the video-documentation of the dissection, and some may find it troubling that patients are being asked to subject themselves to potential risk (from the laparoscopic procedure, especially if the surgeon is inexperienced) without offsetting advantages (because a laparotomy is then performed).

Obesity has not limited our ability to carry out pelvic lymphadenectomy. We have declined only one patient, who weighed 367 pounds, but obesity was only one factor making the patient an inappropriate surgical candidate. She had Stage 1B carcinoma of the cervix, was nulliparous, had a very narrow vagina, and had multiple medical problems. We have carried out laparoscopic pelvic lymphadenectomy in seven women who weighed over 180 pounds, in conjunction with a laparoscopic-vaginal radical hysterectomy for cervix cancer (two cases) or laparoscopic hysterectomy for endometrial carcinoma (five cases). Five women weighed over 200 pounds, and the heaviest weighed 300 pounds.

REFERENCES

1. Dargent D, Salvat J. Envahissement Ganglionnaire Pelvien. Paris: Medsi McGraw Hill, 1988.

2. Reich H, McGlynn F, Wilkie W. Laparoscopic management of Stage I ovarian cancer. A case report. J. Reprod Med 1990;35:601–604.

3. Querleu D, Leblanc E, Castelain B. Laparoscopic lymphadenectomy in the staging of early carcinoma of the cervix. Am J Obstet Gynecol 1991;164:579–581.

4. Schuessler WW, Vancaillie TG, Reich H, Griffith DP. Transperitoneal endosurgical lymphadenectomy in patients with localized prostate cancer. J Urol 1991;145: 988–991.

5. Querleu D. Laparoscopically assisted radical vaginal hysterectomy. Gynecol Oncol 1993;51:248–254.

6. Nezhat CR, Burrell MO, Nezhat FR, Benigno BB, Welander CE. Laparoscopic radical hysterectomy with para-aortic and pelvic lymphadenectomy. Am J Obstet Gynecol 1992;166:864–865.

7. Childers JM, Surwit EA. Combined laparoscopic and vaginal surgery for management of two cases of stage I endometrial cancer. Gynecol Oncol 1992;45:46–51.

8. Childers JM, Hatch K, Surwit EA. The role of laparoscopic lymphadenectomy in the management of cervical carcinoma. Gynecol Oncol 1992;47:38–43.

9. Kadar N. Laparoscopic pelvic lymphadenectomy for the treatment of gynecological malignancies: description of a technique. Gynaecol Endosc 1992;1:79–83.

10. Kadar N, Reich H. Laparoscopically assisted radical Schauta hysterectomy and bilateral pelvic lymphadenectomy for the treatment of bulky stage IB carcinoma of the cervix. Gynaecol Endosc 1993;135–142.

11. Kadar N. Laparoscopic vaginal radical hysterectomy: description of a technique and its evolution. Gynaecol Endosc 1994;3:91-108.

12. Fowler JM, Carter JR, Carlson JW, Maslonkowski R, Byers LJ, Carson LF, Twiggs LB. Lymph node yield from laparoscopic lymphadenectomy in cervical cancer: a comparative study. Gynecol Oncol 1993;51:187–192.

Chapter 22
Laparoscopic Aortic Lymphadenectomy

Not everything that is more difficult is
more meritorious. —Thomas Aquinas

BACKGROUND

Laparoscopic aortic lymphadenectomy does not have the therapeutic credentials of pelvic lymphadenectomy, but if the operation is to be performed at all, the advantages of doing so laparoscopically are arguably greater than for any other gynecological operation. The operation also lacks the historical significance of pelvic lymphadenectomy for its performance entailed no new conceptual breakthrough. Nonetheless, there has been considerable jockeying and even some acrimony (1,2) as to who performed what type of aortic lymphadenectomy first. Childers (3) felt he had been the first to perform this operation, but most of his early procedures were precaval fat pad biopsies ("right-sided aortic lymphadenectomy") (4), and Nezhat (5) preceded Childers both chronologically and in the extensiveness of the operation he performed because he dissected both sides of the aorta in 1989 (although the operation was used inappropriately for Stage IA2 carcinoma of the cervix). Querleu (6) claimed to be the first to have done a "supramesenteric" aortic lymphadenectomy, which is perhaps ironic, for he had earlier noted that "it is impossible at this time to explore para-aortic nodes by laparoscopy" (7), and, not to be outdone, this author could lay claim to have been the first to remove positive lymph nodes fixed to aorta and vena cava laparoscopically (8) and to have the largest series of aortic lymphadenectomies with positive aortic nodes (9).

The most important historic fact about this operation, however, is that Childers and his colleagues, by the sheer volume of their cases and the excellence of their results, managed to persuade gynecologic oncologists in the U.S.A. to accept the operation, so much so that the Gynecologic Oncology Group (GOG) has instigated prospective, limited access studies involving laparoscopic lymphadenectomy in endometrial and cervix cancer. This is a remarkable achievement for which the authors deserve great credit, even if they were not the first either to perform the operation or to do the most extensive type of dissections, and have few patients with aortic lymph node metastases.

REVIEW OF ANATOMY

Para-aortic lymphadenectomy is an unfortunate misnomer for the operative removal of the lumbar lymphatic nodal chain that lies in the retroperitoneum along the course of the great vessels and that serves as the primary lymphatic drainage for the ovaries and kidneys and the secondary drainage site for the pelvic organs and the perineum. Urologists divide the lumbar lymphatic chain into three areas: (1) the left para-aortic nodes, which extend from the front of the aorta to the left ureter, (2) the right paracaval nodes, which extend from the front of the inferior vena cava to the right ureter, and (3) interaortocaval nodes, which extend from the midline of the inferior vena cava to the midline of the aorta (Figure 22.1). These ascending lymphatic channels eventually coalesce to form the thoracic duct behind the aorta and right renal artery in front of L1, and lateral lymph flow between these channels is from right to left.

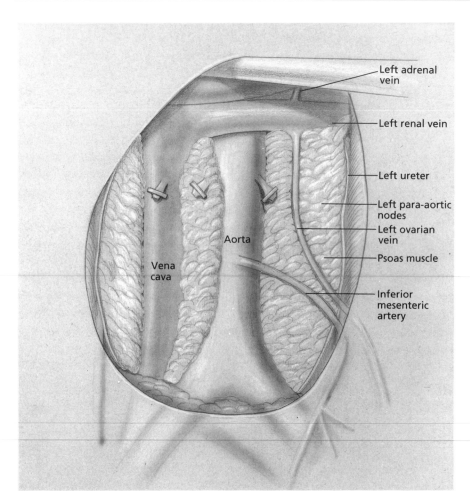

Figure 22.1 The three nodal chains comprising the "para-aortic nodes."

Left adrenal vein

Left renal vein

Left ureter

Left para-aortic nodes

Left ovarian vein

Psoas muscle

Inferior mesenteric artery

Aorta

Vena cava

Careful clinical studies of the pattern of metastases from early testicular tumors have shown that left-sided tumors drain primarily to the left para-aortic nodes, with significant drainage to the interaortocaval region but not to the right paracaval nodes, whereas right-sided tumors drain predominantly into the inter-aortocaval region with significant drainage to right paracaval nodes and a small amount of drainage to the left para-aortic region (10). These studies have provided a rational basis for tailoring the type of lymphadenectomy performed in individual patients. Similar studies have not been carried out to study the pattern of metastases from gynecological malignancies. From the anatomy, it seems reasonable to infer that retroperitoneal lymphadenectomy, at least for ovarian cancer, should extend to the renal vein. Although Burghardt et al. (11) found no aortic lymph node metastases in ovarian cancer in the absence of pelvic nodal disease, the upper limit of their dissection was the inferior mesenteric artery in most cases.

The small bowel mesentery is about 15 cm long and attaches the small bowel (jejunum and ileum) to the posterior abdominal wall along a line extending obliquely downwards from the ligament of Treitz, which lies on the left side of L2, to in front of the right sacroiliac joint. The inferior leaf of the mesentery crosses the aorta just below the third (horizontal) part of the duodenum, which crosses retroperitoneally in front of the great vessels below the origin of the superior mesenteric artery. The third part of the duodenum covers the left renal vein, and, below it, the ovarian arteries, where they arise laterally from the front of the aorta. The lower border of the duodenum also usually covers the origin of the inferior mesenteric artery from the left side of the front of the aorta. The posterior parietal peritoneum is reflected off the posterior abdominal wall to form the lower leaf of the small bowel mesentery at about this level (Figure 22.2). The bifurcation of the aorta is about 4 cm below this point.

The inferior mesenteric artery runs obliquely downwards and to the left in the mesentery of the descending colon, and after giving off the left colic and sigmoid arteries, it crosses the pelvic brim in the base

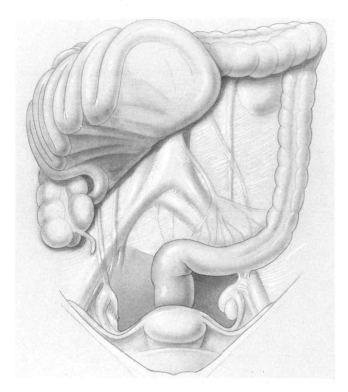

Figure 22.2 *Anatomy of the posterior parietal peritoneum and root of the small bowel mesentery.*

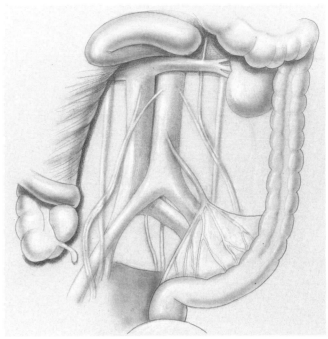

Figure 22.3 *Retroperitoneal structures and the relationship between them.*

of the rectosigmoid mesentery medial to the left ureter, as the superior rectal artery. The left ovarian vessels cross the left ureter just below the origin of the inferior mesenteric artery, which lies medial to the ureter throughout its course. Therefore, above the mesenteric artery, the ovarian vessels will be found medial to the ureter (Figure 22.3).

The left renal vein crosses in front of the aorta on its way from the left kidney to the inferior vena cava, which lies just to the right of the aorta. The left ovarian vein drains at right angles into the lower wall of the left renal vein, approximately 2 cm to the left of the aorta, and the left ureter lies lateral and at a point deep (dorsal) to the ovarian vein. The left adrenal vein drains into the superior wall of the left renal vein directly above its junction with the left ovarian vein (Figure 22.3). It can easily be avulsed if ill-conceived attempts are made to elevate the left renal vein. The left renal vein covers the left renal artery, which is, therefore, usually not seen during aortic lymphadenectomy. Just below where the left renal vein crosses in front of the aorta, the second lumbar artery can be seen arising from the left inferolateral border of the aorta. Rarely, an accessory renal artery can arise at this point, but its origin will be much more anterior. It is important to distinguish this anomaly from the

lumbar artery because, if it is divided, it can lead to infarction of the lower pole of the kidney. The next lumbar artery arises just below the origin of the ovarian artery, and the last one is just above the bifurcation of the aorta. There are four pairs of lumbar arteries corresponding to the first four lumbar vertebrae. The medial member of each pair arises from the right posteriolateral wall of the aorta.

To the right of the aorta lies the inferior vena cava. Apart from the lumbar veins that join its inferoposterior border, the only tributary of the inferior vena cava is the right ovarian vein, which joins the cava at the level of the origin of the ovarian arteries. The right renal vein is very short and, together with the left renal vein and the vena cava itself, covers the right renal artery. Both the right renal artery and vein are covered by the third part of the duodenum and are not exposed during supramesenteric laparoscopic aortic lymphadenectomy for gynecologic malignancies.

OPERATIVE TECHNIQUE

The patient is placed in Allen stirrups, tipped into a steep Trendelenburg position, and rotated slightly to her left. In addition to the four trocars usually used for radical pelvic surgery, a 5-mm trocar is placed in the right upper quadrant, through which a bowel grasper will be introduced into the peritoneal cavity and used to elevate the small bowel mesentery, and, after the retroperitoneum has been entered, the parietal peritoneum. The abdomen and pelvis are inspected in a systematic fashion, washings are taken, and the insertion site of the laparoscope switched to the suprapubic trocar. A second bowel grasper is introduced through the left lower quadrant trocar and used to retract the descending and sigmoid colon laterally. The instruments used for dissection (scissors, spoon forceps, suction-irrigator, bipolar forceps) are inserted through the infraumbilical and the right-sided trocars as needed. The surgeon stands on the patient's right and views the operation on a video monitor placed just above the assistant, i.e., caudad, who stands opposite the surgeon.

Small bowel is first displaced out of the pelvis using the suction-irrigator as a probe, and the root of the mesentery is elevated with the upper bowel grasper. The posterior parietal peritoneum is opened in one of several ways, but we like to pick a spot in front of the aorta, about a centimeter below its reflection onto the posterior abdominal wall (Figure 22.4A). If bowel keeps falling in the way, a more distal site is selected just above the sacral promontory, medial to the sigmoid mesentery (Figure 22.4B). Once the peritoneum has been incised, it can then be elevated and used to keep bowel out of the way (Figure 22.4C). The peritoneum can also be incised over the right common iliac artery or medial to the right ureter, and this may be more natural if a pelvic lymphadenectomy has been carried out.

The peritoneum is picked up with dissecting forceps, desiccated with bipolar forceps, and incised with scissors, the incision extended proximally to the root of the small bowel mesentery and distally to a point in front of the sacral promontory. Using mostly blunt dissection, a plane is developed between the peritoneum and the node-bearing fatty areolar tissue overlying the great vessels. The plane is extended laterally on each side to the ureters, which are elevated with the peritoneum and not mobilized from it (Figure 22.5A). On the left, the dissection is carried under the inferior mesenteric artery, which is elevated with the mesentery of the descending colon (Figure 22.5B). It is important to develop this plane properly and widely before carrying the dissection down to the adventitia of the aorta; otherwise, the nodal tissue may be elevated with the bowel mesentery and retroperitoneal fat during retraction, and the tissue will not be removed. Once the correct plane has been developed,

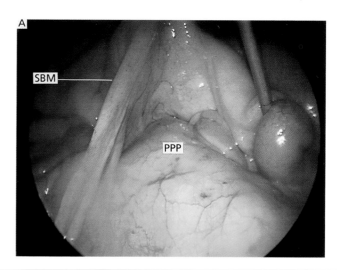

Figure 22.4A Posterior parietal peritoneum is incised just below the root of the small bowel mesentery.

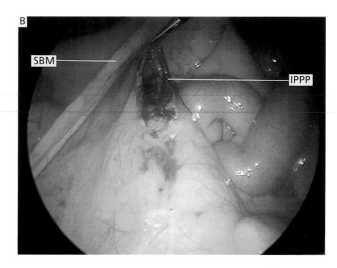

Figure 22.4B More distal incision of the posterior parietal peritoneum.

the duodenum is elevated by blunt dissection with the suction-irrigator or a probe.

The node-bearing areolar tissue in front of the aorta is then incised and the incision is carried down to the adventitia of the aorta. It is not always easy to know where to make one's incision because the great vessels are covered by node-bearing tissue and the aorta can usually only be seen clearly at this stage in thin patients without retroperitoneal pathology. The duodenum and the origin of the inferior mesenteric artery are also usually ill-defined at this point, and the root of the mesentery is elevated to retract the bowel and not in its anatomical position. Thus, there may be no cer-

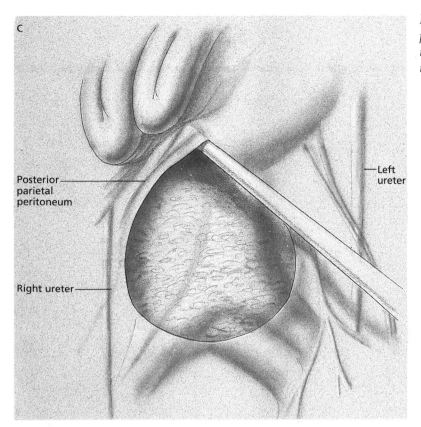

Figure 22.4C The posterior parietal peritoneum is elevated to keep the small bowel out of the pelvis.

Posterior parietal peritoneum

Left ureter

Right ureter

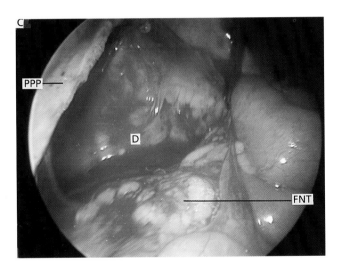

PPP

D

FNT

tain landmarks to orientate the surgeon in the superior-inferior plane. It is usually possible to "feel" the sacrum with a dissecting probe, which serves as a useful guide to the midline, and the pulsations of the aorta can often be "felt" if it is gently pressed with a probe, but much less clearly than one might imagine.

The nodal tissue is incised higher than lower, which is the natural tendency, but below the inferior leaf of the small bowel mesentery. There are no important structures in front of the aorta at this point, and the inferior mesenteric artery is lateral and clearly visible in the mesentery of the colon (Figure 22.6A). On the other hand, if the dissection is started too low, there is a danger of injuring the left common iliac vein below the bifurcation of the aorta. Once the plane between the aorta and the overlying nodal tissue has been developed, however, and the glistening surface of the aorta is seen (Figure 22.6B), the dissection is very

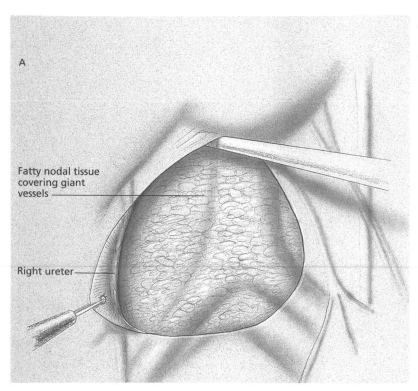

Figure 22.5A *The lateral limits of the dissection are the ureters on either side.*

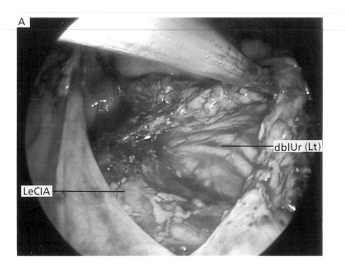

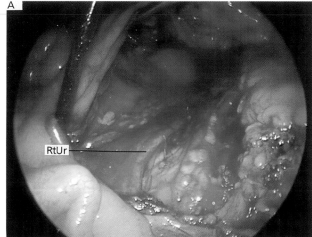

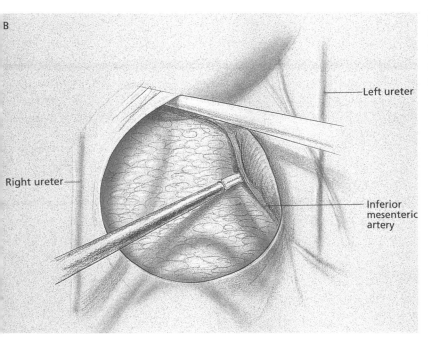

Figure 22.5B The inferior mesenteric artery and sigmoid mesentery are elevated to allow dissection of the left distal aortic and high common iliac nodes.

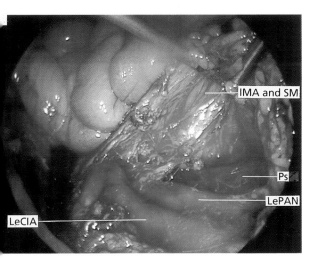

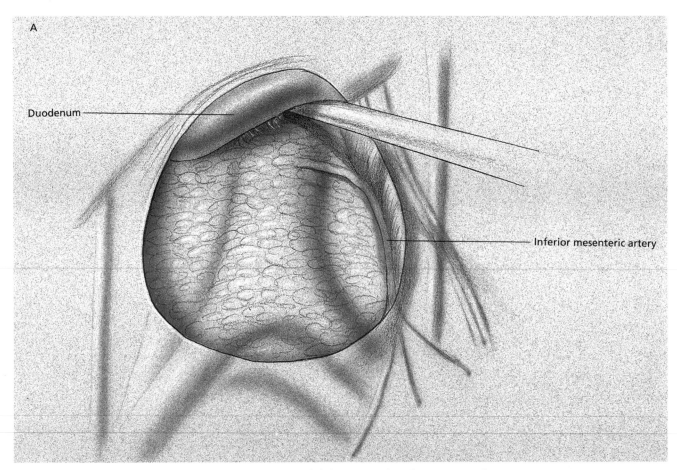

Figure 22.6A Fatty nodal tissue covering the great vessels.

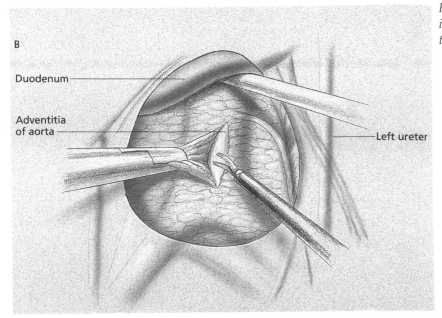

B

Duodenum

Adventitia of aorta

Left ureter

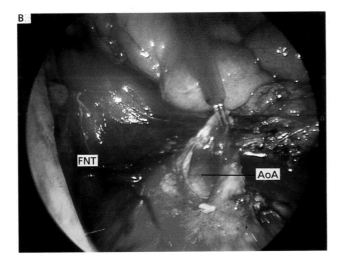

B

FNT

AoA

straightforward, provided one is cautious to coagulate all small vessels that are encountered. The biggest challenge is to keep bowel out of the way. This is done by elevating the posterior parietal peritoneum, and the incision in it must not, therefore, be made too large.

The limits of the dissection are the bifurcation of the aorta inferiorly, the proximal part of the common iliac artery inferolaterally, and the ureters laterally. The superior extent of the dissection is either the third part of the duodenum or the renal vein, in which case the duodenum must be mobilized. The nodal tissue is removed in as systematic a fashion as possible, but the plan of attack often needs to be varied if there is either very little or a great deal of tissue in the area.

We usually start with the left-sided dissection. It is puzzling to this author why the left-sided dissection has been considered to be more difficult than the right by some oncologists (12). It is, in fact, no more difficult and much safer because there are no large veins to contend with. The inferior mesenteric artery does, however, need to be dissected free, and if its origin is lower than usual, this can make exposure more difficult.

Working in a broad plane, the nodal tissue is mobilized "en bloc" from the front of the aorta and upper part of the left common iliac artery and extended as far laterally as possible (Figure 22.7A). The tissue is frequently stuck posteriorly by the left edge of the aorta, and it is often advantageous to "skip" to a more lateral point, identify the left ureter, elevate it on the peritoneum, and dissect the tissue in front of the psoas muscle from lateral to medial to the point of fixity of the tissues by the side of the aorta (Figure 22.7B). The nodal bundle is then transected either proximally or distally, wherever it is most free (usually in front of the common iliac artery), and the tissue teased off the psoas, pushing the wall of the aorta somewhat medially as one goes (Figure 22.7C). One needs to take care not to injure the vertebral arteries and, on no account, pull hard if resistance to the dissection is encountered. If these are injured and retract into the vertebral foramina, laparotomy will be necessary, and, even then, hemostasis may be difficult to secure.

The problem on the right side stems from the inability to see the wall of the inferior vena cava clearly until the areolar sheath investing it has been incised. The wall of the vein merges imperceptibly with the investing tissue, placing it at risk of injury during the initial incision into the sheath. The dissection is, in fact, easier if there is more rather than less tissue in the area because the nodal tissue can then be grasped very superficially and elevated (Figure 22.8A). Cautious dis-

section below the elevated tissue will allow one to enter the caval sheath, and, once the glistening surface of the cava is seen, the incision is extended proximally to the duodenum and inferiorly to the level of the right common iliac artery (Figure 22.8B). Working again in a broad plane, a combination of sharp and blunt dissection is used to clean the cava of fatty areolar tissue, continuing laterally along the psoas muscle as far as the right ureter (Figure 22.8C).

It is a simple matter to extend the dissection under the third part of the duodenum to the left renal vein (Figure 22.9). Blunt dissection is used almost exclusively and the duodenum elevated towards the right using the bowel graspers in the right upper and left lower trocars. The plane of dissection is along the front of the aorta. The left renal vein is cleared of areolar tissue, but it is not elevated. The dissection continues to the left of the aorta, above the inferior mesenteric artery, and nodal tissue is cleared from the front of the psoas muscle. Here one encounters the left ovarian vein medial to the left ureter and, lower down, the left ovarian artery, which usually has to be clipped and divided (Figure 22.10A). On the right side, the vena cava is cleaned of node-bearing tissue as far as the left renal vein, but the right renal vein is not identified. The right ovarian vein in front of the vena cava usually has to be sacrificed, together with the right ovarian artery (Figure 22.10B). The complete dissection is shown in Figure 22.10C.

DISCUSSION

Laparoscopic aortic lymphadenectomy, like its pelvic counterpart, has proved to be a remarkably safe operation that reduces operative morbidity dramatically. Only two cases of caval injury are known to have occurred in almost 100 reported procedures (4,12), and almost all patients have gone home the day after surgery (4,6,8,9,12). This compares with a mean hospital stay of 8 days and a serious acute complication rate of 10–15% (injuries to the great vessels or ureters, postoperative bowel obstruction) following extraperitoneal aortic lymphadenectomy (13,14). The average number of nodes recovered and the frequency of positive nodes can also be at least as high as obtained with an extraperitoneal approach (9,14). Too few patients have had positive aortic nodes and, hence, extended field radiation, to determine how the laparoscopic approach will affect the tolerance of extended field irradiation, if at all. So far, none of our patients who have completed extended field radiation

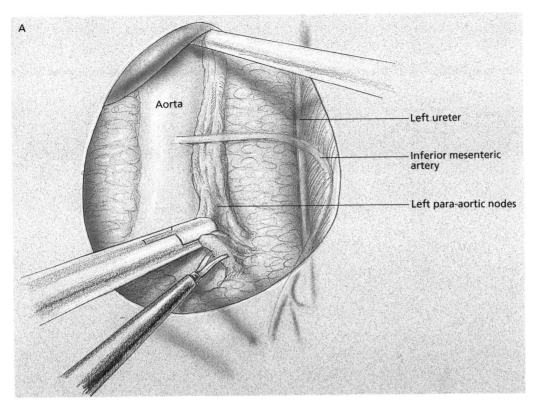

Figure 22.7A *Left side of the aorta being cleaned of node-bearing tissue.*

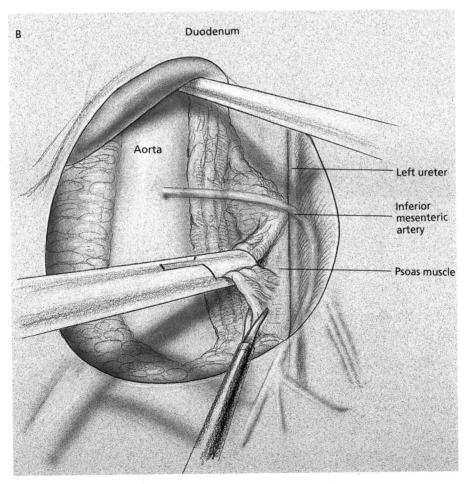

Figure 22.7B *Nodal tissue cleaned from in front of the psoas muscle.*

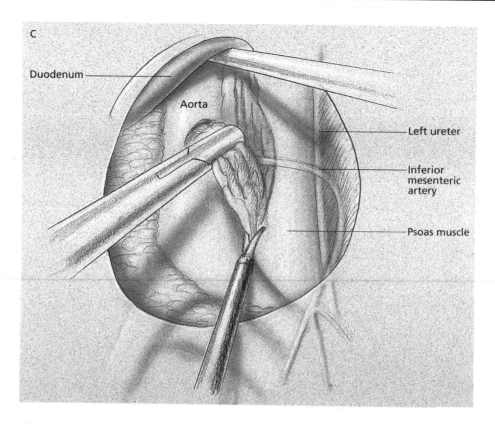

Figure 22.7C *Left aortic nodal bundle is transected in front of the common iliac artery and dissected cephalad.*

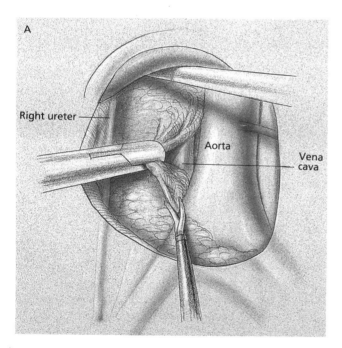

Figure 22.8A *Nodal tissue covering the vena cava is incised.*

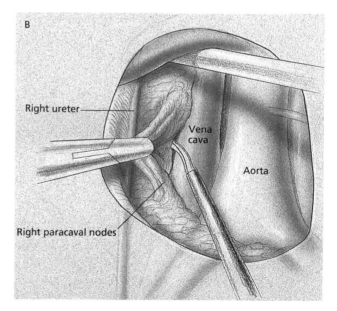

Figure 22.8B *The front of the vena cava is cleaned of node-bearing tissue.*

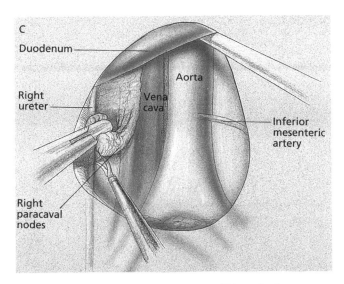

Figure 22.8C Right-sided "paracaval" lymphadenectomy being completed.

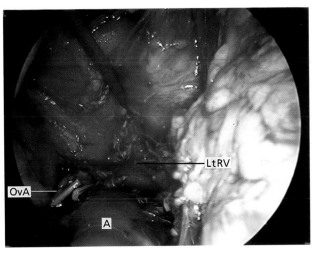

Figure 22.9 The dissection is extended to the left iliac vein.

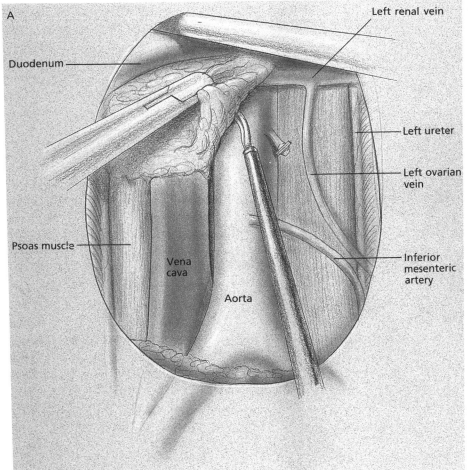

Figure 22.10A The left renal vein is cleaned of node-bearing tissue.

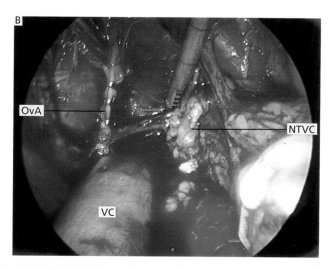

Figure 22.10B *The right ovarian vein is clipped and divided.*

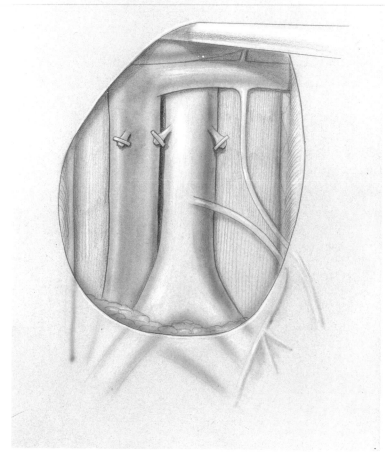

Figure 22.10C *The completed dissection.*

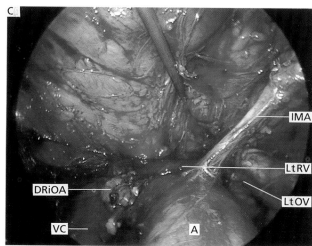

have had any significant toxicity, and all but one received concurrent chemotherapy (9). What was once a questionable staging operation has been transformed into one with about the same morbidity as laparoscopic removal of a tubal pregnancy.

The type of lymphadenectomy to be performed and the indications for the operation remain controversial areas. In this author's opinion, the operation is overused, and a rationale for making it a routine part of radical hysterectomy, for example, cannot be found in the frequency of lymph node metastases in early stage cancer of the cervix (see Chapter 20). The author reserves primary aortic lymphadenectomy for women with advanced cervix cancer, early stage ovarian cancer, or those with early stage cervix and endometrial cancer who are found to have clinically positive pelvic nodes, confirmed by frozen section. In the vast majority of patients with early stage endometrial and cervix cancer, the operation will not be required. We restrict it to those who have positive pelvic nodes and then perform laparoscopic aortic lymphadenectomy as a second operation. This policy has meant that we have done fewer (11 to date) laparoscopic aortic lymphadenectomies than our colleagues, but the proportion of positive nodes among our cases has been much higher (50%).

The most appropriate type of lymphadenectomy to perform has not been established by mapping the pattern of metastases from different gynecological malignancies. The current practice of limiting the dissection to the inframesenteric region of the great vessels appears to have arisen from concern over the potential morbidity of the procedure. If this is the correct explanation, the reduced morbidity associated with laparoscopic aortic lymphadenectomy might give us grounds for attempting a more ambitious retroperitoneal lymphadenectomy in the future.

REFERENCES

1. Nezhat C, Nezhat F. Letter to the editor. Gynecol Oncol 1993;51:292.

2. Childers JM. Reply. Gynecol Oncol 1993;51:292.

3. Childers JM. Laparoscopic para-aortic lymphadenectomy. In: Hulka JF, Reich H, eds. Textbook of Laparoscopy. Philadelphia: W B Saunders, 1993:295–300.

4. Childers JM, Hatch KD, Tran A-N, Surwit EA. Laparoscopic para-aortic lymphadenectomy in gynecologic malignancies. Obstet Gynecol 1993;82:741–747.

5. Nezhat CR, Burrell MO, Nezhat FR, Benigno BB, Welander CE. Laparoscopic radical hysterectomy with para-aortic and pelvic lymphadenectomy. Am J Obstet Gynecol 1992;166:864–865.

6. Querleu D. Laparoscopic para-aortic node sampling in gynecologic oncology: a preliminary experience. Gynecol Oncol 1993;49:24–29.

7. Querleu D, Leblanc E, Castelain B. Laparoscopic lymphadenectomy in the staging of early carcinoma of the cervix. Am J Obstet Gynecol 1991;164:579–581.

8. Kadar N. Laparoscopic resection of fixed and enlarged aortic lymph nodes in patients with advanced cervix cancer. Gynaecol Endosc 1993;2:217–221.

9. Kadar N, Pelosi MA. Can cervix cancer be adequately staged by laparoscopic aorta lymphadenectomy? Gynaecol Endosc (in press).

10 Donohue JP. Retroperitoneal lymphadenectomy. Urol Clin North Am 1977;4:509–521.

11. Burghardt E, Pickel H. Lahousen M. Stettner H. Pelvic lymphadenectomy in operative treatment of ovarian cancer. Am J Obstet Gynecol 1986;155:315–319.

12. Spirtos NM, Schlaerth JB, Spirtos TW, Kimball RE. (Abstract) Laparoscopic bilateral aortic and pelvic lymph node sampling: a new technique. Gynecol Oncol 1993; 49:137–138.

13. Weiser EB, Bundy BN, Hoskins WJ, et al. Extraperitoneal versus transperitoneal selective para-aortic lymphadenectomy in the pretreatment surgical staging of advanced cervix cancer. (A Gynecologic Oncology Group Study). Gynecol Oncol 1989,33:283–289.

14. Gallup DG, King LA, Messing MJ, Talledo OE. Para-aortic lymph node sampling by means of an extraperitoneal approach with supraumbilical transverse "sunrise" incision. Am J Obstet Gynecol 1993;169: 307–312.

Chapter 23
Laparoscopic-Vaginal Radical Hysterectomy

Daring ideas are like chessmen moved forward;
they may be beaten, but they may start a
winning game. —Goethe

HISTORICAL DEVELOPMENT

The first laparoscopic radical hysterectomies for cervix cancer appear to have been performed independently in Professor Bruhat's department in France (1) and by Nezhat et al. (2) in the U.S.A., in 1989. The operations were carried out entirely laparoscopically for Stage IA2 lesions and were not very radical, type II operations at best. A year later, Querleu (3) reported two cases of laparoscopically assisted radical vaginal hysterectomy for Stage IA2 or low-volume (35 mm) Stage IB lesions in the French literature, but initially, Querleu (4), like Dargent (5), favored a two-stage approach, which consisted of laparoscopic pelvic lymphadenectomy and, provided the lymph nodes were negative, a radical vaginal hysterectomy (Schauta-Amreich or Schauta-Stoeckel) at a second operation.

Unaware of this work, a year later, this author, assisted by Reich, performed the first laparoscopically assisted radical vaginal hysterectomy in the U.S.A., which was also the first time a patient with a bulky or frank cervical lesion had been treated by any kind of laparoscopic operation (6). In the technique used for the first two cases, the cardinal and uterosacral ligaments were partly divided laparoscopically using an Endo-GIA stapler, but later, this approach was abandoned in favor of a vaginal approach (7). Dargent (8) subsequently adopted a similar technique and finds it advantageous to divide the cardinal ligaments lap-

aroscopically with an Endo-GIA, as originally performed by this author. However, he restricts the operation to small lesions and to lesions with negative nodes, perhaps a tacit admission that he does not entirely trust his laparoscopic procedure. Querleu (9) recently reported eight cases in which the uterine arteries were divided and ureters unroofed laparoscopically, and the cardinal and uterosacral ligaments were divided vaginally in all but one patient.

Thus, differences between these maturing laparoscopic-vaginal techniques for radical hysterectomy seem to lie principally in the route by which the ureter is unroofed and the cardinal ligament divided. Querleu (9) favors laparoscopic dissection of the ureteric tunnel and vaginal division of the cardinal ligaments, Dargent (8) favors laparoscopic division of the cardinal ligaments and vaginal dissection of the ureteric tunnel, and this author favors the vaginal route for both division of the cardinal ligaments and dissection of the ureteric tunnel, but frees the ureter from the broad ligament and retracts it out of the pelvis laparoscopically throughout the vaginal part of the operation. Another point of difference between these techniques is that both Kadar and Querleu divide the uterine arteries laparoscopically, whereas Dargent divides them vaginally, a reflection, perhaps, of his great experience with the classical radical vaginal operation, prior to the advent of advanced laparoscopic surgery.

OPERATIVE TECHNIQUE

Laparoscopic Phase of the Operation

▶ STEP 1. The cul-de-sac peritoneum is incised.

The pouch of Douglas is incised with dissecting scissors and the incision extended proximally on either side of the rectum, below the uterosacral ligaments. It is much more difficult to carry out this step if it is left to last because the tissues become too slack. A rectal probe developed by Reich is used to displace the rectum to the contralateral side (Figure 23.1). The ureters may or may not be seen in the medial leaf of the broad ligament, but because they always lie above and lateral to the plane of dissection, they are not at risk, and no effort should be expended in trying to identify them at this stage.

▶ STEPS 2–6.

The next steps of the operation have already been described in Chapters 6, 11, and 21 and will only be summarized here. The pelvic sidewall triangles are first opened, and the leaves of the broad ligament separated. The infundibulopelvic ligament is retracted medially and the ureter identified at the pelvic brim. The dissection is then carried under the round ligament, the umbilical ligament identified extraperitoneally, and the paravesical space developed on either side of the umbilical ligament. It is important to open the spaces all the way down to the levator floor. The umbilical ligament is then traced retrogradely to the origin of the uterine artery, and the pararectal space opened by blunt dissection proximal and medial to the artery and cardinal ligament. The dissection must be again carried down to the levator

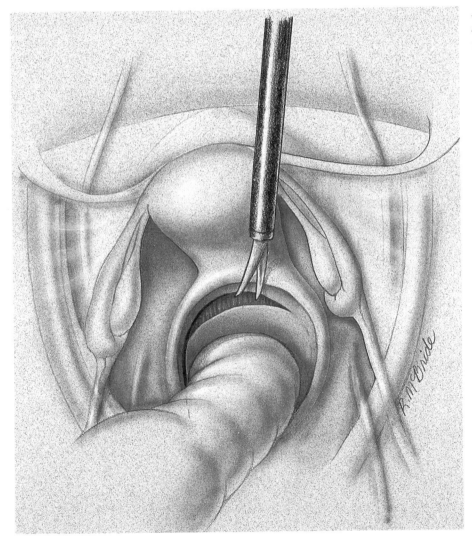

Figure 23.1 *The posterior cul-de-sac peritoneum is incised and the incision extended on either side of the rectum below the uterosacral ligaments.*

floor. Starting at the cardinal ligament, the ureter is reflected off the broad ligament as far as the pelvic brim.

The uterine arteries are freed from the areolar tissue still covering their anterior surfaces, desiccated, clipped, or ligated at their origin, and divided. The proximal stump is then picked up and freed from the underlying areolar tissue by sharp scissor dissection all the way to the uterus. The artery is freed from the underlying ureter, but the ureteric tunnel is not divided. The round ligaments and infundibulopelvic or ovarian ligaments are then desiccated or ligated and divided. After the round ligament is divided, the incision is continued along the anterior leaf of the broad ligament and the bladder peritoneum to the contralateral side, but the bladder is not dissected off the vagina. After the infundibulopelvic or ovarian ligament has been divided, the incision is continued along the medial leaf of the broad ligament to meet the incision in the pouch of Douglas that was made at the start of the procedure (Figures 23.2–23.6). However, the infundibulopelvic ligament is only divided, and the broad ligament is incised after the pelvic lymphadectomy has been completed.

▶ **STEP 7. Bilateral pelvic lymphadenectomy is then carried out as described in Chapter 21.**

▶ **STEP 8. The ureters are retracted out of the pelvis.**

Before proceeding to the vaginal part of the operation, a vessel loop is passed around each ureter and pulled out through the ipsilateral lower quadrant trocar. The best way to do this is to insert both tapes completely into the peritoneal cavity through the

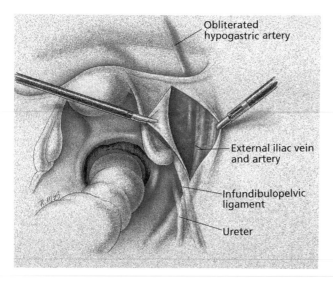

Figure 23.2 The peritoneum of the pelvic sidewall is incised.

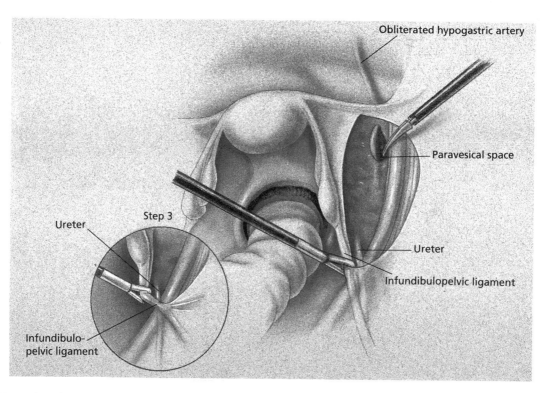

Figure 23.3 The infundibulopelvic ligament is mobilized and pulled medially to expose the ureter at the pelvic brim. The obliterated hypogastric artery is identified under the round ligament.

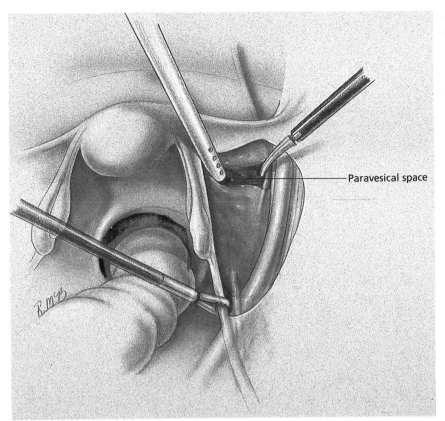

Figure 23.4 The paravesical spaces are developed.

Paravesical space

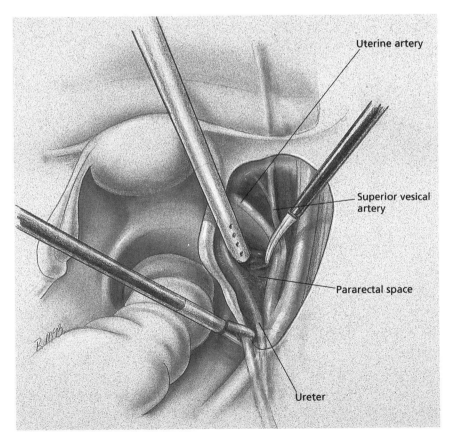

Figure 23.5 The pararectal space is developed just proximal and medial to the uterine artery.

Uterine artery

Superior vesical artery

Pararectal space

Ureter

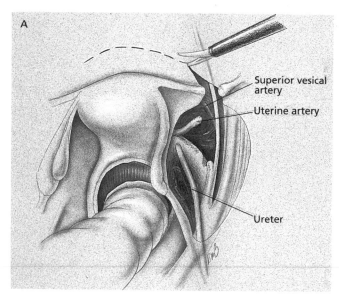
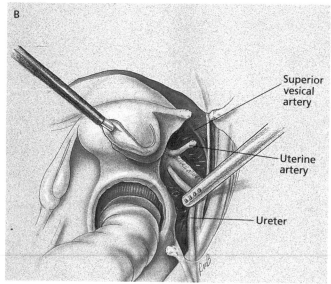

Figure 23.6 *The uterine arteries, round ligament and infundibulopelvic or ovarian ligaments are divided.*

10-mm suprapubic trocar, making sure to direct them to opposite sides of the pelvis so that they do not get entangled. Using the Wolf grasper, the tape is passed around the ureter, both ends grasped, and then pulled out through the ipsilateral trocar. The trocars are then withdrawn and a Kelly clamp placed on the tapes and used to retract the ureters out of the pelvis throughout the vaginal phase of the operation (Figure 23.7).

Vaginal Phase of the Operation

▶ *STEP 9. Formation of the vaginal cuff, division of the supravaginal septum.*

The vagina is grasped with four Kocker clamps at approximately the 10, 2, 4, and 8 o'clock positions, at the level at which the vagina is to be transected (usually mid-vagina, or junction of the middle and upper thirds). If the vagina is redundant, more Kocker clamps may be needed to ensure that it is stretched out flat and there are no ridges in its wall when it is incised. After infiltrating with phenylephrine solution (10 mg/250 ml saline) just under the vaginal fascia, the vagina is incised circumferentially with cutting diathermy (Figures 23.8A,B). The vesicovaginal and rectovaginal spaces are then developed with sharp scissor dissection and the posterior cul-de-sac entered. T-clamps are placed on the distal cut edge of the vagina for traction (usually three or four) and a long weighted Auvard speculum placed in the cul-de-sac.

The anterior dissection proceeds fairly effortlessly until an impasse is reached at the level of the supravaginal septum, which separates the vesicovaginal from the vesicocervical space. The dissection should not be in a plane too close to the vagina; otherwise, there is a danger that the dissection will be under the supravaginal septum and into the superficial layers of the cervix, where the growth is. The tissue is placed on tension by appropriate downward traction on the T-clamps and upward retraction anteriorly. The supravaginal septum is pulled up with forceps and incised. The incision is made approximately a centimeter above the vaginal attachments of the septum, which can usually be discerned. The bladder becomes immediately visible and can be freed further with sharp scissor and then blunt finger dissection to gain entrance into the anterior cul-de-sac (Figures 23.8C,D).

▶ *STEP 10. The paravesical and pararectal spaces are entered, and the vesicocervical ligaments ("bladder pillar") are formed.*

The cut edge of the distal vaginal wall is pulled laterally, i.e., everted, and rendered taut, and the tissue just under the vaginal fascia incised with scissors to gain entrance into the paravesical space (Figure 23.9A). The direction of the correct plane of dissection will be determined by the length of vagina excised. The longer the vaginal cuff, the more vertically orientated should the dissecting scissors be, and the shorter the cuff, the more horizontally. Since the paravesical space has already been opened laparoscopically, this

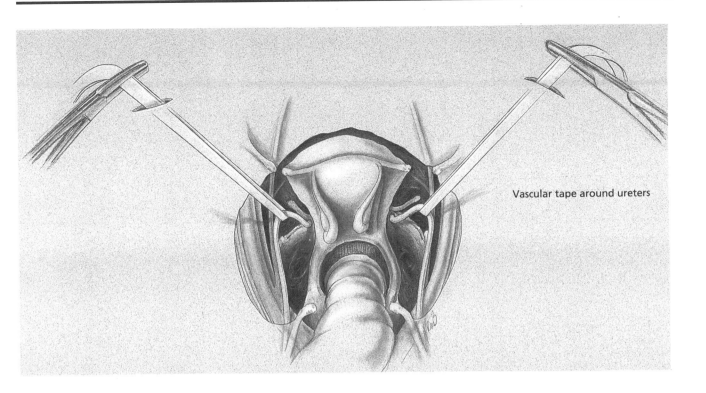

Vascular tape around ureters

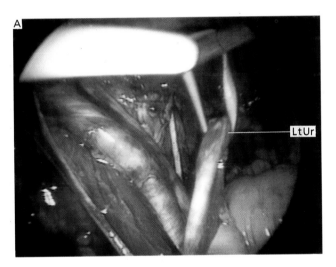

LtUr

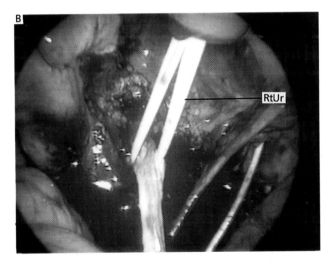

RtUr

Figure 23.7 Vascular tapes are passed around the ureters, and they are retracted out of the pelvis laparoscopically.

is, in fact, a surprisingly easy maneuver. Nevertheless, the position of the pubococcygeus muscle should be checked before making the incision to ensure that the dissection is not too lateral; otherwise, some of the muscle fibers can be pulled medially making the bladder pillars thick and the ureters more difficult to feel. If there is any uncertainty, the pneumoperitoneum can be reestablished and a probe passed laparoscopically into the paravesical space medial to the obliterated hypogastric artery. It will be readily felt vaginally, and the paravesical space can be opened without any further difficulty.

The vaginal incision is then enlarged bluntly with the index fingers and extended posteriorly (Figure 23.9B). The rectum is retracted medially and the pararectal space entered. Usually, quite dense bands of connective tissue separate the paravesical and pararectal spaces (the horizontal fascia), and these need to be divided to unite them (Figure 23.9C). Once the paravesical and pararectal spaces have been united, the entire hand can be placed into the peritoneal cavity, lateral to the uterus and cervix. The paravesical and pararectal spaces on the contralateral side are united and then developed in an identical fashion.

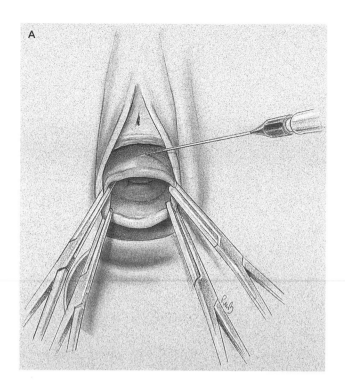

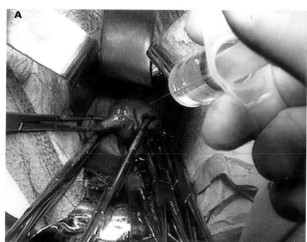

Figure 23.8A The position of the cuff is demarcated with Kocker clamps and the vaginal wall infiltrated with phenylephrine solution.

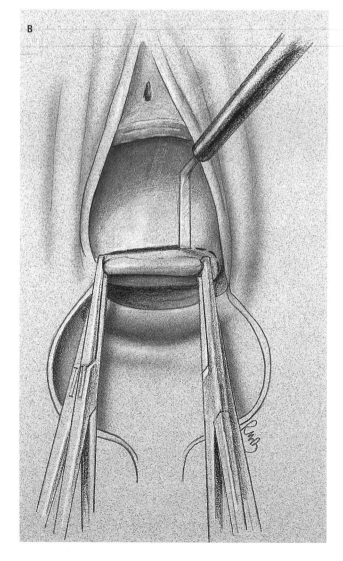

Figure 23.8B The vaginal wall is incised circumferentially with diathermy, using a cutting monopolar current.

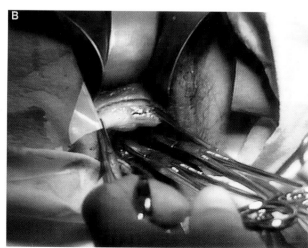

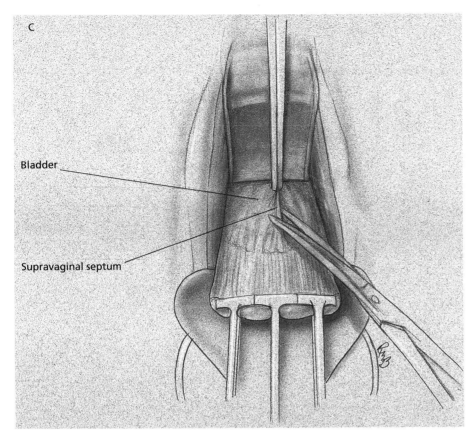

Figure 23.8C *The vesicovaginal and rectovaginal spaces have been developed, the posterior cul-de-sac entered, T-clamps placed on the vaginal cuff, and the supravaginal septum is being incised.*

Bladder

Supravaginal septum

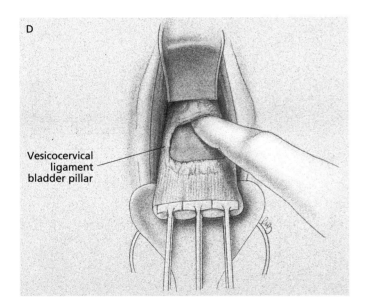

Vesicocervical ligament bladder pillar

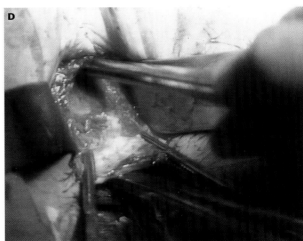

Figure 23.8D *The vesicocervical space is developed with sharp scissor and blunt finger dissection.*

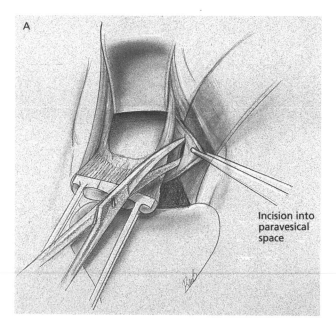

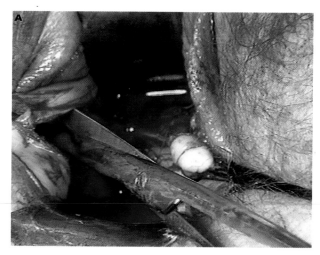

Figure 23.9A The lateral vaginal wall is incised to enter the paravesical space.

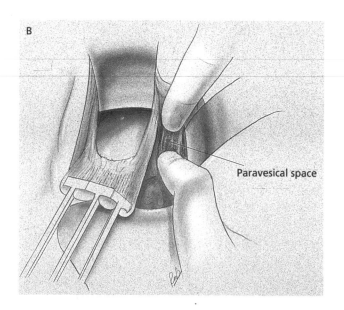

Figure 23.9B The vaginal incision is enlarged.

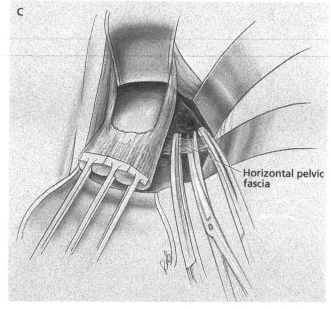

Figure 23.9C The horizontal pelvic fascia is divided.

▶ STEP 11. Division of the uterosacral ligaments (rectal pillars).

Starting on the left side, the uterosacral ligament is placed on tension by pulling the T-clamps upwards and to the right. The rectum is retracted medially, and any remaining peritoneal attachments not freed laparoscopically are divided at this time. The position of the ureter is verified by palpation and the uterosacral ligament clamped close to the rectum with Zeppelin clamps, divided, and suture ligated (Figures 23.10A,B). The right uterosacral ligament is divided in an identical manner. The proximal (superior) portion of the uterosacral ligament will not be reached at this stage, and these will be divided as the last step of the operation.

The uterus is usually rendered quite mobile by division of the rectal pillars, and the operation can pro-

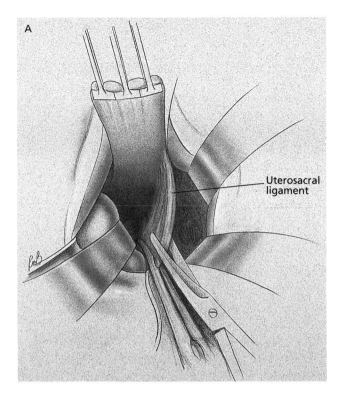

Figure 23.10A *The uterosacral ligament is clamped close to the rectum with Zeppelin clamps, divided, and suture ligated.*

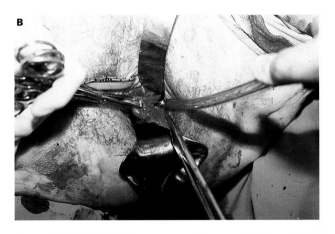

Figure 23.10B *The left uterosacral ligament is being divided.*

ceed with either unroofing of the distal ureters or division of the cardinal ligaments (Figure 23.10C), the sequence that will be described. Although Steps 12 and 13 are usually interchangeable, access to the parametrium after the rectal pillars are divided may still be limited, particularly if vaginal vault is not mobile or if the patient is nulliparous or has had previous vaginal surgery. In these situations, the cardinal ligaments should be divided before the ureters are unroofed (Step 13).

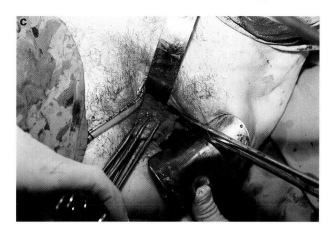

Figure 23.10C *The left cardinal ligament is being divided before the ureters have been unroofed.*

▶ STEP 12. The ureters are freed ("unroofed") from the vesicocervical ligaments.

The left bladder pillar or vesicocervical ligament is placed on tension by pulling the T-clamps downwards and to the right and using suitable retraction in the vesicocervical and paravesical spaces. The ureter can be easily palpated between the middle and forefingers in the upper part of the ligament distally and, lower down, in the ligament more proximally.

The relationship between the ureter and the uterine artery is different in the vaginal and abdominal approaches because, in the vaginal approach, the uterus is pulled downwards rather than upwards and the bladder pushed upwards rather than downwards. A ureteric loop or "knee" is thereby artificially created, through which the uterine artery runs obliquely upwards from the cervix to the hypogastric artery (Figures 23.11A–C).

The ureteric tunnel is entered by gradually snipping away the bladder pillar below the bend in the ureter, and once entered, it is enlarged with finger dissection. The lateral wall of the tunnel is clamped with a fine tonsil clamp, divided, and suture ligated (Figures 23.11D,E). The medial wall is divided without ligation, but the uterine artery is cauterized medial to the ureteric loop to avoid back bleeding. The right ureter, which tends to be higher, is freed in the same way. The distal ureters are then retracted upwards with a right-angled retractor.

▶ STEP 13. Division of the cardinal ligaments.

The fundus is delivered through the anterior vagina, and, starting on the left side, the index and middle fingers are placed on either side of the cardinal ligament, from above if possible, and the uterus and

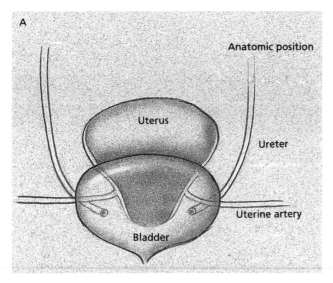

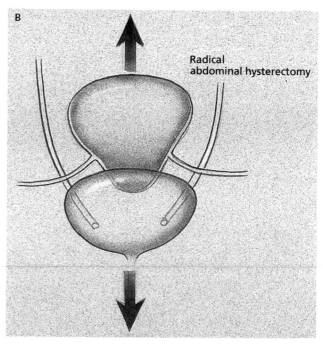

Figure 23.11A The anatomic relationship between the ureter and uterine artery.

Figure 23.11B The relationship between the ureter and uterine artery in an abdominal radical hysterectomy after the uterus is pulled upwards and the bladder pushed downwards.

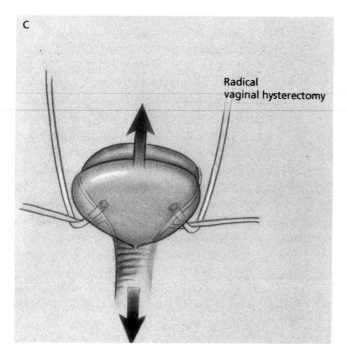

Figure 23.11C The relationship between the ureter and uterine artery in a radical vaginal hysterectomy after the uterus is pulled downwards and the bladder pushed upwards.

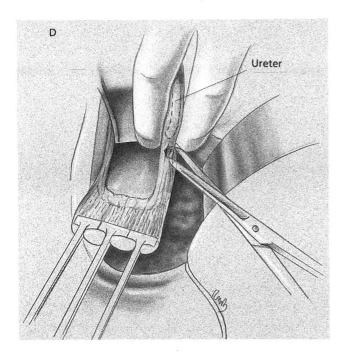

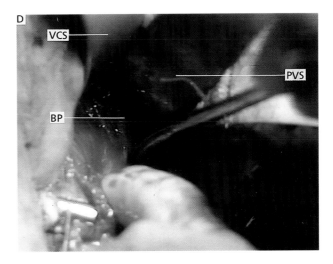

Figure 23.11D The bladder pillar is held between the index and middle fingers just below the ureters and divided in a series of small snips.

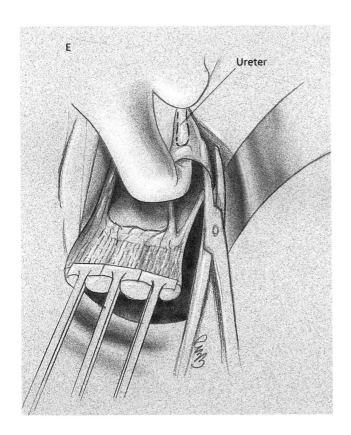

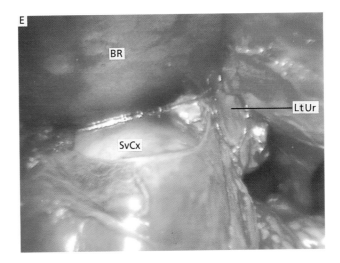

Figure 23.11E The ureteric tunnel is developed bluntly with finger dissection, and its lateral wall clamped and divided.

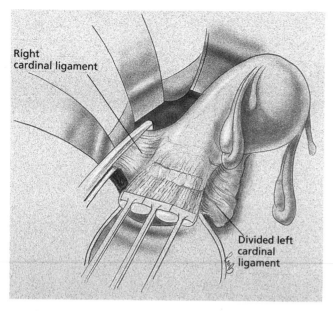

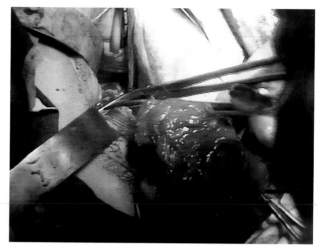

Figure 23.12 The fundus has been delivered through the anterior vagina, and the left cardinal ligament is being divided.

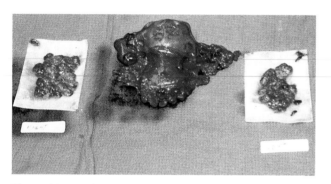

Figure 23.13 The operative specimen; 43 lymph nodes were recovered in this case.

cervix are pulled medially. The bladder and rectum are retracted out of the way, the position of the ureter is checked again, and the ligament clamped at the pelvic sidewall (or closer to the uterus with smaller lesions), divided, and suture ligated (Figure 23.12). The remaining (cephalad) part of the uterosacral and broad ligament on the ipsilateral side is then divided before attention is turned to the contralateral side. The right cardinal ligament is divided in exactly the same way, and it is followed by division of the remaining portion of the uterosacral and broad ligaments, after which the specimen is removed (Figure 23.13).

▶ STEP 14. The cuff is closed, and the pelvis is inspected laparoscopically.

The vagina is closed horizontally with a running, nonlocking chromic suture around a suction drain

(hysterovac), which is removed the next day. The pneumoperitoneum is reestablished and the pelvis irrigated copiously and checked for hemostasis. The operative steps are summarized in Table 23.1.

DISCUSSION

The rationale for a combined laparoscopic and vaginal approach to radical hysterectomy is compelling. Radical vaginal operations for cervix cancer have several advantages over their abdominal counterparts and fell into disuse only because they did not allow removal of the pelvic lymph nodes (10). Mitra (11) tried to correct this deficiency by combining the Schauta-Amreich operation with bilateral extraperitoneal pelvic lymphadenectomy, but his procedure never gained popularity because the reduction in morbidity from the vaginal approach was largely lost. Laparoscopic lymphadenectomy clearly has the potential to complement the operation by correcting its one and only deficiency vis-à-vis the abdominal operation, the inability to remove the pelvic lymph nodes.

However, the laparoscopic component contributes much more to the procedure than the lymphadenectomy for it allows a natural and symbiotic partitioning of the operation into abdominal and vaginal phases. Only those steps of the hysterectomy that are easier to perform vaginally than abdominally are carried out from below—formation of the cuff, division of the cervical ligaments, freeing of the distal ureters—and their execution is greatly facilitated by

Table 23.1 Summary of the operative steps

Laparoscopic Phase

Step 1 The cul-de-sac peritoneum is incised and peritoneal incision is carried proximally along each lateral border of the rectum, below the uterosacral ligaments.

Step 2 The pelvic sidewall triangle is opened.

Step 3 The paravesical and pararectal spaces are developed.

Step 4. The uterine artery and its ureteric branch are coagulated and divided.

Step 5 The ureter is reflected off the broad ligament.

Step 6 The round ligament and adnexal pedicles are coagulated and divided, and the bladder peritoneum is incised.

Step 7 Lymphadenectomy is then performed.

Step 8 Each ureter is tagged with vascular tape and the tape pulled out through the inferior ports.

Vaginal Component

Step 9 The vaginal cuff is formed, rectovaginal and vesicovaginal spaces developed, and supravaginal septum divided.

Step 10 The paravesical and pararectal spaces are developed, the vesicocervical ligament (bladder pillars) formed, the horizontal pelvic fascia divided, and the spaces united.

Step 11 The uterosacral ligaments are divided.

Step 12 The ureters are unroofed and vesicouterine ligament divided.

Step 13 The cardinal ligaments are divided, the residual proximal portions of the broad and uterosacral ligaments are divided, and specimen is removed.

Step 14 The vagina is closed with a running suture around a suction drain (hysterovac), the pelvis inspected and irrigated laparoscopically, and trocars removed.

the preceding abdominal phase of the operation. Strategies that involve either performing the entire hysterectomy laparoscopically (1,2) or following the laparoscopic lymphadenectomy with a radical vaginal hysterectomy (4,5) are, in this author's opinion, ill-conceived because they do not make best use of either the laparoscopic or the vaginal part of the operation, nor exploit the potentially symbiotic relationship between them. This is also true of the author's initial plan to divide the cervical ligaments partly laparoscopically, a tactic that proved to be of no benefit whatsoever (6).

Vaginal entry into the paravesical and pararectal spaces, which can be problematic even for experienced surgeons (12), is very straightforward after these spaces have been developed laparoscopically. Laparoscopic division of uterine vessels makes it easier to unroof the ureters vaginally because it eliminates the need to ligate the vessels repeatedly, at successively more proximal points, as in the Schauta operation. The radical hysterectomy is also facilitated by laparoscopic division of the proximal attachments of the uterus and by freeing the ureters from the broad ligaments. Only distal structures then have to be approached vaginally, and lateral exposure sufficient to divide the cervical ligaments can usually be obtained without a Schuchardt's incision. The ureters can be retracted away from the operative field laparoscopically throughout the vaginal part of the operation (Step 8), making it possible to divide the uterosacral and cardinal ligaments before the distal ureters are freed. This also makes it easier to unroof the ureters and further reduces the need for a Schuchardt's incision.

The major challenge of a laparoscopic-vaginal radical hysterectomy is, in fact, the vaginal part of the procedure, not the laparoscopic component. The laparoscopic component is identical to what is performed during a radical abdominal hysterectomy, with which all gynecologic oncologists are familiar, but the vaginal part is borrowed from a radical operation that is totally unfamiliar to the current generation of gynecologic oncologists, even if they have the writings of their forebears to fall back on (10–12). However, experienced pelvic surgeons adept at radical abdominal hysterectomy, who have studied and thought through the radical vaginal operation and mastered endoscopic techniques, will find the learning curve to be relatively short and, ultimately, rewarding to everyone concerned, especially the patient. Despite the vicissitudes of trying to master a complicated and difficult operation, the potential advantages are so obvious that it can only be a matter of time before many other, if not most, gynecologic oncologists will adopt the approach.

The author's expectation at the outset was that the most difficult part of the operation would be to unroof the ureters and to enter the paravaginal and pararectal spaces, especially if a Schuchardt's incision was not made. In fact, these expectations were not met. Incision of the supravaginal septum, a structure not encountered in the radical abdominal operation, and retraction of the bladder with the anterior cul-de-sac peritoneum intact proved to be most problematic. The first problem resolved itself with experience. The second was resolved by opening the anterior and posterior cul-de-sac peritoneum as soon as the vesicovaginal and rectovaginal spaces are developed, rather than delaying this step as in the Schauta-Amreich operation. The reasons for delaying this step (which caused the bladder to be lacerated with a Deaver retractor in two patients) have never been clear to this author, and the practice was abandoned after the fourth case. The vaginal cuff is also no longer sutured closed but held with (obstetric) T-clamps, which are much better for traction.

The greatest uncertainty during the vaginal part of the operation was caused by the position of the proximal ureter during division of the cervical ligaments, for it cannot be seen or felt as this step is executed as it can be in the abdominal operation. Surgeons who perform radical abdominal hysterectomy grow accustomed to seeing the ureter or feeling it against the hand they use to retract tissues medially as the cervical ligaments are being clamped and divided. This is not possible with the vaginal approach, and after the ureters are unroofed, they are simply retracted away out of the field of vision. The tendency is, therefore, constantly to check and feel for the ureters as the cervical ligaments are being clamped and divided vaginally. Indeed, failure to adequately free or retract the proximal ureter caused the author to cut the left ureter in his second patient, while dividing residual attachments of the broad ligament after the operation was almost complete (6). The problem was resolved by passing a vascular tape around the ureters laparoscopically and retracting them out of the pelvis throughout the vaginal part of the operation. This was the last step to be added to the operation, but it is one of the most helpful. The tags make excellent ureteric retractors and reassure the surgeon about their safety.

Laparoscopic retraction of the ureters is helpful for another reason; it allows the ureters to be unroofed after the cervical ligaments are divided, as in Okabayashi's modification of the abdominal operation. It is believed that this tactic, together with laparoscopic division of the proximal attachments of the uterus will make it possible to avoid a Schuchardt's incision in most patients. Thus, the only modification to the vaginal part of the operation (dividing the cervical ligaments before freeing the ureter from its tunnel) has been made possible by the laparoscopic technique that precedes it.

It is obviously too early to try to assess the results obtained with this operation, but the success of radical vaginal hysterectomy in a previous era coupled with the remarkable success of laparoscopic lymphadenectomies, both pelvic and aortic, make it inconceivable to this author that the radical abdominal operation will survive much longer as the standard operative approach to early invasive cancer of the cervix.

The author has treated twelve patients with Stage IA2-IIA carcinoma of the cervix with a laparoscopic-vaginal radical hysterectomy. The patients were unselected. Three had Stage IA2 lesions, six Stage IB lesions, and three Stage IIA lesions. Four patients had bulky (>5 cm) tumors. One of these patients weighed 239 pounds; one had old bilateral tubo-ovarian abscesses; one had a previous anterior-posterior repair, was apareunic, and had a very narrow vagina; and one patient had extensive pelvic adhesions and an 18-week-size uterus weighing 480 grams. There was one ureteric injury in the author's second case (6). Querleu (9) reported no complications in eight cases, and Hatch has had one ureteric injury in his first eleven cases (Hatch, personal communications). These complications, however, represent lack of experience with the operation rather than any inherent limitation of the technique. Indeed, once the techniques have been mas-

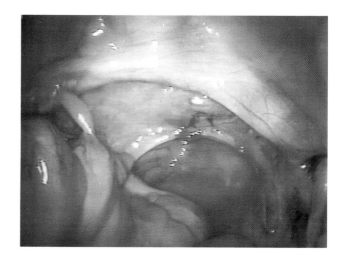

Figure 23.14 Appearance of the pelvis 4 weeks after laparoscopic-vaginal radical hysterectomy.

tered, fistula rates are likely to be lower than with the abdominal operation. Bladder dysfunction remains a major potential problem after radical surgery for invasive cancer of the cervix, which a laparoscopic-vaginal approach is unlikely to eliminate. However, there is no objective evidence of which this author is aware that bladder dysfunction after radical vaginal hysterectomy is greater than it is after radical abdominal hysterectomy, even though Barclay is of the opinion that it is (Barclay, personal communications).

Laparoscopic aortic lymphadenectomy was carried out in one patient who had three positive pelvic nodes, and inspection of the pelvis revealed no bowel adhesions whatsoever (Figure 23.14). Clearly, if this case is representative of patients undergoing laparoscopic-vaginal radical hysterectomy, bowel complications from postoperative radiation therapy are likely to be reduced compared with an abdominal radical hysterectomy (13).

REFERENCES

1. Canis M, Mage G, Wattiez A, Pouly JL, Mahnes H, Bruhat MA. La Chirurgie endoscopique a-t-elle une place dans la chirurgie radicale du cancer du col uterin. J Gynecol Obstet Biol Reprod 1990;19:921.

2. Nehzat C, Nehzat F, Welander C, Burrell M. Laparoscopic radical hysterectomy and pelvic and para-aortic lymphadenectomy in the treatment of carcinoma of the cervix. Am J Obstet Gynecol 1992;166:864–865.

3. Querleu D. Hysterectomies enlargies de Schauta-Amreich et Schauta-Stoeckel assistées par coelioscopie. J Gynecol Obstet Biol Reprod 1991;20:747–748.

4. Querleu D, Leblanc E, Castelain B. Laparoscopic lymphadenectomy in the staging of early carcinoma of the cervix. Am J Obstet Gynecol 1991;164:579–581.

5. Dargent D, Roy M, Keita N, Mathevet P, Adeleine P. The Schauta operation: its place in the management of cervical cancer. Gynecol Oncol (Abstract) 1993;49:109–110.

6. Kadar N, Reich H. laparoscopically assisted radical Schauta hysterectomy and bilateral pelvic lymphadenectomy for the treatment of bulky stage IB carcinoma of the cervix. Gynaecol Endosc 1993;2:135–142.

7. Kadar N. Laparoscopic-vaginal radical hysterectomy: description of a technique and its evoluton. Gynaecol Endosc 1994;3:109–122.

8. Dargent D, Mathevet P. Hysterectomie enlargie laparoscopico-vaginale. J Gynecol Obstet Biol Reprod 1992;21:709–710.

9. Querleu D. Laparoscopically assisted radical vaginal hysterectomy. Gynecol Oncol 1993;51:248–254.

10. Feroze R. Radical vaginal operations. In: Coppelson M, ed. Gynecologic Oncology. Edinburgh: Churchill-Livingstone, 1981, pp 840–853.

11. Mitra S. The Schauta operation. In: Meigs JV, ed. Surgical Treatment of Cancer of the Cervix. New York: Grune & Stratton, 1954:267–280.

12. Reiffenstuhl G, Platzer W. Atlas of Vaginal Surgery. Philadelphia: WB Saunders, 1975.

Part E
Miscellaneous Topics

Chapter 24
Credentialing and Training Guidelines

Mistakes are always initial. —Pavese

The mechanisms for credentialing and licensing medical practitioners vary with local customs and practices as well as with the law of the land. The most important factor in achieving the right result, however, is the integrity of the individual physician, which is not a matter for legislation. Ideally, credentialing guidelines should be informative and summarize what has been found to be necessary to achieve competence at a new surgical technique. In our view, these are best arrived at by dividing what has to be learned to perform laparoscopic surgery into its component parts.

The most important factor is a sound basic surgical training that consists of a thorough knowledge of anatomy and the pathological process being treated, an understanding of the operation being performed, and the use of sound surgical techniques of dissection. In short, one has to be able to perform the intended endoscopic operation by laparotomy under the right circumstances using good techniques of dissection. The gynecologist, whose main technique of dissection involves pushing structures with a large "sponge-stick" or who has never dissected the retroperitoneum, will have difficulty adapting to this type of surgery, and the root of difficulty will not be lack of familiarity with endoscopic instruments. He or she will, to some extent, have to relearn how to operate by sharp dissection.

The next phase is to learn how to manipulate and control endoscopic instruments while watching a video camera, to become familiar with basic equipment, such as trocars, suction-irrigation systems, insufflators, cameras, and monitors, and to understand electrosurgery (other energy sources being en-

tirely optional). This can and must be learned outside of the operating room. If the previous phase of the process is in place and the gynecologist is a good surgeon, this stage of endoscopic surgery is much easier to master than is popularly believed. However, to learn it requires access to an animal laboratory and approximately 8–12 hours of practice for a complete novice.

The purpose of the laboratory training should not be to carry out specific operations in an animal whose anatomy bears no resemblance to the human, nor should the session be devoted to learning how to use the sponsoring manufacturer's products. Under no circumstances should the surgeon waste time trying to suture or tie knots at this stage of his or her surgical development because endoscopic operations can be carried out without the need to suture. Suturing is an advanced technique; no one can do it without having had considerable practice of endoscopic surgery, and no one will (and certainly should not) use these techniques until they are proficient at techniques of dissection. Suturing should be learned as a separate activity in the laboratory, and it, too, requires about 6–12 hours of separate practice. I have seen gynecologists waste hours of precious time and become increasingly frustrated as they have been asked to tie intracorporeal knots with inappropriate grasping instruments simply to become familiar with a manufacturer's endoscopic suture products. This is totally inappropriate and detracts from the physician's training.

The surgeon should go into the animal laboratory and simply practice picking up tissues, cutting them, and coagulating them until he or she has complete control over the surgical instruments and can manipulate them watching video monitors. Once this is mastered, the surgeon should be allowed to tackle operations he or she is qualified to perform by laparotomy, although, obviously, everyone should start with simpler operations and not attempt too much too soon. Most will benefit from watching videos of operations and from watching other surgeons operate "live" in the operating room. Whether a formal system of prosectorship is necessary or better than an informal system that leaves asking colleagues for assistance up to the individual surgeon is open to question, and having witnessed first hand the abuses it has generated, I have my doubts. Besides misuse, prosectorship carries the risk of perpetuating faulty techniques.

The next component of laparoscopic surgery involves understanding instrumentation and operating room setup. The difficulty here is that the surgeon is not in full control of his environment but dependent on a number of individuals for the proper working of the equipment and to achieve optimal working conditions. The cooperation of such ancillary personnel, unfortunately, cannot be relied upon. Anesthetists may not cooperate with positioning the patient, the nursing staff may be completely unfamiliar with the equipment, or the hospital may refuse to purchase essential instruments or, worse still, force the surgeon to use vital equipment he or she may feel uncomfortable using. In an attempt to feign objectivity, operating rooms often conduct seemingly democratic surveys, only to come up with highly undemocratic decisions. Mechanisms must be developed to protect surgeons and patients from these kinds of commercially motivated machinations.

A sense of chaos surrounds laparoscopic surgery at many hospitals at the present time. Everyone, regardless of experience or knowledge, seems to have an opinion about how useful and safe these techniques are (1), and its advantages and disadvantages are being debated in the lay press and the media. Bad outcomes are taken out of context and rarely discussed in an atmosphere conducive to learning something from these unfortunate events. The inevitable response is to question the training and the credentialing of the surgeon. Although this is right and proper and necessary, insufficient attention has been paid to the environment in which laparoscopic surgeons generally have to operate, their dependence on that environ-

ment, and the potential of that dependence to adversely affect outcome. If hospitals are permitted to advertise their capacity to provide "minimally invasive therapy," then surely there must be some scrutiny of whether they can, in fact, provide the service they are touting and they have taken the necessary provisions that patients cared for in their facility will be cared for safely, efficiently, and properly. This involves far more than simply how good or experienced the surgeon doing the operation has to be before he or she is permitted to do an operation laparoscopically. It seems appropriate to this author, given the complex nature of laparoscopic surgery and the lack of an existing structure to integrate its various facets, for regulatory agencies that oversee hospitals to enact requirements that will ensure that laparoscopic operations can be carried out safely in a facility in the way that has been done for the use of lasers.

Our approach at a local level has been to institute a departmental committee charged with reviewing instrumentation and results. We have also suggested that a form be made out for each laparoscopic case that is designed to identify any technical difficulties that the surgeon may have experienced with anesthesia, nursing, equipment, and pathology/anatomy. Clearly, as endoscopic surgery becomes the standard way to perform most operations, questions of credentialing will recede and merge imperceptibly with the general methods used to ensure that surgeons have received proper surgical training. The American Association of Gynecologic Laparoscopists will also soon offer formal credentialing in laparoscopic and hysteroscopic surgery based on examinations similar to the board examinations of other organizations. This is clearly a bold, characteristically constructive, and much needed initiative.

Finally, there is an equally pressing need to credential endoscopic courses to ensure that they provide adequate training for physicians. Training courses will continue to be necessary for some time to come, and physicians must have a way to ensure that they will be participating in an educational activity useful to them rather than to instrument manufacturers or the faculty, department, or facility that sponsors the course.

REFERENCE

1. Chandler JA. Laparoscopic pelvic surgery. Better? Safer? Am J Obstet Gynecol 1994;170:253–254.

▼   ▼   ▼   ▼   ▼   ▼   ▼   ▼   ▼

Chapter 25
Randomized Clinical Trials

*Any mental activity is easy if it need not take
reality into account. —Proust*

A chapter on randomized trials in a surgical atlas is probably unprecedented but so is the orchestrated attack on laparoscopic surgery. A justification for this truly shocking policy in an epoch that has celebrated the triumph of democracy over demagoguery has apparently been found in the randomized clinical trial, which is seen as the only certain way to prove that new forms of medical therapy are effective, despite the fact that penicillin and Pap smears, for example, were never shown to be effective by this means.

This is obviously not a book about clinical trials, but many have attempted to discredit laparoscopic surgery by making unthinking calls for randomized trials in the belief that they are somehow serving a higher scientific purpose than the remarkable individuals who developed these surgical techniques. My purpose in analyzing their arguments and in highlighting the limitations of randomized trials is not to suggest that we should either seek or accept a lower scientific standard but simply to remind the reader as well as the critics of these techniques, that, in the final analysis, science is about seeking the truth. The tacit, and sometimes the explicit, suggestion that randomized trials provide the only valid means of learning the truth is not only a grotesque hyperbole, but it is a view that impedes scientific progress and obfuscates the truth. There is no question that if a properly designed clinical trial is feasible and will generate results that are useful and clinically relevant, it is an analytical approach that is to be preferred over all others. However, meaningful clinical trials are frequently impossible to carry out. The technique, in general, is not well-suited

to resolve complex clinical questions, nor was it designed for this purpose. Therefore, to ignore these practical realities and press on regardless, demanding that clinical trials that are bound to end in failure be carried out, is not clever or profound, and does not further the cause of science or understanding; it is simply a waste of time and money.

WHAT IS THE PURPOSE OF A CLINICAL TRIAL?

Conceptually, clinical trials had their origins in the elegant experimental designs Fisher and Yates developed for agricultural and industrial work. Although these designs were directed at much more complicated questions than which of two or more treatments worked better, *clinical trials,* in general, *have one and only one purpose, to eliminate bias from treatment comparisons.*

Treatment comparisons can be biased because factors besides treatment, such as patient characteristics or features of the disease, can affect outcome. The unequal distribution of these factors between patients receiving different treatments, rather than the true difference between the treatments, may, therefore, account for any difference in outcome observed after therapy. To ensure that treatment comparisons are unbiased, it is necessary to (1) select study patients randomly from the population to which the results of the trial are to be applied, (2) assign the treatments to be compared randomly to these patients, and (3) "blind" both the patient and the physician to the treatment received by a particular patient, although this last requirement can be relaxed when the outcome is objective, e.g., survival. *These conditions are never fully met in clinical practice.*

A PRIORI LIMITATIONS OF CLINICAL TRIALS

Inability to Generalize the Results

Unlike the experimental units used in agricultural or industrial experiments, patients are never selected at random for inclusion into trials, and they may not, therefore, be representative of the population to which the results of the study are to be applied. This does not create a problem if the purpose of the study is simply to determine whether a new drug is effective or not, for a positive result would demonstrate conclusively that it was effective in at least some patients. However, difficulties arise as soon as we try to extrapolate the results to patients not enrolled in the study for we can only be certain that the results are applicable to them if the study patients were a random sample of the population to which the results are to be applied, which they never are. We cannot assume that therapy will be equally effective in all segments of a diseased population. Consequently, a treatment that is found not to be effective in the study sample may nonetheless be effective in the diseased population and vice versa.

Thus, *clinical trials are always flawed* to some extent from the outset. Whether the departure from theoretical requirements vitiates the legitimacy of a particular trial is, unfortunately, always unknown and unknowable. There is no way to test whether a particular trial is or is not biased, and the *rules for conducting clinical trials simply reflect the conditions under which bias cannot exist.* If the rules are broken, bias may or may not exist, and there is no way to know.

The inability to generalize the results of a randomized trial is even more problematic when the treatment involved is operator-dependent, as when treatment is an operation, especially if the techniques are still evolving, as is true for many laparoscopic operations. For example, Grimes claimed that there was "an epidemic of surgical morbidity and mortality related to laparoscopic cholecystectomy now unfolding in New York State" (5). Yet, Coletta and Rose (8) found no increase in minor morbidity and a decrease in major morbidity from laparoscopic cholecystectomies. Now, those who have criticized laparoscopic procedures would not accept this as proof of the operation's safety because the investigators did not carry out a random-

ized trial. What they fail to appreciate, however, is that even if they had and had obtained the same result, this would have neither reassured us about nor altered the outcome from the procedure in New York State, for those poor outcomes are attributable not to any deficiencies inherent in laparoscopic cholecystectomy but to the poor training and preparation of those who undertook them. As if to underscore this fact, the state's legislators responded to these calamities not by proscribing the use of laparoscopic cholecystectomy or restricting its use to patients enrolled in a randomized trial, but by setting rules for its use that would ensure that only those with sufficient training and experience could undertake the procedure in the future.

The uncertainty over whether or not the results of a trial are applicable to nontrial patients is a limitation common to all randomized clinical trials. Other limitations apply only to some trials, but these include almost all trials involving laparoscopic surgery.

Inability to Assign Treatment Randomly

The second difficulty that may be encountered in clinical trials but not in designed experiments is the inability to assign "treatments" randomly to patients for ethical reasons. This makes it simply impossible to study some clinical problems by a randomized clinical trial. An obvious and relevant example would be whether cyst rupture affects prognosis in Stage I carcinoma of the ovary.

Inability to Blind the Study

The third requirement can also seriously vitiate many clinical trials because bias from failure to blind either the physician or the patient to the treatment received by a patient can be at least as great as the bias from nonrandom treatment assignment. This is true whenever outcome or its measurement can be influenced by knowledge of the treatment received. Clearly, no trial involving a comparison between laparoscopic surgery and laparotomy can ever be blinded, and elimination of bias cannot, therefore, be guaranteed unless the outcome of interest is an objective measure, such as survival, pulmonary embolus, etc. But, in almost all instances in which it is used, laparoscopic surgery is undertaken to reduce morbidity. Thus, the outcome of interest is usually some subjective measure, such as length of hospital stay, return to work or normal function, postoperative pain, and so on. Clearly, these kinds of measures can be greatly influenced by knowing which treatment the patient received, and the inability to blind the study renders randomized trials incapable of eliminating bias from treatment comparisons. A good example of an unblinded randomized study that was highly biased was discussed in Chapter 13, and the difficulties that the inability to blind create for trials involving laparoscopic hysterectomy were discussed in Chapter 10.

WHY ARE RANDOMIZED TRIALS NECESSARY TO ELIMINATE BIAS?

One only needs to attend grand rounds or scientific meetings on a regular basis to discover that, to all intents and purposes, randomized clinical trials are regarded as the only certain means of learning the truth about medical therapy. In many other walks of life, the idea of experimentation is meaningless because controlled experiments are impossible to carry out, yet stochastic phenomena have been profitably studied by probability models. Examples include industrial accidents, economic phenomena, geographical events, and the weather. In all these cases, cause-and-effect relationships have been fruitfully studied by probability models, and the same is, in fact, true of the medical field. Governmental agencies and insurance companies rely heavily on statistical models to determine what are appropriate patterns of care and outcomes after medical therapy. They employ statisticians to model such important variables as the expected length of hospital stay after different operations, expected mortality among hospital admissions, and the cesarian section rate. If current views about randomized trials were correct, one cannot help but wonder why statisticians would engage in creating such an edifice of falsehood.

Enormous advances have taken place in statistical theory over the past 25 years and entire new classes of analytic techniques have been developed that enable us to adjust treatment comparisons for covariate effects, i.e., factors besides treatment that might affect outcome, regardless of whether the outcome of interest is a proportion, involves time to an event ("survival" analysis), or is a quantitative measure (weight, height, serum hCG concentration). The advances in computer technology and programming have played an integral part in making such undertakings a practical reality, and in fact, many years elapsed before problems that were solved at a theoretical level found practical applications in the analysis of clinical data. For example, Cox's proportional hazards model was derived in 1972, but most investigators did not have access to software that enabled the model to be ap-

plied easily or on a regular basis until as recently as 10 years ago.

Many of the statistical techniques for data analysis that are available today were simply unknown when the randomized clinical trial was introduced into clinical medicine by Hill in the 1950s. At that time, comparisons between different treatments simply meant comparing the results obtained with each treatment without regard to other factors that could affect outcome. This was the meaning of "historical controls," and such comparisons would be considered pointless, if not frankly absurd, today, unless, as we shall see, therapy produces very large effects. However, at that time, the only alternative to these crude comparisons was the randomized clinical trial, and it is little wonder that they were looked upon as the only means to save us from futile comparisons that often provided illusory results.

But, things have changed since Hill's day. Probability models are now available that enable treatment comparisons to be controlled for known risk factors regardless of the nature of the response variable. We have powerful computers that would enable vast data banks to be developed and institutions to share data. We have software that could ensure uniform data collection. These facilities provide mathematicians with untold opportunities to develop a whole array of simulation and combinatorial techniques in a way unimaginable before. It is inconceivable to this author that with the use of these techniques new and more fruitful approaches to clinical research could not be developed. All that is required is a change in philosophy so that individuals who have the ability to tackle such an undertaking are inspired and properly funded to do so.

CASE AGAINST STATISTICAL CONTROL

If treatment is not selected randomly, there will usually be an association between the treatment given and the prognostic factors that affect outcome from therapy. It will not be possible to disentangle these effects if most patients with the same risk factors receive the same treatment. For example, although proof that pelvic radiation affects survival in endometrial carcinoma is lacking, many patients with adverse risk factors, such as deep myometrial invasion, receive radiation therapy. It would clearly be impossible to disentangle the effects of radiation therapy and deep myometrial invasion on survival if at least some women with deep myometrial invasion did not receive radiation therapy. Large computerized data banks would, however, almost certainly resolve this problem. Subset data from single institutions, representing perhaps 5–10% of the database, are usually too small to obtain stable estimates of treatment effects, but a 5–10% segment of a database, consisting of, say, 100,000 cases, would provide a very sizable subset for statistical analysis.

The theoretical argument against statistical adjustment of observational data relies on the proposition that treatment comparison can still be biased because other unrecognized and, hence, unadjusted-for prognostic factors may be unequally distributed between the two treatment groups. Although this is true, large differences become progressively less likely if the same findings are repeatedly confirmed in large separate similarly adjusted data sets. Moreover, these same unknown prognostic factors are just as likely to be unequally distributed between the patients in a randomized trial, and the population to which the trial's results are to be applied for study patients are not selected randomly from the population. Therefore, the same argument would equally invalidate randomized trials for we cannot assume that the results of a randomized trial apply to the population (see above), especially if these putative factors have a large effect on outcome.

This argument also ignores some practical realities. Risk factors are usually interrelated, and many variables that individually exert a significant effect on outcome cease to have an important effect after outcome is adjusted for the effects of other variables. Thus, we may start with 20 "significant" variables but end up with a model containing five. It is unlikely that unrecognized risk factors will have a large effect on outcome independently of known prognostic factors unless little is known about the condition being investigated. For example, risk factors in endometrial cancer have been the subject of many studies, and it is simply implausible that an unrecognized variable exists that influences survival to any great extent independently of other known risk factors. If little is known about the phenomenon under study, useful probability models obviously cannot be developed, nor can effective randomized trials be designed.

CASE FOR CLINICAL TRIALS

The case for clinical trials is, in fact, entirely presumptive and theoretical. There is no acceptable evidence that I am aware of from either simulation studies or actual trials to demonstrate that randomized trials yield more accurate information about treatment effects than statistically adjusted observational data. The argument *for* randomized trials is based on demonstrating the deficiencies of retrospective studies rather than the virtues of clinical trials themselves, and it must be said that the examples used by proponents of randomized trials make sorry reading. Almost all the trials they cite are uncontrolled observational studies from the 1960s that did not adjust treatment comparisons statistically for known prognostic factors.

Grimes' Argument

In the absence of randomized trials, well-intentioned physicians have provided many worthless or harmful therapies. This is Grimes' argument (4–6), but it contains two fallacies. First, it assumes that the only alternative to clinical trials is to compare treatments using happenstance data without controlling for known prognostic factors. Second, the argument relies on the faulty syllogism, (1) there have been many useless therapies, (2) they were not subjected to randomized clinical trials, (3) therefore, useless therapies can be prevented by randomized clinical trials. However, the futile therapies Grimes cites were not supported by well-designed retrospective studies either, and on this logic, an equally strong case could be made for conducting properly designed retrospective studies.

Pitkin's Argument

Retrospective studies yield positive results far more often than randomized trials, the implication being that the retrospective studies, not the clinical trials, are "wrong." This is Pitkin's argument (2), but it has at least two fallacies.

First, clinical trials are usually not repeated and certainly not as often as retrospective studies. Therefore, the opportunity for disagreements between clinical trials to arise is much less than it is for retrospective studies. Nonetheless, many large randomized clinical trials have yielded diametrically opposite results, some examples being trials involving mammography, management of postdate pregnancies, and nitroprusside therapy (8).

Second, and much more fundamental, clinical trials are designed with a built-in bias to yield null results, because the values assigned to the α and β errors are *never* equal. Typical values used are 0.05 for the α error and 0.2 for the β error, *which render clinical trials four times more likely to miss a real treatment effect than to detect an effect that is not real,* i.e., due to chance. Since the odds are stacked against a positive result, it is hardly surprising that clinical trials are less likely to yield positive results than studies that are not biased in this way. Most trials that yield null results are insensitive, and it is impossible to know whether the result simply reflects this insensitivity or that the treatment studied was ineffective. For example, Sacks et al. (9) found that the sensitivity of randomized clinical trials ranged between 0% and 27% (mean 12%)!

Pocock's Argument

If the same control treatment is used in different randomized trials, it can yield results that differ to a statistically significant extent (a finding that simply reflects lack of random selection of control subjects). The implication here is that if historical controls are used for comparative studies, the results obtained will depend on which control subjects are selected for study. This is Pocock's argument (10), but it is one, like Pitkin's and Grimes', that ignores the fact that happenstance data can always be adjusted statistically for known prognostic factors before treatments are compared.

Chalmers' Argument

Randomized trials will prevent the adoption of useless therapies and minimize the exposure of patients to therapies that are harmful. This is Chalmers' argument (11), but it is one that is deceptively mendacious.

The frequency of side effects is never the endpoint of a clinical trial, and the frequency of unrecognized serious side effects is always low; otherwise, they would have been detected in the developmental stage of the drug. The cause-and-effect relationship between drug and side effect is not established on the basis of a randomized trial but by observing a certain number of events that allow us to attribute the side effect to the drug rather than to chance, whereupon the drug is withdrawn. The number of patients that will need to be exposed to the drug before a sufficient number of side effects is observed for the drug to be withdrawn depends on the frequency of the side effect, but, clearly, this number will be the same regardless of whether the drug is administered as part of a trial or off trial.

The other aspect of Chalmers' argument relies on the totally unrealistic belief that if a certain treatment for a given condition is believed to be effective from basic principles or on the basis of uncontrolled or statistically controlled observations, then a single randomized study with a null result will dissuade clinicians from the belief that the therapy, in fact, works. The real world is simply not like that, as reflected by the recent trials involving thrombolytic therapy after heart attacks. Randomized trials initially showed no difference between TPA and streptokinase, but there was good reason to believe that this was in fact a false negative result. Therefore, the manufacturers mounted a truly massive trial costing some 50 million dollars to demonstrate that TPA did, in fact, confer a small but definite survival advantage over streptokinase.

One might, of course, argue that individuals who do not readily accept null results are simply ones who are not easily persuaded by facts. This, too, is an untenable proposition because many factors besides the effectiveness of therapy determine whether or not statistical significance will be achieved in a particular trial. These factors are well known and include the effect size one wishes to detect, the degree of confidence with which one wishes to detect it, and how willing one is to falsely accept a result as being significant. Given the many uncertainties that surround the results of a randomized trial, to suggest that they provide such conclusive evidence about treatment efficacy that clinicians will disregard all other evidence pertaining to the effect of therapy is not only naive and unrealistic, it is, curiously enough, highly unscientific. To pursue this argument would take us into the realm of Baysian statistics, which is outside the scope of our present intent.

PRACTICAL LIMITATIONS OF CLINICAL TRIALS

In addition to the *a priori* limitations already discussed, randomized trials are capable of providing only limited information about treatment effects because there is a limit to the number of patients that can be enrolled in a particular trial. In principle, some trials can be identified ahead of time as being impossible to carry out, but, frequently, unrealistic assumptions are made about accrual rates and the trial is initiated and cannot be completed. For example, the Gynecologic Oncology Group (GOG) has been conducting a trial in which patients with cervix cancer and positive pelvic nodes are randomized to whole pelvic radiation or no further treatment after radical hysterectomy. This trial has still not been completed after 8 years because of poor patient accrual, and there is little prospect that it will ever be completed.

Clinical problems cannot, however, be easily dichotomized into whether or not they are amenable to study by a prospective randomized clinical trial on the basis of sample size requirements. The effect of sample size is much more pervasive, and it more often determines trial sensitivity than trial feasibility. What happens in practice is that compromises are made between what is desirable and what is feasible, and investigators relax the effect size they are prepared to accept as significant or sacrifice the power of the study. This leads to some glaring inconsistencies.

For example, chemotherapeutic trials in ovarian cancer conducted by the GOG are generally designed to detect a 15% difference in survival with 80% power and an α error of 5%, yet trials involving early stage endometrial and cervix cancer require aortic lymph node dissection, even though the frequency of aortic lymph node metastases in early stage disease is only about 5%, and, at most, only 40% of women with aortic lymph node metastases are cured of their disease. Clearly, if it is meaningful to undertake therapy that is likely to benefit only 2% of women with endometrial or cervix cancer, it must also be meaningful to try to secure the same survival advantage in women with ovarian cancer. The only reason that trials are not designed to detect such small differences is that the sample size required to detect them would be prohibitive. But, is it legitimate, ethical, or, indeed, "scientific" to withhold treatment we suspect might be better (from first principles or the findings of a retrospective study) on the grounds that we are, let us say, 35% sure it does not improve survival by more than 5%?

Careful scrutiny of some of the randomized trials that have been actually carried out and reflection on the conclusions drawn from their results leave the dispassionate observer with the indelible impression that, often, the overriding concern seems to have been to carry out the trial rather than be useful or produce meaningful results. A good example is provided by a study recently published in the *New England Journal of Medicine* that purported to show that in patients with grade I, Stage IA and IB ovarian carcinoma, adjunctive therapy with oral melphalan does not significantly improve survival (12). What the results of this widely quoted study, which was initiated in 1976, actually showed was that the 5-year disease-free survival of patients receiving melphalan was 98%, whereas that of patients not receiving melphalan was 91% (P = 0.41). Now, 43 patients received melphalan and 38 did not. The probability that this trial would detect a real difference in 5-year survival of 7% was about 10%. In other words, the trial found a 7% difference in 5-year survival favoring treatment; there is a 40% chance that this was a chance difference and a 90% chance that if this difference was real, the trial failed to detect it statistically.

It is unclear to this author by what logic it is considered "scientific" to accept a false negative rate that is more than double the false positive rate and, therefore, to interpret such trials as showing that therapy is ineffective rather than effective, given that the study is not going to be simply discarded as being utterly meaningless (which is, of course, the correct interpretation of the findings). Those who would blithely reply that the study was simply too small should reflect on the fact that this was a collaborative effort involving some of the leading authorities in gynecologic oncology in the United States that took 6–8 years to carry out and 12–14 years to report, during which time, three new chemotherapeutic agents active in ovarian cancer (at least two of which are more active than melphalan) received FDA approval.

COMMENT

Randomized clinical trials have enjoyed great success in the evaluation of new drugs because, in this setting, interest primarily centers on a single and simple question, "Does the drug work?" Before reaching trial stage, new drugs undergo extensive testing in Phase I and Phase II trials, and only those shown to produce the desired effect are considered for Phase III clinical trials. Moreover, all that is required for approval of a new drug is evidence of efficacy, not proof that the new drug is better than an old one. For example, carboplatin was approved for use in ovarian cancer on the basis of evidence showing that it produced results equivalent, not superior, to cisplatin. Therefore, the prior probability is high that when it is used to evaluate the effectiveness of a new drug, a clinical trial will yield a useful answer, even if the results of the trial are null.

Clinical trials have met with considerably less success when applied to more complex questions. Examples from our specialty include induction of labor in postdates pregnancy, inhibition of premature labor, use of fetal heart rate monitoring, forceps, or breech deliveries, surgical staging of cervix cancer, postoperative radiation therapy in endometrial and cervix cancer, and so on. In all these cases, we know that the treatment is effective in a narrow cause-and-effect sense. Labor can be induced in postdates pregnancies (in most cases), premature labors can be stopped (at least for a while), babies can be delivered by forceps and breeches by the vaginal route, aortic metastasis can be detected by surgical staging, and radiation does kill endometrial and cervical cancer cells. Whether these treatments should be used, however, is quite another matter, one on which clinical trials have generally not shed much light.

The reasons are usually attributable to one or more of the following: (1) many factors affect outcome, (2) there is more than one outcome of interest, (3) the outcome of interest is rare, (4) small treatment effects are of interest, and (5) the undesirable effects of therapy may be as great or frequent as the beneficial effects. These factors alone or in combination militate against a successful trial. A null result is usually obtained, but the trial is so insensitive that little meaning can be attached to the result (10).

It is becoming increasingly clear to clinicians who have experience conducting clinical trials that other methods are required to investigate complex clinical questions. Unfortunately, however, a double standard has been applied to research on randomized trials and retrospective studies. The discrepant results of small poorly controlled retrospective studies that would not get a hearing today are used to condemn all such studies and to make sweeping generalizations about a methodology that is in its infancy for lack of support. But, despite many failures, unsuccessful trials have not caused the method to be questioned or alternative strategies to be sought but have simply evinced the response that the cases in question were simply bad trials. A point must surely come, however, when investigators begin to question the value of an analytical tool that cannot be used to study practical clinical questions because of an inability to (1) assign treatment randomly, (2) blind the study, and (3) accrue enough patients, and when they think they can study a problem, end up with a

study that is too small, a result that is out of date, and an answer that is uncertain.

Why has this state of affairs been allowed to develop, and why do trials, such as the recent RADIUS study (13), that consume vast amounts of public funds and simply generate results that are highly controversial, do not alter clinical practice, and are hotly debated by experts, continue to be carried out? The explanation probably lies in the fact that, as Alvan Feinstein put it, an industry has grown up around the randomized clinical trial. Many trials are funded by the pharmaceutical industry, and physicians are usually paid handsomely for putting patients onto these trials. After the results are known (and provided they are favorable), the investigators are further sponsored by the pharmaceutical industry to make the findings of the trial known by way of lectures. Even participation in trials funded by NIH involves the receipt of funds of some sort. Collaborative groups have a contract with the NIH, and to ensure continued receipt of funds, trials must be in place as soon as existing ones are closed. This means that trials are designed before the results of the trials they are replacing are known, which is hardly conducive to optimal study design. Randomized clinical trials are also highly undemocratic. Most are designed by committees, and, as in all committees, there is much jockeying between the members to ensure ascendancy of their individual points of view. Those best placed to analyze the problem at hand or to design a trial to solve it may not be members of the committee. With so much vested interest in randomized clinical trials, it is, perhaps, hardly surprising that few are clamoring for change.

Be that as it may, it is critical to the development of laparoscopic surgery that it does not become embroiled in highly questionable clinical trials. Throughout this text, we have had occasions to point out why laparoscopic surgery is particularly unsuitable to be investigated by this means. Let us end by summarizing these:

1. Treatment effects are often so large that controlled studies are not required to demonstrate a benefit from the laparoscopic approach. For example, most women can be discharged the day after a laparoscopic aortic lymphadenec-

COMMENT

tomy, which is simply impossible after an open operation.

2. Treatment cannot be blinded and bias cannot be eliminated from treatment comparisons when the endpoint is subjective, e.g., time to full recovery.

3. The frequency of the outcome of interest is so low that a meaningful trial cannot be carried out. Some examples would be the frequency of

serious side effects (ureteric injury, pulmonary embolus) after surgery and the frequency of lymph node metastasis after laparoscopic and conventional lymph-adenectomy (pelvic and aortic).

4. Some of the techniques are still evolving and the results could not be generalized for they would be highly operator dependent.

REFERENCES

1. Pitkin RM. Operative laparoscopy: surgical advance or technical gimmick? Obstet Gynecol 1992;72:441–442.

2. Pitkin RM. Operative laparoscopy: surgical advance or technical gimmick? Keynote address, 21st Annual Meeting of the American Association of Gynecologic Laparoscopists, Chicago, September, 1992.

3. Trope C, Inversen T. Laparoscopic radical hysterectomy: technical gimmick or surgical advance? Gynaecol Endosc 1993;2:83–84.

4. Grimes DA. Frontiers of operative laparoscopy: a review and critique of the evidence. Am J Obstet Gynecol 1992;166:1062–1071.

5. Grimes DA. Laparoscopic surgery: experiment or expedient. Reply to letter. Am J Obstet Gynecol 1993; 168:1333–1334.

6. Grimes DA. Technology follies. JAMA 1993;269: 3030–3032.

7. Chandler JA. Laparoscopic pelvic surgery. Am J Obstet Gynecol (in press).

8. Kadar N. The operative laparoscopy debate: technology assessment or statistical Jezebel? Biomed Pharmacotherapie 1993;47:201–206.

9. Sacks HS. Chalmers TC, Smith H. Sensitivity and specificity of clinical trials. Arch Int Med 1983;143:753–755.

10. Pocock SJ. Clinical trials. A practical approach. Chichester, U.K.: John Wiley & Sons, 1983.

11. Chalmers I. Evaluating the effects of care during pregnancy and childbirth. In: Chalmers I, Enkin M, Keirse MJNC, eds. Pregnancy and Childbirth. Oxford: Oxford University Press, 1991, pp 3–38.

12. Young RC, Walton LA, Ellenberg SS, et al. Adjuvant therapy in Stage I and Stage II ovarian cancer. Results of two prospective randomized trials. N Engl J Med 1991; 322:102–114.

13. Goncalves LF, Romero R. A critical appraisal of the RADIUS study. The Fetus 1993;3:1–18.

▼ ▼ ▼ ▼ ▼ ▼ ▼ ▼ ▼

Epilogue

Technological progress has made advanced laparoscopic surgery possible, and it is to technology that we must look to develop our craft further. But, technology means different things to different people. To some, it means ever more sophisticated lasers that can peel away tissue micron by micron; to others, it means the prospect of virtual reality, remote control surgery, and three-dimensional images. As we ponder the import of these fantastic possibilities, it is all too easy to lose sight of the fact that however an operation is performed, the surgeon will still need to know the anatomy, understand the pathology being treated, dissect with a meticulous technique, and be able to see what he or she is doing. This is why traditional surgical principles and techniques have been the leitmotif of this atlas, not because we do not recognize the importance of technology to our field.

But, if progress is to be made, technology must serve the needs of the surgeon, not the creative needs of engineers or the commercial needs of large corporations. We need better trocars that are sharp, require minimal force to insert, have a protective safety shield, maintain their position in the abdominal wall, and do not pull out or work their way into the abdomen. We need to see better. This requires not only more sensitive cameras with better image processing and iris mechanisms to eliminate glare and darkness that all too frequently impede our work, but also systems that automatically rid the peritoneal cavity of all the endoscopic pollution that our energy sources create so that the tempo of surgery is not interrupted by the need to suction out smoke and plume and to reestablish the pneumoperitoneum that is lost in the process. We need to be in control of our environment from the sterile field, and with a press of a button, be able to alter camera settings, the position of the operating table, and, with a system of levers, move the laparoscope into any position. Finally, we need to devise an entirely different system of suturing that allows us to place stitches without the need to pick up a needle, pass it through tissues, release it, pick it up again, and then tie knots. No amount of engineering will speed up the process significantly until these steps are eliminated, and one can think of many ways in which this might be done.

If we focus on what is within our reach rather than on what is currently available to us, it is not difficult to see that most operations will be carried out laparoscopically by the beginning of the next century. This is the prospect that has kept most of us going when the road uphill seemed impossibly steep, the knowledge that by remaining faithful to the principles of surgery and harnessing it to the right kind of technology, the laparoscopic surgeon could continue to blur the line between endoscopic and conventional methods of surgical therapy.

Index